CLINICAL ASSESSMENT OF CHILDREN

CLINICAL ASSESSMENT OF CHILDREN:

A Comprehensive Approach to Primary Pediatric Care

J. DEBORAH LOTT FERHOLT, M.D.

Associate Professor of Pediatric Nursing
Yale University School of Nursing

Associate Clinical Professor of Pediatrics
Yale University School of Medicine

J. B. LIPPINCOTT COMPANY
Philadelphia   Toronto

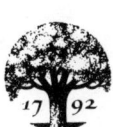

Copyright © 1980 by J. B. Lippincott Company

This book is fully protected by copyright and, with the exception of brief excerpts for review, no part of it may be reproduced in any form by print, photoprint, microfilm, or by any other means without the written permission of the publishers.

ISBN 0-397-54329-8

Library of Congress Catalog Card Number 79-19625

Printed in the United States of America

9 8 7 6 5 4 3 2 1

Library of Congress Cataloging in Publication Data
Ferholt, J.   Deborah Lott.
    Clinical assessment of children.

    Includes bibliographies and index.
    1. Children—Medical examinations. 2. Children—Diseases—Diagnosis. I. Title. [DNLM: 1. Primary health care. 2. Pediatrics. 3. Child, Hospitalized. WS200.3 F355c]
RJ50.F47   618.9′2007′5   79-19625
ISBN 0-397-54329-8

Dedicated to my husband Julian

Preface

This book is a general introduction to the clinical assessment of children. Its focus is on primary health care, but the comprehensive approach offered here is also relevant to pediatric subspecialties and to the care of hospitalized children.

The perspective of this book is broad. It provides a discussion of how clinicians can collect the information they need in order to foster both the physical and mental health of children in the context of their families and communities. Throughout, the major concern is with clinical practice—specifically, with presenting an approach to clinical work that encourages practitioners to think about how their pediatric patients and families experience the office visit and examination. I believe that this approach greatly facilitates the gathering of information that clinicians need in order to form a sound impression of a child's health status and to discuss the assessment with the family in a supportive way.

The approach itself does not change in the face of new scientific discoveries, development of new diagnostic tools, and changes in both preventive measures and management of illness. It remains central to good clinical practice and must be mastered if the clinician is to succeed in delivering effective health care. I stress that throughout the visit, practitioners should keep in mind that they are building—via their approach—a relationship with the child and family which must be based on respect and caring if it is to succeed in promoting healthy growth and development. To put it starkly: I believe that building such a relationship is crucial for successful health care.

This book presents the comprehensive approach and includes sufficient details and illustrative material to help the student understand how to operationalize the principles. It is intended to help students integrate the personal side of the clinical relationship with the scientific and technical aspects of health assessment and management. It is not a textbook on physical diagnosis, a manual on child development, nor a book on the management of common pediatric problems.

This book, which has evolved from ten years of teaching and clinical practice, was written mainly for primary care clinicians including pediatric and family nurse practitioners, pediatricians and family physicians, and physicians' assistants. However, because of the overlap with general pediatric care, pediatric subspecialists in both medicine and nursing, and clinicians engaged in mental health work with children will also find this book useful in their practice.

In the context of the developing and changing roles of health care providers, it is difficult to choose professional labels which avoid traditional bias toward medicine on the one hand or nursing on the other. Therefore, "clinician," "examiner," and "practitioner" are used interchangeably in this book without reference to any one training or discipline. Emphasis is on their approach, rather than on their role definitions. However, specific titles are sometimes used in examples to illustrate particular points about health care delivery.

Comprehensive pediatrics is not a new concept; there is a long tradition of collaboration between pediatricians and mental health professionals in an effort to integrate the general medical care of children with preventive mental health care. Training programs in behavioral and developmental pediatrics were begun in many medical centers in the late 1920s, and they included famous teachers of pediatrics and psychiatry. Since that time every generation of pediatric clinicians has had strong advocates for comprehensive pediatrics and humanistic care. The principles of comprehensive pediatrics espoused in this book are my own synthesis of the ideas of those pediatric teachers and selected relevant concepts from psychoanalysis, psychiatry, psychology, social work, early childhood education, and anthropology.

Over the past ten years I have participated in the development of a graduate program for pediatric nurses at the Yale University School of Nursing. As the primary pediatrician on the faculty, I have planned, taught, and evaluated training for masters degree pediatric nurse practitioners and specialists. Concurrently, I have taught primary pediatric care to medical students and pediatric house officers at the Yale University School of Medicine. The ideas in this book are the outcome of years of work to provide patients and families with scientifically competent and humane pediatric care, to answer the probing questions of students and colleagues, and to conceptualize why some things succeed in practice and others do not. Pursuing the ideas presented here has been very rewarding, but the greatest reward has been the experience of putting them to use in primary pediatric care.

J. Deborah Lott Ferholt, M.D.

Acknowledgments

Many people have helped in the preparation of this book. Their encouragement, interest and work were invaluable to me. I wish, at this time, to take the author's prerogative of acknowledging them by name. My husband Julian and our friend David were by far the most important.

Julian Ferholt, M.D., Director of the Child Development Unit at the Yale Child Study Center, provided essential assistance by taking on a great deal of responsibility of a busy household with two young children. Further, he critiqued the manuscript in all its drafts and contributed his extensive knowledge of child psychiatry and child development.

David E. Hunter, Ph.D., Research Associate at the Yale University Child Study Center, was personally supportive and also an important consultant. He applied his skills as an experienced writer to the difficult task of editing and rewriting the early drafts, and in addition he contributed his expertise as an anthropologist by continually examining many of the conceptual issues. He approached this task with the devotion of a good friend and a commitment to improving health services for children.

Walter Anyan, M.D., Director of the Medical Program for Adolescents at Yale University, generously provided the original materials on adolescent care.

William J. Grego produced the excellent photographs.

A number of individuals gave generously of their time to critique many parts of the manuscript. In particular, I wish to thank Katherine B. Nuckolls, M.S.N., Ph.D., Thomas Dolan, M.D., Sally Provence, M.D., Albert J. Solnit, M.D., Jane Milberg, M.S.N., Diane Rotnam, M.S.N., and Elsa Stone, M.D. Also, Donna Diers, M.S.N., Dean of the Yale University School of Nursing, provided important support and advice.

At the J. B. Lippincott Company, Mary Ann Whitemore and David Miller were most helpful editors and advisors.

Susan Hurst did a wonderful job of typing and retyping a sometimes difficult to read manuscript.

Several colleagues, teachers, and students have supported the growth and development of the ideas in the book. Katherine B. Nuckolls has been both my mentor and colleague in teaching primary pediatric care for many years. Several of my teachers at the University of Rochester Medical School had a major influence on me. George Engel taught the comprehensive clinical approach to the adult patient; Robert Haggerty taught about the pediatric patient in the context of the family and society; and Evan Charney was a superb teacher of pediatrics and a personal mentor. While I was a resident in pediatrics, Cecil Bruckman encouraged me to specialize in ambulatory pediatrics; Sally Provence nurtured my interest in child development; Pete Rowe taught me a great deal about primary pediatric care; and Ray Duff encouraged me to think critically about the effectiveness of patient care.

Finally, I wish to express my deepest appreciation to my daughters, Beth Rachel and Sarah Rebecca for teaching me more than anyone else about children and about being a parent; to my mother Rose Lott, without whom I would never have become the person I am; and to Rose, Julian, and Ruth and Ray Leopold for their practical support and confidence in me throughout the writing of this book.

Contents

UNIT ONE

    1. Comprehensive Pediatric Care   1

UNIT TWO   The Data Base: Foundation of Clinical Practice   17

    2. The History   21
    3. The Physical Examination: An Outline   50
    4. Screening   62

UNIT THREE   Clinical Assessment: Sources for the Data Base   77

    5. The Interview   79
    6. Evaluation of a Complaint or Concern   116
    7. Developmental Assessment   131
    8. The History of One Day   173
    9. The Art of the Physical Examination   184
    10. The Art of Performing Painful Procedures   226

UNIT FOUR   The Clinical Summary   239

    11. General Principles and the Typical Clinical Summary with No Problems   241
    12. The Clinical Summary with Minor Problems   251
    13. The Clinical Summary with Major Problems   262
    14. Consultation   280

UNIT FIVE

    15. The Annotated Interview and Write-Up   289

INDEX   319

CLINICAL ASSESSMENT OF CHILDREN

UNIT ONE

Comprehensive Pediatric Care

CHAPTER 1

Comprehensive Pediatric Care

The Changing Face of Pediatric Health Care
Comprehensive Primary Care Defined
The Personal Relationship as a Tool in Comprehensive Care
Making Decisions in Pediatric Practice
The Setting in Pediatric Health Care
Time and Clinical Practice
Society and Health Care Delivery
Comprehensive Pediatric Care: Ideal and Challenge

THE CHANGING FACE OF PEDIATRIC HEALTH CARE

Pediatrics, as a differentiated domain of clinical practice, is only some 50 years old. Originally it was conceived of as a subspecialty of medical practice; but in the last 30 years it has emerged as a rather distinct and quite separate branch of health care service. This has as much to do with the nature of children themselves as it does with the politics of health care.

Children have two outstanding characteristics that make them qualitatively different from adults—especially in their health care needs. First, children are in a state of rapid flux: both in body and mind, children are constantly growing and developing. The physical, cognitive, and emotional problems that children face vary greatly from one developmental stage to another, which in practice frequently means from one year, month, or week to the next. This rapid change poses many challenges to the pediatric practitioner, who must constantly assess the course of these developments and evaluate them with a flexible notion of what is "normal" for a given child at any point in his or her life.

Secondly, children are by their very nature extraordinarily dependent on their caregivers. Indeed, this is so much the case that in practice a complete assessment of a child will inevitably include an assessment of the child's ongoing relationships with his or her most important caregivers, usually the parents. Further, for clinical intervention to be successful, it is crucial for the clinician to form a supportive alliance with the caregivers. This means that clinicians must develop effective ways of communicating both with children (the patients) and adults (their caregivers). Each level of communication poses its own problems, but both are essential for building helpful, ongoing relationships.

There are other differences between child and adult health care practice. Most are obvious and need not be dwelt on here. Two do bear separate mention, however. The first has to do with a major orientation of pediatric practice: it is directed far more than adult care toward long-range planning and preventive intervention. The early years are obviously very important for future health and development and the pediatric health practitioner must therefore always assess how present circumstances may affect later physical and psychological health.

Another consideration of clinical practice with children is the issue of advocacy. Whereas for the most part it is assumed that adults can make adequate arrangements for their own care, this is not the case with children. Nor can the pediatric practitioner assume that a child's parents necessarily will do an adequate job of promoting and protecting the child's growth and development. Every family must be evaluated with regard to the physical, emotional, and intellectual environment it provides for each child. And when ever it appears that a child is being maltreated, neglected, or abused, the pediatric clinician must find ways to intervene effectively on behalf of the patient. Such intervention is always difficult and involves weighing and balancing a large number of very complicated factors.

Finally, there are limits to the resources that any individual family —and society at large—can allocate to health care for its members. In a sense all individuals are in competition with each other for the health maintenance resources of our society. Families must make decisions about the priorities they assign to expenditures on health care for each member of the family. In the wider society, diverse interest groups are at work lobbying for funds to support their particular health care needs. Children are least able to promote their needs and interest by themselves; they must depend on concerned adults to work on their behalf, both within families and through the political apparatuses of local, state, and national government. Pediatric health care practitioners inevitably become enmeshed in some of these battles. Consequently, pediatric clinicians often find that increasing amounts of their time must be spent on advocacy. These are just some of the characteristics of pediatric health care that set it apart from adult health care work.

Even in its brief tenure of existence, pediatric practice has changed enormously. This has come about because of a number of factors, not the least important of which is the fact that the problems faced by children in this country have changed dramatically over the years. In the early part of this century clinicians had to be most concerned with infectious, often life-threatening, diseases, and with problems of infant nutrition. Now, with easy availability of immunizations and antibiotics, acute infectious diseases are no longer a significant threat in the technologically developed world. And, with improved public health measures, severe nutritional problems are rare in infants. Consequently, at least half of the modern primary pediatric clinician's time is spent in preventive health care. A slightly smaller portion is spent in dealing with acute illness, most of which is not serious. Also, practitioners spend a much larger proportion of time addressing psychological, developmental, and social problems. Although the time spent in caring for children with chronic illness has also increased, it is still only a small part of a general pediatric practice.

In the early years, pediatricians acted primarily as specialized consultants to general practitioners. Over the years the focus has changed, and pediatric clinicians most frequently have become generalists who care for children. Increasing concern with prevention of illness and the promotion of health, and also the rise of knowledge about psychological, developmental, and social problems, have broadened the pediatric domain of primary care. This "new pediatrics" is often called "comprehensive care," and demands a sophisticated approach that goes quite far beyond evaluation and treatment of individual medical problems.

At the same time, an opposite trend away from general practice in pediatrics has asserted itself. The rapid emergence, in the past two decades, of new information and technology which pertain to the diagnosis and treatment of disease, has led to increasing subspecialization in both pediatric nursing and medicine. Because of these scientific advances, those rare children with serious acute illnesses, and also children with chronic diseases, are often cared for by a pediatric subspecialist rather than by the child's primary clinician. This is especially true in urban areas. As many have pointed out, teachers of future primary care pediatric clinicians must find a way to instruct on the scientific and technical advances of pediatrics, and at the same time to give sufficient emphasis to the special skills and orientation which are necessary for good comprehensive primary care.

In the past two decades there has been a tremendous increase in the number and variety of health care professionals. A contemporary pediatric clinician may be a nurse who has become a nurse practitioner or a clinical nurse specialist, a pediatrician who has decided to specialize in the primary care of children, or someone who has pursued an educational program to become a child health associate, school health associate, or a physician's assistant.

Economic pressures have been among the most significant factors stimulating the development of many new training programs for nonphysician health care professionals. In recent years increased emphasis has been placed on supplying adequate health care to all children, especially children of the poor. This has given impetus to the movement to train many nonmedical clinicians, because such training is much less expensive than a traditional medical education but nevertheless develops clinicians who are competent to deliver high quality primary pediatric care.

The growth in the variety of health care providers is also closely related to the role expansion of the professional nurse. Nurses are now learning to do many of the activities previously only performed by physicians, as well as expanding patient services to include more education and counseling related to health care. There is, in fact, some overlap among members of the primary health care team so that gathering data, making diagnoses, and planning and implementing care are all done by the nurse practitioner, physician's assistant, and physician. Careful planning and continuing dialogue are necessary for the team to work together in the best interests of the patients. Recent experience has shown that a team of medical and nonmedical clinicians can be acceptable to patients and their families, and that such teams can provide a safe and effective way to deliver primary health care—for both preventive and acute illness intervention.

Comprehensive primary care for children, as an approach to health maintenance, remains the same for all clinicians, regardless of their professional discipline or level of expertise. This book is about that approach. Throughout, the examples have been chosen to illustrate the ways in which many different clinicians can work together in the delivery of pediatric health care. Consequently, although this text is intended to teach students about clinical assessment in pediatric practice, it also is a treatise on the comprehensive approach to primary care in general.

COMPREHENSIVE PRIMARY CARE DEFINED

The term "comprehensive care" is used to highlight an approach in health care practice which rejects a narrow focus on pathology and medical intervention and emphasizes the broad scope of health care, including the physical, emotional, cognitive, and social well-being of the patient. Further, it encompasses the view that clinicians should not confine themselves to assessing and treating just the patient, but rather should pay attention to the family and the community as well.

In pediatric practice the family is especially important because the young child alone cannot provide sufficient data for diagnosis, nor can a child carry out a health management plan without support from the family. In addition, the child's physical, cognitive, and emotional development all depend on the nurturing environment provided in the family, both nuclear and extended. The psychological statuses of a child's primary caregivers (usually the parents) have a tremendous effect on the child's development. For example, a seriously depressed mother is not able to provide an appropriate, stimulating environment for her infant. Therefore the child may become apathetic, may be delayed in cognitive and emotional development, and may even develop serious physical problems such as failure to grow properly. For the older child (especially the adolescent), the clinician must be concerned with social forces outside the family, such as the school and peer group. Occasionally, state agencies mandated to promote and protect children's interests are also involved.

Comprehensive primary care is focused on health promotion, not just the treatment of illness. It includes health maintenance and the prevention of possible future health problems. Since the effects, both positive and negative, of early experiences continue to be important through adolescence and even adulthood, the practitioner must consider the long-range effects of both the physical environment and the family situation. It is likely that more and more factors in the early years will be discovered to be related to later physical and emotional problems. The education of the child and parents about the importance of preventive health care, immunizations, good nutrition, and dental care, as well as counseling about child-rearing and other aspects of family life are essential.

Good comprehensive primary care requires the integration of mental health care with physical health care. Paying attention to the quality of the child's emotional life, including relationships to parents, siblings, and people outside the nuclear family is as important as noting his or her height, weight, and immunization status.

One of the most important concepts underlying good comprehensive health care is that psychological and physical factors are closely related to each other. The child's body and mind are interdependent and therefore affect each other. This is most critically true for infants and very young children, and remains true through adolescence. There are many physical illnesses that affect a child's psychological development and, conversely, many psychological problems that can affect the child's physical growth and maturation. Often, these two processes of development are closely intertwined, and manifestations of physical and mental problems occur together.

It is absolutely necessary for the clinician who gives comprehensive pediatric care to have a good working knowledge of children's psychological and cognitive development. Normal development is very complex, and abnormalities are caused by many factors. The clinician should be careful not to flee from the complexity by subscribing dogmatically to any one simple theory of development. As in other areas of practice, clinicians need to maintain a thoughtful, empirical attitude about developmental problems and their management. Just as the promotion of physical health requires prevention and screening for early detection of problems, so too does the promotion of mental health. Emotional and cognitive problems must be identified as early as possible to avoid serious or irreversible damage. Often, the primary pediatric clinician is the first person in our society to have the data necessary for recognizing the presence of emotional problems. This is especially true for children before they enter day care, nursery, or elementary school. However, all through the patient's childhood the pediatric clinician should continue in this role.

THE PERSONAL RELATIONSHIP AS A TOOL IN COMPREHENSIVE PEDIATRIC CARE

In order to be successful in promoting their patients' health, pediatric clinicians must be able to identify and nurture the strengths of each child and family; they should not merely focus on problems. This requires an interest in learning about the psychological, social, ethnic, and cultural background of each family, as well as collecting all the "medical" data on the physical aspects of the child's health. In its essence, the delivery of such broad, comprehensive care depends on the clinician's deliberate building of a relationship with each family. This takes a very clearly thought out and introspective approach to the details of the clinician's behavior, a willingness to set aside the necessary time, and a mastery of communication skills.

The fact that comprehensive pediatric practice depends on the building of an enduring relationship between the clinician and family members raises some very important issues. The family grants the clinician access to what is often very private information and the right to examine the child's body. Naturally the family and the patient can reasonably expect that the clinician will use the information thus gained to promote their own—and not the clinician's—interests. They can also expect the information to be kept confidential. In addition, there are situations when the child does not want the clinician to share certain information with the parent. This concern with privacy may be experienced most intensely by adolescents.

Sometimes there appears to be a conflict of interest between what the clinician believes is good for the child and what other family members believe to be best. The pediatric health practitioner must always remember to be first and above all an advocate for the child. Therefore, if the family does not behave positively toward the child, the practitioner must recognize the situation and pursue the best possible evaluation and management in the context of an honest, caring relationship with the parents. The clinician's concerns cannot be evaded in order to protect the parents' feelings. The most difficult situations through which to sustain a constructive relationship with the parents are cases of overt child abuse, when the clinician must confront the family with the implications of their behavior and report to the authorities. A similar problem presents itself in situations of child neglect or "psychological abuse," which occur much more frequently.

Primary pediatric clinicians must have especially good insight into their own emotional reactions. It is all too easy for clinicians to identify with a child against the parents, to side with the parents against a child, or with one parent against the other. Clearly, the better clinicians understand their own feelings, the better they will be able to intervene as effective advocates for the child.

MAKING DECISIONS IN PEDIATRIC PRACTICE

An important aspect of the approach to clinical practice which practitioners should strive toward is a skeptical stance with regard to current fashions in management. There are few truths in medicine and nursing, but there are many opinions. A person may argue persuasively that a particular opinion is the only correct one. However, tomorrow, or next month, there may be new evidence that will require a change in that "correct" opinion.

The uncertainty and gaps in our knowledge are disconcerting, particularly to student clinicians. We all want to know what is right and how to implement it. However, there is almost always more than one "correct" way to manage a problem. Rather than be disheartened by this situation, I encourage students to view it as one of the aspects of primary health care that make it exciting and challenging. As clinicians become more highly trained and experienced and gain confidence in their own competence, these uncertainties are less frustrating and even come to be appreciated as the substance for serious intellectual work. An attitude that combines humility and confidence will allow new practitioners to practice safely and also to enjoy the pleasures and challenges of clinical care.

One point that cannot be stressed too much in this regard is that all clinicians encounter situations in which they do not have adequate knowledge to make informed decisions. Also, all clinicians sometimes make mistakes. In fact, patients are more likely to trust clinicians who make honest acknowledgments of their personal limitations. This trust is well-founded when clinicians who know and acknowledge their limitations also have a sincere interest in continuing to learn. Furthermore, it is not necessary for primary clinicians always to provide solutions for problems that families present. It is very constructive for health practitioners to encourage families to come up with their own solutions, especially for psychological problems, using the clinician as a concerned consultant. It is not good for families to be too dependent on their primary clinicians; a clinician who "has all the answers" may foster such dependency, to the detriment of the clinical relationship and the family's ability to function.

THE SETTING IN PEDIATRIC HEALTH CARE

No matter how thoughtful and self-aware a practitioner is, the ability to provide good comprehensive care will be diminished if the clinical setting is inadequate. There are several important features that a good clinical setting should provide. First, there must be enough time for each family to feel that the clinician can listen to them talk about their concerns. There should be adequate time for any examination or procedures, and, last but not at all least, time for the clinician to review comfortably the findings and proposals in the clinical summary.

Continuity of care is another crucial component of a good pediatric health care setting. This means that the same clinician should be taking care of a child over an extended period of time. Ideally, a family would live in the same location for most of a child's life, and clinicians would never move away. In reality, of course, because of the mobility of the American family, few clinician relationships continue for more than a few years. Nevertheless, even a few years represent significant continuity, particularly with infants and young children who are seen several times a year for health promotion. When the primary care work is done by a team, such as one consisting of a physician and a nurse practitioner, it is quite possible that even if one member of the team leaves, the family will still have one familiar clinician with whom to continue their care. This is also helpful when student clinicians (who usually do not stay in one clinical facility for very long) work closely with a clinician teacher who knows the patients.

The main reason why continuity is a very important factor in a clinical relationship is that it promotes the building of rapport, which is necessary for good comprehensive care. When continuity is minimal, or absent, patients and their families or caregivers will not develop sufficient trust in the clinician to ask worrisome questions or to confide their fears. For the disturbed parent or the wary adolescent, lack of continuity is an insurmountable barrier to adequate care.

The attitude of the staff in the clinical setting is a third factor which plays a very important role in determining the quality of the clinical relationship. This attitude, however subtly communicated, provides a powerful context that inevitably shapes patients' and their families' experiences of their visits and also affects how they perceive the behavior, intentions, and attitudes of the clinicians who are working with them. If staff members are curt, abrupt, and inconsiderate, they communicate that they do not value the patients' and families' right to be respected and treated courteously. Such a lack of respect erodes the clinician-client relationship because patients and parents are especially vulnerable in health care settings, where so much of their well-being is at stake. As a result, health care consumers feel dependent and are afraid that if they challenge the way they are treated, their health care will be compromised. Although this is a harsh statement of the situation, we all know how difficult it is to "talk back" to people in authority.

The physical environment, although secondary to the attitudes of the clinicians and staff is significant for the same reason: it reflects whether the people who are responsible for the facility respect their clients. The physical environment should convey that patients and their families are people with sensitivities who deserve to receive care in pleasant surroundings. The waiting room, office, and examining area should be light and not too noisy, and should have appropriate furniture for both children and adults. It is very important to provide toys which are maintained in good working order and stored so that they are easily accessible. Toys can also serve as an educational tool for parents, who may learn by example about toys that are safe and appropriate for a particular age or interest, and that toys serve an educational as well as an entertainment function.

The final requirement of a good clinical setting that will be listed here is the presence of a practical record system. The Problem Oriented Medical Record (POMR)* is a fairly new tool which is very helpful to clinicians in this regard. It serves the important function of helping the

---

* L.L. Weed, *Medical Records, Medical Education, and Patient Care: The Problem-Oriented Record as a Basic Tool*. Cleveland, Case Western Reserve University Press, 1969.

practitioner to organize the extensive data base (see Chapters 2, 3, and 4) into a usable format. It can be adapted for outpatient or inpatient work, for adult and pediatric patients, and for physical and mental problems. This book will not describe the POMR in any detail, but the case write-up in Chapter 15 illustrates a modified Problem Oriented Medical Record. The POMR is especially helpful to students in providing them with a framework for usefully organizing the information gathered during the assessment; and it provides a way for teachers to learn how students formulate their cases. This format is also most helpful in the care of a patient with many serious problems, all of which need monitoring and ongoing data gathering by a variety of people on the health team, and in clinical research where computerized records are utilized.

TIME AND CLINICAL PRACTICE

Time is a crucial commodity in health care, just as it is in any other endeavor. How much time is available—and how that time is used—has great impact on the success of health care. Not of least importance is the fact that the use of clients' time during their visits to the health care site reflects whether their clinician respects the clients' time as much as his or her own.

The length of a visit should take into account what must be learned, what it would be nice to learn, and the time available—both to the patient and family and to the clinician. The time it takes to see a child can vary: from 10 minutes for a case of acute otitis media to one hour for a new patient. In many practices, a new patient is given 30 to 45 minutes for the first visit and 30 minutes for routine health assessments thereafter. A typical visit for an acute problem lasts about 15 minutes.

Although these times are approximate and represent common practice, the practitioner has the responsibility to set individual priorities and to use available time accordingly. If a family has significant social or financial problems, a 15-minute visit concerning a rash may have to be lengthened to a 45-minute visit in order to assess and address all the other problems. Often, such global problems cannot be anticipated when the appointment is made, and adjustments in the clinician's schedule must be made as needed. Likewise, a seriously ill child may need urgent care, and concurrent routine appointments for other patients will have to be postponed.

Practitioners should also be flexible about how they use the time available for a given visit. If, for example, a parent must have forms for a day-care center filled out in order to start a new job, this will take precedence over the important but secondary goal of gathering a thorough social history.

SOCIETY AND HEALTH CARE DELIVERY

There are many complex factors in the health care delivery system of our society which influence the quality of health care that patients and their families receive in every clinical setting. Although it is not within the scope of this book to discuss these factors in any depth, they are mentioned here in order to raise them for thoughtful consideration by newcomers to pediatric health care practice.

Even the most altruistic and energetic clinicians cannot deliver quality care if economic support is lacking. In this country economic factors should not block people from receiving health care, but they may prevent many children from receiving *continuity* of care, and may jeopardize the *quality* of care which they receive as well. Understaffed, overworked health care workers become disgruntled and less effective, and inadequate funds often result in unpleasant surroundings. An understaffed and poorly equipped clinic cannot provide adequate care, nor can a private office operated as a high volume business to increase profits, for such a practice also deprives families of adequate time and attention.

In the United States, the most acutely ill people receive a very large proportion of all funds available for health care. Further, an astoundingly large portion of the health care dollar goes into expensive equipment and procedures, hospital contruction and upkeep, basic science research, and training in the physical aspects of medical care. In medicine as in so many areas of our competitive, materialistic society, active procedures, new machines, and scientific facts have been highly valued, while nurturing care, honest communication, and empathetic understanding have been denigrated. As a result, clinical practice has become increasingly dehumanized. Since most children are not seriously ill and a very large proportion of their needs involve preventive care, only when society allocates far more funds to train and provide comprehensive primary care clinicians will it be possible to bring adequate care to all children. Consequently, both consumers and providers of pediatric health care should work together in the political arena to increase the allocation of resources for comprehensive primary care of children.

COMPREHENSIVE PEDIATRIC CARE: IDEAL AND CHALLENGE

The body of this book is aimed at teaching student clinicians how to think critically about comprehensive health assessment in primary pediatric care and how to incorporate an attitude of respect and caring into daily practice. Included are: a discussion of the data necessary for adequate assessment; considerations in talking with children and their parents; the integration of developmental assessment into routine health appraisals; how to perform a complete physical examination and other procedures in a way that is psychologically as comfortable as possible; and how to present conclusions arising from the assessment to both the child and the family. Successful health care requires the clinician to perform the technical aspects of pediatric care in an individualized and flexible manner, while simultaneously building a relationship that can be used to promote good health, growth, and development in children and their families. Therefore, the term "comprehensive pediatric care" represents not only an ideal for the quality of care that every child should receive but also a personal challenge to all clinicians who have chosen to devote their professional work to the care of children. This text is intended to communicate both the ideal and the challenge to students of pediatric health care, and to provide them with a reliable guide for the initial stages of their journey.

Suggested Readings
Unit I: Comprehensive Pediatric Care

Chapter 1: Comprehensive Pediatric Care

Alpert, J., et al. Delivery of health care for children: report of an experiment. *Pediatrics* 57: 917–930, 1976.

Brown, K.C. The nurse practitioner in a private group practice. *Nurs. Outlook* 22: 108–113, Feb. 1974.

Chappell, J.A. and Droges, P.A. Evaluation of infant health center care by a nurse practitioner. *Pediatrics* 49: 871–877, 1972.

Charney, E., and Kitzman, H. The child health nurses (pediatric nurse practitioner) in private practice—a controlled trial. *New Eng. J. Med.* 285: 1353–1358, 1971.

Claiborn, S.A. and Walton, W. Pediatricians' acceptance of PNPs. *Am. J. Nurs.* 79(2), Feb. 1979.

Day, L.R., Egli, R., and Silver, H.K. Acceptance of pediatric nurse practitioners. *Am. J. Dis. Child.* 119: 204–208, 1970.

Deisher, R.W., Engel, W.L., Speilholz, R. and Standfast, S.T. Mothers' opinions on their pediatric care. *Pediatrics* 35: 82–90, 1965.

DeTornyay, R. and Bergman, A.B. Two views on the latest manpower issue; Part 2. Expanding the nurse's role does not make her a physician's assistant. *Am. J. Nurs.* 71, May 1971.

Duncan, R., Smith, A.N., and Silver, H.K. Comparison of the physical assessment of children by pediatric nurse practitioners and pediatricians. *Am. J. Pub. Health* 61: 1170–1176, 1971.

Ford, L. The changing role of the nurse in child health care. *Am. J. Dis. Child.* 127: 543–545, 1974.

Green, M., and Haggerty, R.L. Child health services and the clinician. Pp. 1–10 in *Ambulatory Pediatrics II*. Philadelphia, W.B. Saunders, 1977.

Haggerty, R.L. The changing role of the pediatrician in child health care. *Am. J. Dis. Child.* 127: 545–549, 1974.

Hoekelman, R.A. What consititutes adequate well-baby care? *Pediatrics* 55: 313, 1975.

Jordan, J.D. Nurse practitioner in group practice *Am. J. Nurs.* 74: 1447–1449, Aug. 1974.

Knafl, K.A. How nurse practitioner students construct their role. *Nurs. Outlook*, 26: 650–653, Oct. 1978.

Korsch, B.M., Negrete, V.F., Mercer, A.S., and Freeman, B. How comprehensive are well child visits? *Am. J. Dis. Child.* 122: 483–488, 1971(b).

Shetland, M.L. An approach to role expansion—the elaborate network. *Am. J. Pub. Health* 61: 1959–1964, Oct. 1971.

Silver, H.K., Ford, L.C., and Day, L.R. The pediatric nurse practitioner program. *JAMA* 204: 298–302, 1968.

Starfield, B., Birkowf, S. Physican's recognition of complaints by parents about their children's health. *Pediatrics* 43: 168–172, 1969.

White, K. Health care organization. *Am. J. Dis. Child.* 127: 549–553, 1974.

Wise, Harold. Making health teams work. *Am. J. Dis. Child.* 127: 537–542, 1974.

UNIT TWO

The Data Base: Foundation of Clinical Practice

INTRODUCTION

The data base consists of the information about a child and family to which the primary care clinician should have access during each examination, whether for the health maintenance of a well child or the evaluation and treatment of a sick child. Its content is now fairly standard as a result of several generations of pediatric practice. It includes information from the history, physical examination, developmental assessment, screening tests, and laboratory procedures. These data should be collected during the earliest contacts with the child and family, since they provide baseline information against which to measure and assess the significance of change. The clinician uses the data base to develop a plan for health maintenance and to manage problems as they arise.

The clinical interview is a crucial source of many kinds of data, including answers to direct questions, information spontaneously offered by the child and parents, sequences of communication, and observations of nonverbal communication. We must stress that all of these aspects offer valuable information. Therefore, an adequate data base could never be gathered simply by using a questionnaire or by asking direct questions; skillful, nonstructured but standardized interviewing and observation techniques are essential. (See chapters on the Interview, Physical Examination, and Developmental Assessment.)

The process by which the information is obtained is as important as the data collected. The professional relationship which is essential for adequate comprehensive care is built on the personal interactions that take place in the data collection process. This is especially true when the clinician and family are getting to know each other, in the course of which both the child and the parents will inevitably reveal personal information—including fears, feelings, and values. The practitioner, in turn, should express understanding and interest.

A common error is the failure to complete the data base during the initial visit; it is very easy to "never quite get around to it" subsequently. So, if a complaint or some other concern monopolizes the initial visit, the clinician should arrange another visit for the specific purpose of completing the data base. This base should be expanded as the child grows and develops, since there will be important changes in his or her psychological and social life. Some of the more typical situations which require additions to the data base include: the child attending a new school; the birth of a sibling; a serious illness striking the family; a change in a parent's work; divorce of the parents; the child developing new eating and sleep patterns; and the emergence of a new developmental achievement, such as learning to walk. Of course, should abnormalities arise, new information must be collected and evaluated along with what is known from the data base.

An example may illustrate one kind of situation requiring an expansion of the data base. Sally, a 5-year-old girl, comes for a prekindergarten health evaluation. In response to the question "How have things been?" the practitioner learns from Sally's parents that her 20-year-old uncle, who lives with her family, had meningitis six weeks ago. Although her uncle has recovered, and the parents report that "everything is back to normal," the clinician should be aware of the seriousness of the disease and its potential effect on the family. It is appropriate for the clinician to ask about the uncle's relationship to the family, where he was hospitalized, what the 5-year-old girl was told, what questions she asked, how she appeared to react to the event, how the uncle is currently functioning, and how his illness is affecting the family life. This information may not be recorded under a separate problem heading, but it does need to be in the chart under the family medical history.

Another example is the case of a 13-year-old boy whose family has just moved into the community from a different school district. The boy comes for evaluation of an earache, but the practitioner learns about the recent move when asking "How have things been?" Although moves to new homes and new schools are not necessarily so difficult that they should be considered problems, they are always stressful. Thus, in this case the practitioner should inquire about the family's adjustment in general and about how the patient has been adjusting to the new neighborhood and school. Such information should be recorded as new social history.

This unit and the succeeding one will discuss the contents of an extremely thorough data base. *In practice, this very comprehensive model is adapted or abbreviated to suit the needs of patient, clinician, and institution.* However, if the student first masters the entire format, then she or he can alter it to suit the demands of a given situation—and be confident that nothing essential is being overlooked.

It is important to record the data base in a systematic, comprehensive form; this ensures that information may be easily retrieved for such purposes as patient care, teaching, and clinical research. Information hidden in the cobwebs of someone's memory or lost in an obscure part of the record is useless. Different clinicians caring for a patient at various times depend on the medical record for accurate, concise information. In any clinical setting, the written record is still the most reliable means of communication between colleagues. Careful recording of information helps foster clear thinking—whereas careless, incomplete records predispose to inadequate identification of problems, poor formulation of management, and lack of follow-up.

Parenthetically, students also benefit from conscientious recording. Students' records provide their instructors with material to use in assessing their progress in developing methodology and skills. Further, should the student wish to undertake research, she or he will find that complete, well-organized data are crucial to all research—be it retrospective, ongoing, or prospective.

In a good medical record the information is well organized. This means that the data should be separated according to their content: for example, history, physical examination, and laboratory tests. Needless to say, within each of these categories, uniform, precise subject headings are essential.

CHAPTER 2

The History

Identifying Data
Chief Complaint
Historians (Sources)
Sources of Health Care
Present Problem(s) or Current Status
Past Health
    Birth History
        Maternal obstetric history
        Pregnancy
        Labor and delivery
        Patient's condition at birth
        Immediate postpartum period for the mother
        Neonatal period for the infant
    Early Infancy
    Childhood and Adolescent Health
        Common childhood illnesses
        Serious illnesses
        Surgical procedures
        Obstetric history
        Accidents and injuries
        Allergies
        Immunizations
Patient Profile
    Current Life Situation (the Social History)
        Household members
        Physical characteristics of the home
        Primary caregivers at home
        School

                    Economic situation
                    Agencies
                Development
                    General description
                    Affect, energy, and fears
                    Child's relationship with family members
                    Habits
                    Child-school relationships
                    Play
                    Language and communication
                    Motor skills
                    Adaptive or problem-solving ability
            Family Medical History
            Review of Systems

IDENTIFYING DATA

This section should include only a restricted range of information; its purpose is to provide clinicians an orienting context for interpreting a medical record. The identifying statement should be concise and should contain only essential information.

This section should always include the patient's *age* and *sex*. The names, addresses, and telephone numbers of the child and the parents are usually provided on an addressograph plate or the front page of the chart.

Frequently, the patient's presumed *race* is included. However, this is rarely useful information, and it too often leads to prejudiced views about the patient. In fact, racial labels are arbitrary and capricious, and are not an accurate way to indicate a patient's genetic makeup. However, a number of diseases such as sickle cell hemoglobin, glucose-6-phosphate-dehydrogenase (G-6-P-D) deficiency, and thalassemia all require special tests for detection, and occur much more frequently in dark-skinned people of Mediterranean, African, and Arab ancestry. For this reason, significant characteristics such as skin color and the geographic origins of the child's ancestors should appear in the identifying data *if* they are relevant to the particular patient.

Sometimes it is wise to include other kinds of information in the identifying data as well. These might include religion, marital status, number of children, presence of an important (usually chronic) disease, primary language, country of origin, and cultural background.

Religion sometimes influences people's views of health practices; it may happen that the patient and/or parents do not share the values of the attending health care professionals. For instance, a Jehovah's Witness may not be willing to accept a blood transfusion; a Catholic may not want to use birth control; a Jew or Muslim may have special dietary restrictions. In pediatrics, the problem is most serious when parents withhold livesaving treatment from the child. Occasionally, clinicians feel called upon to obtain a court order to allow a treatment to proceed in spite of the parents' objections.

Marital status and *number of children* are important in adolescent pediatrics. Adolescent patients may be married or living away from their families with other adolescents or adults, and even may have children of their own.

Serious and *chronic illnesses* always have profound effects on the physical, developmental, medical, social, and psychological aspects of the patient's life. The clinician and other health team members need to be informed of such facts at the beginning of the medical record. For example, if the patient has cystic fibrosis, it is important that this fact be indicated briefly in this section. Then the details of that problem can be spelled out in that portion of the record which is appropriate; i.e., under Chief Complaint or Present Problems.

The patient's *primary language* will influence her or his health care. A patient who does not speak English faces many difficulties living in an English-speaking country and may have difficulty obtaining adequate health care if the practitioner or supporting health care workers are not fluent in his or her language. Frequently, a patient, although not fluent in English, can use the language to some extent. But this also may cause problems, since the health team members may think that the patient is quite fluent in English because she or he seems to grasp all that is said—whereas in fact the patient only understands some small portion of the whole interaction. (Patients are often reluctant to let clinicians know how little they understand.) In any event, it pays to be very alert to language and communication. If problems arise, this fact should be mentioned in the Identifying Data, along with concise explanations. One might say that the patient is "a 6-year-old boy who speaks only Spanish" or "a 12-year-old Portuguese-speaking girl who also manages to communicate in English." If an interpreter assisted in the health care visit, this should be indicated in the section entitled Historian.

Country of origin is included in the identifying statement if the patient recently immigrated to the country where the clinician is practicing, or if the influence of the original nationality is still very strong even though the immigration occurred many years earlier.

Several vignettes follow, with appropriate identifying statements for each situation.

> George is a 12-year-old boy who immigrated to the United States with his parents from Greece when he was 2 years old. Currently, he views himself as American, and has no significant family ties in Greece.

In this case, the country of origin would be omitted from the identifying statement, but this information would be recorded briefly in the Patient Profile.

> Juan is a 4-year-old boy who came with his mother from Chile 6 months ago, and now lives with his aunt and uncle in Chicago. Juan's mother does not get along well with his aunt and uncle. His father is in prison in Chile, and Juan witnessed much street fighting and violence before he left. He has had enuresis and night terrors since he arrived.

In this case the identifying statement would include the information that Juan is a four-year-old boy from Chile. The description of the current family situation would be recorded with the family social history. Enuresis and night terrors would be described as complaints in the data base and would be listed as problems in the problem list.

> Joann is a 7-year-old who was born and raised on a Navajo Indian reservation in the Southwestern United States. For the last year she has been living with her parents in Phoenix, Arizona. Her parents are active in the Native American civil rights movement, and the family cultural identity is strongly Navajo.

The identifying statement would include that the patient is a 7-year-old Navajo girl. Details about the parents' occupations and cultural identity would be included in the family social history.

CHIEF COMPLAINT

This section includes a brief description of the patient's perception of the primary *reason* for the visit to the health care facility. Usually it is important to note the *duration* of the symptoms that led up to the visit. This may be an outpatient visit to an office, clinic, or emergency room; or it may be a hospital admission. Record the complaint briefly, using a few of the patient's own words whenever possible. Readers will have a more precise idea of the situation if they know the complaint as the patient or parent explained it than if they have only a revised version in the words of the receptionist, admitting clerk, or other health professional. Explanatory details do not belong in this section. Common chief complaints in pediatric practice include the following: "checkup," "baby shots," "earache," "fever," "school problems," "vomiting," "eating paint," "stomachache."

A brief note on terminology is needed here. "Well-child care" is sometimes used to refer to a checkup or to routine preventive care. "Health maintenance" is both more technical and more precise; it designates management of routine preventive care, including counseling about growth, development, and common health practices, and advice about minor concerns or deviations from "normal."

The *duration* of the symptoms that are the cause of the complaint should be noted, except when the visit is for health maintenance. This may tell whoever is reading the medical record whether the problem is acute or chronic and is also useful for evaluating the severity of the problem. Examples in which knowing duration is particularly helpful are complaints described as "fever for two months," "headaches for three weeks," "vomiting for one day." The duration may suggest that there is an additional underlying reason for the visit, especially if the duration of the complaint and urgency of presentation do not seem to be appropriately related to each other. For instance, if a patient comes to the emergency room at midnight with "headaches for five years," it is productive to note the incongruity between the duration of the headache and the urgency of the request for care. In such a case, clinicians should ask the patient exploratory questions that will reveal the "true" reasons for the patient's visit to the emergency room at this particular time. Frequently, there are a number of serious problems in the patient's life, and the headaches serve only as a way to gain access to help.

Clinicians working in emergency rooms have noted a more subtle but very serious example of incongruity. A parent will bring in an apparently well infant at 3:00 A.M. and complain, "The kid is always crying and I can't handle her." Many an actual or potential case of child abuse has been picked up by alert clinicians in such contexts.

HISTORIANS (SOURCES)

The patient and the adult(s) accompanying the patient are the primary sources of data for the medical history. However, information may be gleaned from additional sources including: adults not present at the visit, medical records, and letters from schools, consultants, and other agencies. Any person providing historical data is termed a historian and should be described by name and/or relationship to the patient. It is not uncommon for different family members to accompany the patient on different visits and for adolescents to be accompanied by friends rather than parents. Clinicians often forget who came with the patient at the previous visit, and frequently a different member of the health care team takes care of the patient at a subsequent visit. Therefore, it is quite helpful to identify each historian explicitly. When medical records or letters are a source, the name of the institution or health care professional from whom they came should be indicated.

It is important to record whether or not one believes that the historians are *reliable*; that is, that their reports are complete and accurate. Any inadequacies should be clearly identified, and the nature of the inadequacies should be mentioned. For example, the information may be incomplete, vague, or disorganized. It may be presented in a chronological order that does not seem logical, or be distorted in another consistent or significantly patterned way. Also, the reasons for the problem should be noted, if known. Some parents say "I don't know" as a way to avoid discussing personal or upsetting issues. For others, the inadequate information they offer may be a result of intellectual limitation, psychological problems (psychosis, depression, anxiety), or drugs, alcohol, or other organic brain problems which interfere with perception and recall. Additionally, the stress of the health care visit itself may interfere with the child's or parents' motivation or attention; for instance, they may be frightened or angry.

The following vignettes illustrate diverse situations and how to record them concisely in the medical record.

> Eric is a 4-year-old boy who comes for a health evaluation with his father. The father gives a complete history which seems accurate. He is relaxed, willing to answer questions about the family, and does not seem to avoid topics or fabricate the data.

The entry in the medical record could simply be "Historian: father, reliable."

> Sarah is a 10-year-old girl who comes for a health evaluation required by the school. Her 16-year-old sister accompanies her because both parents are working. Sarah and her sister seem comfortable, pleasant, and intelligent, but they do not know very much about Sarah's past medical history or early childhood. They do, however, present a complete picture of Sarah's current life and health.

The entry in the record might read "Historians: patient, and 16-year-old sister; both reliable, but data incomplete, especially past history." The clinician will have to contact the parents in order to complete the data base. This should be listed in the plan at the end of the note for this visit.

> Jonathan is a 14-year-old boy who comes for a health evaluation with his foster mother, Mrs. Roberts, and the social worker from Protective Services, Mr. Jonah Perkins. Jonathan is angry, unhappy, and uncooperative in giving any history. He was placed with Mrs. Roberts only 2 weeks prior to this visit, so she knows very little about him. Mr. Perkins has information about the reasons for placement in a foster home, but has little to contribute about the boy's past health.

The entry might read: "Historians: patient, uncooperative in giving information; foster mother, Mrs. Roberts, cooperative about placement period of the past two weeks, but knows no past history; Mr. Jonah Perkins, social worker from Protective Services, helpful with social information, but knows no past medical history." As in the previous example, one of the first items in the plan would be to complete the data base by contacting the patient's family, if possible, and obtaining previous records from other health care facilities.

Margot is a 7-year-old girl who has been referred to you by the local visiting nurse for evaluation of frequent school absences and an unstable home situation. She is accompanied by her mother, Mrs. Smith, and her 3 younger siblings. Margot seems very mature and is able to give a great deal of current history about herself and her family. Her mother is very disorganized, easily upset to the point of tears, and unable to give a coherent account of Margot's health or family life. Mrs. Smith has the odor of alcohol on her breath, and admits readily that she has a drinking problem.

The record might read: "Historians: patient, reliable and unusually competent for her age, but with imcomplete information about past history; mother, acutely intoxicated with alcohol, and unable to give a coherent history." The plan at the end of the note would include contact with the Visiting Nurse Association for more data about the family problems and for Margot's medical history. In this case Margot would not be the only focus for care. Her mother, and even other family members, should be offered a health plan.

SOURCES OF HEALTH CARE

In this section the clinician should record the usual or prior *sources* of health care, and also the *reasons* why the client(s) changed to this new health care site. The names and addresses of the other health care institutions and professionals should be listed, so that information can be obtained from them if necessary. There are many reasons why clients change their health care sites, including dissatisfaction with previous health care, the cost of services, or simply a move to a new city. Parents are sometimes reluctant to tell the new health care professionals about their dissatisfaction with their previous health care institutions. However, if the parents are encouraged to talk about such dissatisfaction, the new clinicians can understand better how that family uses health care services; and they should consequently be better able to satisfy the client's needs. This discussion can also serve to demonstrate a great deal about the clinician's respect for the patients as well as their own self-respect and confidence.

PRESENT PROBLEM(S) OR CURRENT STATUS

This section includes any present problem(s) needing evaluation. The following narrative illustrates how a current problem might be recorded in the chart:

> Three-week history of right knee pain. Onset after a fall while playing hockey. No obvious bruise, swelling, redness or heat at that time or subsequently. Aching pain daily, not at night. Pain localized to knee. Some relief with aspirin, heat, and rest. Clearly worse after walking or any exercise and at end of day. Pain increasingly persistent over last 7 to 10 days. Patient well otherwise; no other joint symptoms. Patient without past history of joint problems; negative family history.

The discussion of how to evaluate a problem is detailed in the chapter on the interview. If there are no problems identified and the purpose of the visit is for health promotion (sometimes called well-child care), it is appropriate to write a short section about the child's current status. The emphasis will vary with the age of the child. For an infant or young child, details about diet, sleep, elimination habits, and current developmental adjustment and achievements are appropriate. For the older child, information about diet, relationships with family and friends, and school performance would be emphasized. In this situation, the early section on current health would be followed by the traditional data base.

PAST HEALTH

Birth history

This section should be a well-organized, concise but detailed presentation of the patient's neonatal history and the mother's obstetric history. Events during the pregnancy and perinatal period have long-range organic and psychological effects which frequently go unnoticed by parents. It is very important to know the medical and psychological details of the birth history in order to evaluate the child's health accurately and to plan health maintenance and problem management. *If the patient is a school-age child or adolescent and has had no serious medical or psychological problems, clinicians need not pursue questions about the perinatal period in detail. Rather, they should ask selected, open-ended questions. Only the birth weight and the fact that there were no reports of problems during the pregnancy or in the perinatal period need be recorded.*

Literary style is not an important consideration in recording the history. Accuracy and completeness are. Although grammatically incorrect, a series of phrases is usually the most succinct and clear format for recording and retrieving information. On occasion it may be useful to quote the child or parents, and this should be indicated with quotation marks. Also, any discrepancies between the history being elicited from the patient and the previous medical record should be noted and resolved if possible. (These principles are relevant to the entire medical record. However, in an oral presentation, one should use complete sentences.)

MATERNAL OBSTETRIC HISTORY:
This section of the record should include the mother's age at the time of the patient's birth, previous pregnancies and their outcomes (including miscarriages, abortions, and premature births), and the number of living children. Also, if any children died after the neonatal period, this should be indicated. Each hospital uses its own abbreviated forms of nomenclature to record the obstetric history of a patient. For example, in one hospital "G3,2,2" means "three pregnancies, two live births, and two living children." Presumably, one pregnancy ended in a miscarriage or a stillbirth. These abbreviations vary greatly, so we will not elaborate on them any further.

PREGNANCY:
This section should include details about the conception. Typically, examiners record answers to questions like, "Was the pregnancy planned?" and "How long did it take for you to become pregnant?" It is very important to include illnesses and symptoms of the mother: for example, vaginal bleeding, fevers, rashes, hospitalizations, weight gain, weight loss, vomiting (including any mild first trimester morning sickness), hypertension, proteinuria, preeclampsia, general infections, and (in particular) urinary tract infections.

   The clinician should be sure to ask specifically about drugs. Did the mother take any medications? Did she use over-the-counter pills? Did she take "uppers," "downers," or any other such substances? Did she smoke marijuana? How much alcohol did she drink? (People often overlook their use of alcohol, and do not consider it a drug.)

   It is also important to find out if the mother had any x-rays (either diagnostic or therapeutic) during the pregnancy, and whether she was exposed to injurious chemicals or other agents.

   For any of the items relevant to the mother's health during the pregnancy, details such as time of occurrence during pregnancy, diagnostic tests, final diagnosis, course, and treatment should be recorded. Also, details of the mother's prenatal care should be described, including the name of the physician, midwife, nurse practitioner, or clinic; the time in the pregnancy when care was initiated; and whether the patient had care regularly. Attendance at prenatal classes should be recorded with a brief description of the content. It also is important to note whether the father or another person participated in the classes with the mother.

LABOR AND DELIVERY:
This section should include the number of weeks of gestation before labor began; the place (name and address of hospital or home) where the patient was born; length of labor in hours; when the membranes ruptured in relation to delivery; whether the membranes ruptured spontaneously

or if they were artificially ruptured; whether labor was induced and, if so, for what reason. Information about the delivery must include whether it was vaginal or by cesarean section. If cesarean delivery was used, the reason should be specified; if vaginal, whether it was vertex or breech. It is very important to find out what kind of analgesia and anesthesia were used and when during the labor they were administered. The parents' memory of their personal experience of labor and delivery are also worthy of note, because these subjective experiences sometimes have long-range effects on the parents' view of the child and on the mother's feeling about her own competence. It is frequently helpful to ask, "Was the labor difficult?" "Were the labor and delivery what you expected?" Asking the parents to elaborate will provide important data for insight into their views of the birth and the parenting process and will help them to feel supported. It is interesting to note whether or not the father or a friend was present during the birth process and what first impressions the father and mother each had of their newborn child.

PATIENTS CONDITION AT BIRTH:
If no medical record is available to provide details of the child's health at birth, the following questions are helpful: "What was Michele's weight?" "What color was her skin (pink or blue)?" "Did she cry soon after she was born?" "Did you want to hold her right away?" "Were you (the mother) allowed to hold her in the delivery room?" If the mother did hold the infant very soon after delivery, it probably means the infant's condition was stable, the mother was awake, she wanted and was able to hold the baby, and the personnel involved in the delivery encouraged early contact of the mother and the infant. The clinician should also ask whether the father wanted and was able to hold Michele soon after she was born.

Even if a medical record is available, it is useful to ask a brief open-ended question such as "How was Freddy right after he was born?" Occasionally the parents will have a particularly distorted view of the child's condition at birth. They may exaggerate the seriousness of a benign situation, such as an umbilical cord being loosely wrapped around the child's neck, or they may forget a potentially serious problem such as inadequate respiration after birth. Such distorted perceptions may point to severe problems in the family and may later develop into psychological problems for the child.

IMMEDIATE POSTPARTUM PERIOD FOR THE MOTHER:
The clinician should ask if there were any problems for the mother, either physical or emotional. It is quite important to ascertain whether or not she had a rooming-in arrangement with the baby, and if not, why not, as well as the quality and amount of time of her interactions with the baby. (It may not have been available in the place where she delivered.) It

is also important to note whether or not the father was available to visit and support the mother during this period, his interaction with the baby, and his psychological reactions.

NEONATAL PERIOD FOR THE INFANT:
This section concerns information about the child's health during the first days of life. If the medical record is not available, the following questions are particulary helpful: "Did the baby have any problems in the hospital?" "Was the child in a special care nursery for observation or treatment?" If the child was in a special nursery, the clinician should ask why and for how long. Specific questions about respiratory problems, jaundice, and treatment such as phototherapy ("special lights") and exchange transfusion may yield important information.

The clinician should also inquire about the patient's discharge from the hospital. Some helpful questions are: "How many days old was Ruthie when she went home from the nursery?" "Did you (the mother) and baby go home together?" If the answer is negative, the clinician should inquire about the details of the situation. For example, when an infant is well but premature, she or he might be kept in the hospital to mature and gain weight after the mother has been discharged. If the child did stay after the mother's discharge, the clinician should find out if the parents visited the child in the nursery, whether they held and fed the infant in the hospital, and how they felt about having the baby in the hospital. Another reason for the mother's being discharged before the child is that the mother is not physically or emotionally ready to care for the infant, and the hospital serves as a temporary home for the child. Again, all the medical and behavioral specifics of the situation should be described, including the quantity and quality of the contacts between parents and child and how the parents felt about the complicating circumstance.

Early infancy

This section includes a description of the child's health and behavior during early infancy, as well as the family's adjustment during the first weeks after birth. The examiner should ask about any illnesses at this time and should elicit information about the child's daily routines of eating and sleeping. Some specific questions are: "How was Tommy?" "Was it easy or difficult to comfort him?" "Was he an irritable baby?" "Did Tommy develop a regular pattern of eating and sleeping?" "Was he *too* good (demanded little or no care)?" "Did he smile and make eye contact?" "Was he alert?" If any problems were present, details of the problems, courses, treatments, and outcomes should be noted.

Adjustment to a new infant is a challenge for all members of the household. Here are some questions which can help the clinician assess whether there were any unusual stresses during this time: "How did the members of the household adjust to the new baby?" "Were there any surprises?" "What was most enjoyable?" "What was most difficult?" "How did you feel about Tommy?" "How did his father feel about the child?" "Did the siblings show any signs of being jealous?" "How did they demonstrate it?" "How did you and your husband handle the jealousy?"

If the patient is an older child and there were no problems during early infancy, some brief, general comments about this period are sufficient. However, it may be necessary to return to this part of the history if a psychological problem does develop later. In any case, some broad, open-ended questions about early infancy and family adjustment should always be included in the data base.

Early infancy is singled out for specific and detailed questions because this is a difficult time for most parents. Also, it is becoming increasingly evident that family problems during this period often have long-lasting and extensive effects on the child's subsequent development. An account of the child's physical and emotional health will develop during the rest of the interview.

Childhood and adolescent health

This section presents an organized body of important information about the child's past physical and emotional health. It is usually not a very long section, and most of the details come from the historian rather than from the medical record. However, if the patient has a chronic illness and many complicated hospitalizations, it is prudent to be particularly conscientious in obtaining that information from medical records.

COMMON CHILDHOOD ILLNESSES:
This section is a simple list. It should include the name of any disease, the year and child's age at the time of the occurrence, and any known complications. Examples are: "(1) Mumps, 1965, age three years, no complications. (2) Chickenpox, 1974, age four years; secondary skin infection with some scarring."

SERIOUS ILLNESSES:
This section includes all serious illnesses, including those treated in hospitals and those treated at home. The clinician should obtain details such as the name and address of the hospital or of the health care practitioner who cared for the patient at home; length of hospital stay; diagnosis; complications; course of illness; and medications or treatment continued after discharge.

An experience with a serious illness always influences people's attitudes about health care professionals and hospitals. It is important to be alert to such attitudes, for they may cause parents and other caregivers to have distorted perceptions or false assumptions about the patient's stamina and overall state of health. For instance, sometimes a serious illness is completely cured, but parents, patient, or teachers still think of the child as vulnerable or handicapped and so unnecessarily limit his or her activity and independence. Here are some examples of serious illnesses and how they might be written up in a chart:

> 1. *Hepatitis*, 1974, age 3 years. Treated at home with limited diet to alleviate vomiting and diarrhea. Followed by Dr. Rosemary Jones in New Haven, Ct., with "Blood tests for his liver." Acute illness over in 10 days, blood tests "OK" in 4 weeks. No residual problems, is "healthy and active." Contact for the hepatitis was a nursery school classmate.
>
> 2. *Fractured femur*, 1975, age 7 years, secondary to bicycle accident. Treated at Eastern Hospital, Yorktown, Ct., by Dr. Robert Smith. Hospitalized for 2 weeks and at home in a cast for 6 weeks. Was able to attend school wearing cast. "All healed on the x-ray in 3 months." No other fractures before or since. Patient did well in hospital, no major regression after hospitalization. Resumed usual active life after cast removed.
>
> 3. *Psychological problems*: 1965 to 1967, age 5 to 7 years, treated as an outpatient at the New London Child Guidance Clinic by Dr. Ellen Parker for night terrors, enuresis, and school problems. Counseling of parents was included. Good result from treatment, with resolution of night terrors and enuresis, and much improved school situation, both in social adjustment and ability to learn. Patient is still a "sensitive child," but seems "happy and functioning well." (See chart under Development for current psychological data.)

SURGICAL PROCEDURES:
These should be described using the format provided for serious illnesses. Surgical procedures do not have to be listed separately from serious illnesses, but it is sometimes convenient to classify them this way. Occasionally patients and parents forget to mention elective surgery such as a herniorrhaphy or tonsillectomy. This category serves as a reminder to the clinician to ask specifically about both elective and nonelective surgery.

OBSTETRIC HISTORY:
Pediatric clinicians generally omit this section. However, practice settings usually include adolescent patients, and teenage pregnancies are not uncommon. The clinician needs to know whether an adolescent has been pregnant and what the outcome of each pregnancy was. It is useful to know whether previous pregnancies were carried to term; the source and use of prenatal care; course of each pregnancy; complications during pregnancy, labor and delivery, and the postpartum period; and emotional reactions to the pregnancy and its outcome. Similarly, with previous abortions, a concise summary of the patient's expectations, experiences, and feelings is most helpful to the primary health professional caring for

the adolescent. Past decisions to continue a pregnancy to term or to interrupt it can be reviewed in terms of such factors as the adolescent's plan or wish to have a baby, her view of the impact it would have on her future, and the reactions voiced by her family and friends. When an adolescent has had an abortion, her reaction must be assessed in light of the supportive care available to her as well as her subsequent sexual activity and contraceptive practices.

If the adolescent patient is pregnant at the time of the visit, this should be recorded as an active problem rather than part of the past medical history. Even when the visit is for another purpose or concern, information about the current pregnancy should be noted in the history of the present illness.

It is convenient to note current sexual activity and birth control methods in this section, although they may be listed instead in the Review of Systems.

If the patient is a father, information about his parenting is usually recorded in the social history.

ACCIDENTS AND INJURIES:

This section overlaps the previous sections on serious illnesses and surgical procedures. However, parents and patients frequently forget about accidents and injuries unless the clinician specifically asks about them. One way to obtain this information is to inquire "Did Ellen ever break any bones or have any serious accidents?" "Did she have emergency room visits for accidents or ever need stitches?" "Did Ellen ever swallow anything dangerous?" If there are any positive responses, then the clinician should proceed with more specific questions.

A history with many accidents and/or ingestions should alert the clinician, since it suggests a major problem. The causes are usually complex, but such a history does involve poor supervision by parents and perhaps even neglect or abuse. It is easy to miss this important information if one does not ask specific questions. (Many health care professionals are personally upset by indications of child abuse or neglect and defensively "overlook" data indicating the presence of such problems. Clinicians must guard against this possibility and evaluate the situation just as they would for any other serious symptom.) In situations of neglect or abuse, one must pursue the problem further and often must obtain consultation from a social worker and/or psychiatrist to provide long-term follow-up.

ALLERGIES:

This section includes details about symptoms, course, etiology (if known), treatment, and results. An example:

> *Penicillin allergy*, 1972, age 5 years; occurred 3 days after beginning course of treatment for otitis media. Developed pruritic rash with some hives; itching partially relieved with Benadryl. Rash faded in 4 days, after

penicillin was discontinued. No other allergies. No penicillin since. Family history of "hay fever" in mother and maternal uncle.

IMMUNIZATIONS:

This section should include the name of the preparation, amount given for DPT immunizations, who (person or institution) gave it, and what reaction, if any, occurred. Usually there is a separate place in the medical record for listing this information. Parents should be asked whether they have a card or book in which the child's immunizations are listed. Such a record should be filled in at the time of an immunization. It can also be used to provide data for an incomplete medical record.

Here is an example for a six-year-old child born on January 2, 1971:

DPT (0.5 cc) 3/3/71
DPT (0.5 cc) 5/7/71—high fever to 105°F
DPT (0.25 cc) 7/7/71
DPT (0.25 cc) 9/15/71

DPT booster (0.25 cc) 9/17/72
DPT booster (0.25 cc) 10/23/72

DPT booster (0.25 cc) 11/6/75
DPT booster (0.25 cc) 1/7/76

OPV 3/3/71, 5/7/71, 7/7/71
OPV booster 9/17/72
OPV booster 11/6/75

MMR 7/7/72 Reaction seven days after MMR received; rash over entire body and fever of 101°F. Rash and fever spontaneously resolved in two days.

DPT means the immunization for diphtheria, pertussis, and tetanus. The usual dose is 0.5 cc. In our example the patient had a high fever following the second DPT injection. Subsequent DPT immunizations were divided, as indicated, into doses of 0.25 cc each to reduce the likelihood of severe febrile reactions.

OPV means oral polio vaccine. Currently, trivalent oral polio vaccine is used. In the 1950s, when the polio vaccine was first introduced, the vaccination was given by injection. Subsequently, oral monovalent preparations were used. These were replaced by the current trivalent preparation. In an older patient's immunization record there may be entries such as Salk polio (injection) or OPV-I, OPV-III, and OPV-II. All three strains were given separately, usually in the order indicated above.

MMR means the combined measles, mumps, rubella injection. In years past, these three immunizations were given separately rather than in combination. The record in those cases would indicate which component was given on a particular date. There are preparations with two of the components, such as measles-mumps, measles-rubella, and mumps-rubella. These are given if the patient has had one of the diseases or if she or he has been immunized previously with one antigen and the clinician prefers to complete the immunizations with only one injection.

PATIENT PROFILE

This section should present the reader with an organized, concise picture of the child's current life situation, including both psychological and developmental status and an appreciation for the quality of his or her relationships with other people. In addition, the examiner should assess how both the child and other family members handle and adjust to stressful situations. It is advisable to ask clearly worded questions which lead to detailed answers about the patient's life. Vague generalizations about the patient often gloss over significant social, developmental, or psychological problems, so one should take care in the phrasing of questions. Sometimes both patient and parents do not really understand a question; sometimes they do not recognize that problems exist; and sometimes they do not think the interviewer is really interested. It might well happen, for example, that when one asks of an older child "Are you under any psychological stress?" the patient answers "No." In fact, if the same child were asked how she or he is feeling about other family members, and how members of the family are getting along with each other, the answer might reveal significant family conflict and "acting out" behavior.

Each institution has its own format for recording such patient profile information. Too often, in order to expedite the interview, clinicians use prearranged forms, which do not allow sufficient time or space for the child and parents to elaborate on this information. It is, of course, useful to utilize forms to aid in the recording of information, but if the forms do not provide sufficient space for wide-ranging information, one should always feel free to write in margins or on the overleaves to note detailed descriptions of important circumstances and feelings. If a form is used in the medical record, this information should also be supplemented by a brief narrative which gives the reader some impression about the quality of the patient's life.

One suggested format follows. (Information recorded earlier in Current Health Status or Present Problem for a well child would *not* be repeated here.) Space for complex descriptions or comments should be used whenever needed.

Current life situation (the social history)

HOUSEHOLD MEMBERS:
This section should list names, ages, and relationships of household members, including both biological relatives and unrelated members. If both parents do not live in the home, the examiner should elaborate on the situation and describe any visiting arrangements and their effects upon the child. For example:

John (patient) 5 years
Mother—Susan Hodge, 35 years

Sister—Monica, 4 years
Half-brothers, twins—Robert, 7 years
             Michael, 7 years
Maternal uncle—Chris, 23 years
Maternal grandmother—Mrs. Anna Olson, 65 years
Maternal grandfather—Mr. John Olson, 66 years
Father—Eric Hodge, 39 years. Not living at home since parents separated 2 years ago; lives in New York City, visits semimonthly on weekends; arrangement stable and "works out well."

Note: As the clinician learns more about the family, the parents' separation should be described further. This information would be recorded in the section Current Life Situation or Social History in subsequent notes.

PHYSICAL CHARACTERISTICS OF THE HOME:
This section describes the home in terms of its location, type of neighborhood, number of rooms, type of water supply and sewage system (if not city water and sewage). For instance:

> Second floor apartment of a 2-family house in a semirural suburb of New Haven. Six rooms, 3 bedrooms, porch, and yard. City water and septic system.

PRIMARY CAREGIVERS AT HOME:
This section should indicate who is involved in the child's care and supervision. The amount of time each person spends with the patient should be noted when this is pertinent, and the clinician should inquire into the stability of the arrangements and how the child and parents feel about them. For example:

> Mother and father give primary care; father very involved. Supplemented by morning care (about 20 hours per week) by baby-sitter in patient's home while mother is at work. Same sitter for 2 years; parents and child very comfortable with arrangements. Maternal grandparents help once or twice a week, also.

SCHOOL:
This section should include the name and address of the school, the teacher's name, and the child's grade. "School" is used here to mean all educational settings outside the home which the child regularly attends. Other useful details are how the child gets to and from school and the hours attended. If the patient attends a school for children with special physical or emotional needs, details should be elicited and recorded. If the child is attending a day care center or nursery school, this should be elaborated upon here. Similarly, the clinician might note whether the child also attends music school, religious school, or after-school day care. Some examples follow:

> Elm Street school, Mr. Hopkins, second grade. School is part of public school system; John (patient) is in a special class for children with learning

disabilities. Attends Neighborhood Music School for rhythm and music appreciation class with sister, once a week.

Center Street Day Care Center, Mr. Thomas, director; 9–3, group day care, 3 teachers for 15 children from 3–5 years of age, good physical facilities and qualified staff.

ECONOMIC SITUATION:

This section describes the occupations of the parents, their job security, satisfaction with their work, level of education, source of payment for medical care, type of medical insurance, eligibility and use of welfare, food stamps, and other government aid. The parents' occupations, participation in welfare programs, and sources of payment for medical care have first priority. Other information is useful but frequently is not discussed at the first visit. Some families are eligible for government assistance but do not want to accept it. Others are alienated by bureaucracies or lack the skills and knowledge to negotiate their way through the various bureaucratic channels to avail themselves of aid. Here is an example of such an entry:

Father: skilled auto mechanic, owns garage with a partner, stable business for 10 years, likes his work and feels successful; high school education. Mother: experienced legal secretary, working half-time since youngest child entered school 2 years ago, enjoys her work; high school education plus 1 year of business school. Medical insurance through father's group plan from fraternal organization.

AGENCIES:

This section should list agency names, addresses, telephone numbers, and names of all personnel involved with the patient and family. This list should be supplemented with additional data including: dates of involvement; why the relationship ended, if relevant; kinds of services rendered; how the patient and parents feel about the agency; and whether the patient and parents are willing to have the clinician contact the agency. The source of this information should be documented. If the source is not the historian, it is useful to specify exactly how the clinician obtained the data—e.g., through a letter from the agency to the clinician or a telephone call from a teacher. Some examples follow:

1. New York City VNA (Visiting Nurse Association), Ms. Robinson, R.N., visited monthly when children were young to teach mother and supervise home for basic health and safety requirements. Contacts stopped in 1974 because the home situation was satisfactory. Information from VNA reports in old hospital chart.

2. New Haven Child Guidance Clinic, telephone 773–0176, Dr. Jefferson, from 1975 to present. Weekly treatment with the patient for his emotional problems and monthly sessions with parents for same. Parents very pleased with their child's progress and willing for us to contact Dr. Jefferson.

Development

The most productive way to obtain an accurate and complete picture of the patient's past and current developmental status is to combine a developmental history with structured and unstructured observations. The history should consist of a series of carefully planned but open-ended questions which cover both developmental tasks and interpersonal relationships. The structured tasks are usually presented to the patient between the history and the physical examination in an office setting. They can also be presented at home or in a day-care center. Evaluations done when a patient is in the hospital are problematic and must be interpreted by taking into account the stress placed on the patient by the situation.

Clinicians frequently place a great deal of emphasis on developmental landmarks such as the age when the child first sat, walked, talked, or was toilet trained. This turns out to be rather a waste of time. Not only are parents' memories of questionable accuracy but the information itself is far less important in assessing the child's development than is evaluating his or her current capabilities. It is rare to find a child who had extremely unusual (usually delayed) landmarks in infancy and early childhood and is completely within the normal range at a later age. It is much more useful to gather a thorough data base about the child's current developmental functioning. Naturally, when current abnormalities are found, it is important to ask about past development in order to obtain additional data.

The following outline is suggested as a way to organize the developmental data. The questions may be altered to suit the age of the patient. A more complete discussion about concepts of development, the 24-hour format, and use of structured tasks is presented in Chapter 7 on Developmental Assessment.

GENERAL DESCRIPTION:
This section should provide a general picture of the child's personality. The clinician needs to know if the child has any particular sensitivities or any characteristics which the parents view as weaknesses. But it is also important to note strengths. The following questions are helpful in assembling a description: "How would you describe your child to a person who did not know her well?" "Does your child have any characteristics which you see as weaknesses or problems?" "What are the most enjoyable things about your child?" "What are the most difficult things about him?" "How does she compare with her siblings?" "How is he, compared with other children his age?" There are specific characteristics which the parents may mention or the clinician may want to ask about, such as confidence, insecurity, stubbornness, flexibility, kindness, and hostility. Other qualities are shyness, assertiveness, impulsivity, reflectiveness, ac-

tivity, and passivity. This section of the medical record should reflect both the information supplied by the parents and the clinician's observations of the child.

AFFECT, ENERGY, AND FEARS:
This section should include information about the child's moods, fears, and anxieties. Mood can be assessed by asking the parents to describe their child's usual moods and also by asking if the child's present behavior during the health evaluation is typical. One might ask "What things make Susan sad, anxious, or fearful?" "How does she show these feelings?" Some children use words to express their feelings, some become irritable, while younger children often cling to their parents more than usual or regress in other ways. Other specific questions include "How does Susan respond to new situations?" "How does she respond to separation from people she knows well?" "How long do those responses last?" "What do you do to help with difficult changes?"

CHILD'S RELATIONSHIP WITH FAMILY MEMBERS:
This section should include a description of the quality of the child's relationship with his or her parents, siblings, and other household members. It is important to know both how they behave with each other and how they feel about each other. The feelings affect the tone of the behavioral interactions in a way which may determine their impact. A spanking with a loving tone is less rejecting than a calm lecture about behavior by a furious parent. If the child is young (for example, not yet six years old), a simple question such as "How does John get along with you?" is adequate as a first inquiry. However, a simple "OK" is not a sufficient answer and must be followed up with more penetrating questions. If the child is older, the clinician can also ask, "How did Alice get along with the family when she was younger?" Specific questions about siblings, grandparents, and others are often very useful.

The examiner should always use this context to ascertain how the parents set limits for the child and how they use praise and discipline or punishment to mold behavior. Again, a general opening question should be followed by specific ones. It is useful to ask "How do you and your husband discipline Sarah?" "In what situations do you feel the need to discipline her?" "Does that method work?" "How often do you need to do that?" "Do you and your wife agree about it?" "How were the two of you disciplined when you were younger?" "Do you ever resort to punishment?" "When?" "What form does it take?" The emotional tone of the discipline should be ascertained. "How do you feel when you have to discipline John?" "How does John respond?"

HABITS:

   1. **Feeding:** This section should focus specifically on the emotional environment in which the patient eats. The content of the child's diet is usually recorded in the Current Health History or occasionally in the Review of Systems, but it may be included in this section. Difficulties with feeding and eating are among the most frequent parental concerns with babies and young children and may be crucial symptoms in making the diagnosis of psychological and organic problems. In a young child, abnormal eating behavior on the child's part—or unrealistic expectations or demands on the parents' part—are often symptoms indicating severe psychological difficulties between parents and child. In an older child, serious difficulties with eating usually accompany other signs of developmental or organic problems.

   The clinician can learn about eating patterns by asking direct questions: "How is Robert's eating?" "When does Robert eat?" "Does he eat when you do, or at a separate time?" Parents usually will mention problems with feeding and eating during the discussion of eating patterns. However, if they do not mention problems, the examiner should ask "Are there any problems with eating?" or "Has eating ever been a problem for Susan?" Other useful questions are "Do you think she eats enough?" "Do you think she eats too much?" "Do Susan's eating problems upset the rest of the family?" What does your spouse think about it?" "How do you handle the problem?"

   2. **Sleeping:** The examiner should ask for a description of sleeping arrangements and patterns and also whether there are any problems in this area. Some useful questions are: "Does Charles have his own bed?" If not, "With whom does he sleep?" "Who shares the bedroom?" "Are these arrangements OK with you?" (This is addressed to both parents and also to the patient, if she or he is old enough.) "How much sleep does Charles usually get at night?" "When does he usually go to bed?" "Does he sleep all the way through the night?" "Does he sleep soundly?" "Have there been any problems with Charles's sleep?" If there have been, ask both the parents and the child to describe what happens and how they handle it. For the preschool-age child also ask "Does he take a nap?" "How long does he nap?" "How do you know when he is tired?"

   This information may have been included under Current Health at the beginning of the data base for a child who comes for health promotion rather than for a problem. If that is the case, the information would not be recorded here.

   3. **Toileting:** For a younger child, the clinician should find out at what age the child was toilet trained, how this was accomplished, and whether there were any difficulties with the training. For an older child the frequency of toilet use, and of course the presence of enuresis, daytime wetting, and poor control of bowel movements should be noted. If

there are problems, it is always important to ask how these problems have been and are currently being handled by the parents, teachers, peers, and (very important!) the child as well.

CHILD-SCHOOL RELATIONSHIPS:
This section should include data on the child's adjustment to the school setting, the quality of the patient's relationship with peers and teachers, the presence of any separation problems, and an assessment of the child's attention span and academic performance. If is often helpful to ask the child directly what she or he likes most and least about school.

PLAY:
This section should describe the content and quality of the child's play and leisure activities. Again, this information is best obtained by asking both the patient and parents to describe in some detail what the child does and how the child feels. For example: "What kinds of play does Michael enjoy?" "Which adults and children play with him?" "Describe what he does when he plays with them" (such as being bossy, fearful, competitive). "Does Kate play alone?" "What is that play like?"

The kinds of questions addressed to children depend very much on their age. In general, they are asked what they like to do best, with others and alone.

LANGUAGE AND COMMUNICATION:
This section should describe how the child communicates feelings, needs, and wants and how the child indicates comprehension of communication. It should of course also include the child's skills in vocalization, expressive language, and comprehension of language. The ability to use these skills for communication and the pleasure the child gets from them are equally important.

 1. Infants and toddlers: The examiner can ask "How does Anne let you know what she wants or how she feels?" In addition, there are important specific questions that should be asked according to the patient's age, such as whether the child uses single and combined vowel sounds, simple consonants, jargon, and specific words and phrases. With good humor and patience the clinician will be able to test comprehension in a young child by asking the child to "play games" like naming or identifying body parts, following simple directions, and describing pictures in a book.

 2. Older children: The examiner should evaluate whether the patient's language is intelligible and whether it is age-appropriate. Specific details to be noted include the quality of enunciation, ability to form grammatically correct sentences, any difficulties in speech production, and the presence of stuttering. Most children will talk to the examiner after their initial anxiety has eased off, although sometimes it is helpful to ask the parents to step outside for a few moments before engaging the child in conversation. The clinician thus can assess the child's speech from their interchanges. If the child remains too shy to talk during the visit, one may resort to asking the parents to describe the child's speech and language and to give examples. It is also important always to ask about the child's ability to read and write if the child is attending school.

MOTOR SKILLS:
This section should describe the child's physical abilities, the ways he or she uses these skills, and the pleasure the child gets from them. For example, the fact that a toddler moves an adult chair to a counter and climbs up on it to get a piece of fruit is a more useful piece of information than knowing only that the child can climb up on an adult-sized chair.

    1. **Fine motor:** This refers to the use of hand muscles for the manipulation of small objects. For the young child, it is important to ask about (and—if it is practical—test) a child's eye-hand coordination; ability to grasp, hold, and release objects; and aptitude for completing complex tasks such as block building, drawing, screwing and unscrewing, buttoning, tying shoelaces, and the like.

    2. **Gross motor:** This refers to the use of large muscles of the limbs and trunk. The clinician should observe the child's movements if possible. Then the parents should be asked what skills the patient has, whether they are age-appropriate, and whether the patient can modulate his or her activity. It is important to find out if the child is impulsive or driven while active.

ADAPTIVE OR PROBLEM-SOLVING ABILITY:
This information is derived largely through evaluating the child's performance of structured tasks presented by the examiner. The contents of this section overlap information about the child's play and school performance. With preschool children, the clinician can ask a child to draw or copy geometric figures such as a circle, cross, square, triangle, or diamond. The child's knowledge of colors, use of numbers, and ability to complete puzzles should also be evaluated. Details of developmental assessment are discussed in Chapter 7.

FAMILY MEDICAL HISTORY

This section should document significant features of the medical history of all immediate family members. The clinician should take care to note diseases with a strong genetic component and those that are highly infectious. If a genetic disease is present in the family history, the examiner should elicit a pedigree of at least three generations. If serious contagious disease is found to have been present, details about the diagnosis, course,

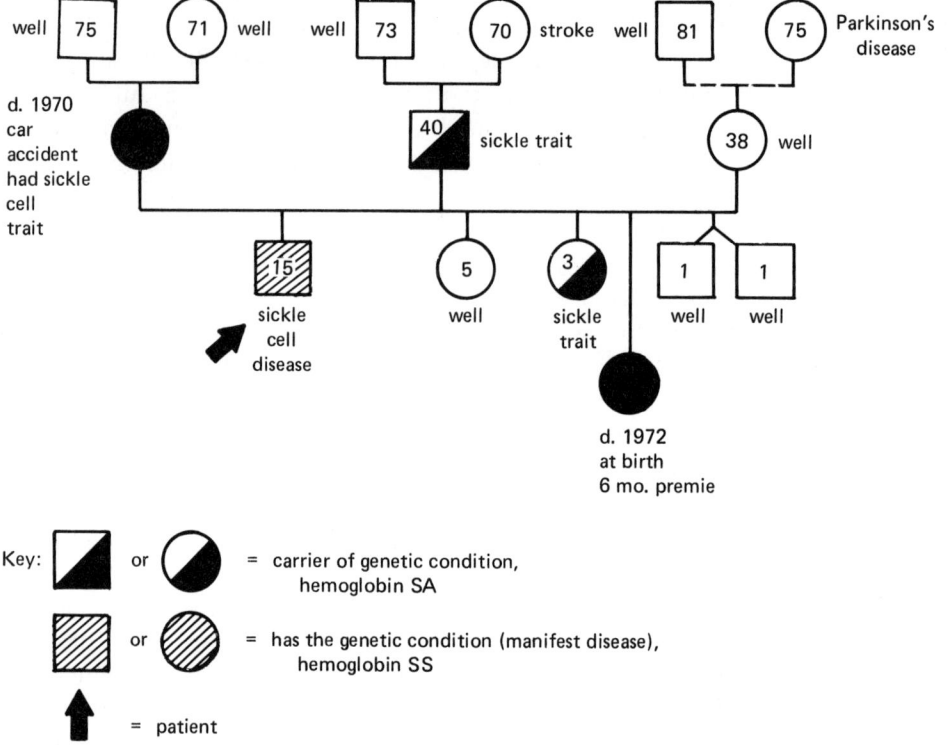

Figure 2-1. *An example of a medical genealogy.*
Note: *Grandparents were not available for hemoglobin electrophoresis testing.*
Additional data: (written out and keyed to specific diseases)
    1. Tuberculosis: maternal aunt; died 20 years ago; no other TB; patient's mother checked regularly with chest x-rays, always negative
    2. Cancer of stomach: paternal uncle
    3. Diabetes mellitus: paternal aunt
(Note: *the use of written entries such as those included under "Additional data" above, keeps the genealogical tree simple and easy to read.*)

The following key is presented for the reader of this book, but would *not* be written in the medical record since it is commonly used:

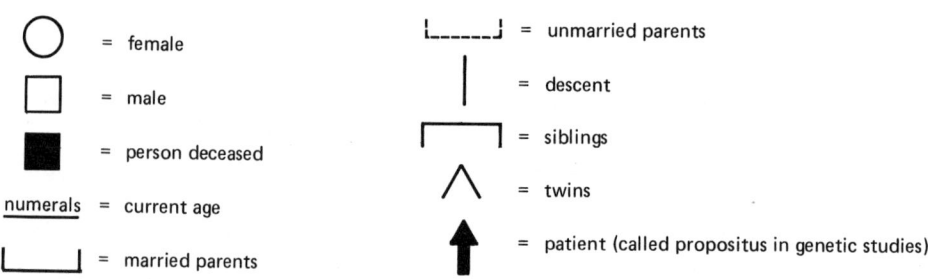

44

and treatment should be elaborated. The best example of this is tuberculosis. If a contact patient is identified, or if one member of the household has a positive screening test, then everyone else in the household should be screened and appropriate treatment instituted.

The family medical history frequently has important psychological ramifications, especially for parents of pediatric patients. For instance, a father whose brother died of leukemia may be extremely concerned when his own child has bruises on her legs. These bruises may be the result of "normal" trauma from play, but the father or both parents may worry that the child has leukemia. The parents may not be able to state this explicitly, but an astute clinician will realize the emotional significance of the bruises in relation to the family medical history—even if they are perfectly innocent.

One should choose a format which provides a concise, complete presentation of both the medical data and the relevant genealogy. A rendering of the family tree that is supplemented by a list or narrative is particularly well suited for this purpose. One example of this format is presented in Fig. 2-1. In any such display it is very important to provide the reader with a key, in which graphic symbols are explained clearly. This is necessary because use of symbols varies widely and is frequently quite idiosyncratic.

REVIEW OF SYSTEMS

This section is essentially a thorough checklist of questions about recent symptoms. Clinicians use it to remind themselves and historians of all possible topics that need covering and to ensure that no problem is omitted from the history. Not infrequently, the review of systems will bring to light information which elucidates a previously identified problem.

The review presents a list of symptoms relevant to the proper functioning of each system. If the historian indicates that some symptoms are present, it is most practical to gather additional information according to the format used for a chief complaint. This should include duration, frequency, intensity, time course, and other specifics about the symptom, associated factors, and results of treatment.

Thoroughness is of the utmost importance when going through the review of systems; however, it is only necessary to *record* the significant positive responses. In practice, one asks only a few carefully chosen questions in each category and pursues the whole list only in those areas where one has reason to suspect an abnormality. For example, under *Respiratory*, one might ask: "Does Eric have any problems with his chest or breathing?" "Has he ever had asthma or pneumonia?" There is no need to ask further questions in this category if the responses are negative.

Occasionally, information is obtained from the review of systems which should be recorded under another heading. For instance, if in the course of questioning about earaches a complex history of repeated ear infections with extensive evaluation and treatment is discovered, this fact should be recorded in the section Past Medical History.

Here is a suggested outline for the review of systems:

1. GENERAL HEALTH AND GROWTH: The examiner usually asks about general health at the beginning of the interview. If this has been overlooked, it can be discussed during the review of systems. The question "How would you describe Nancy's usual state of health?" can be quite revealing. (The question should also be addressed directly to any patient over nine or ten years of age.) If the answer does not correspond with the facts already recorded in the history, this discrepancy must be pursued further. For example, the parents of a child with a functional heart murmur may treat the child as a "cardiac cripple" by limiting his or her activities far more than is called for medically, which interferes with the child's independence and healthy development.

It is also convenient to discuss the child's growth at this point in the process. Asking the parents to estimate whether the child has been growing adequately and comparing this to the known height and weight can elicit important attitudes and possible distortions of perceptions on the part of the parents.

2. DIET: In most cases it is adequate to ascertain and record whether the diet seems to meet average (American) daily requirements for protein, carbohydrate, fat, iron, calcium, vitamins, and trace minerals. If the child is consuming an unusual diet (e.g., not eating meat), this should be noted in the record. Whenever diet is a major problem, a complete diet history should be recorded as a separate section under the Present Illness or Chief Complaint.

3. SKIN: Dry or oily skin; changes in color and texture; rashes in patients of all ages; and the appearance of acne (pimples, blackheads, "zits") in the adolescent who may not consider acne a "rash."

4. HAIR: Loss; changes in texture; excessive growth of fine body hair; hirsutism.

5. NAILS: Changes; abnormalities; nail biting.

6. HEAD AND FACE: Headache; pain; injuries.

7. EARS: Pain; infections; drainage; hearing; tinnitus.

8. EYES: Pain; infections; discharge; vision problems; strabismus; date of last vision test and results. If the patient wears glasses, when and by whom were they prescribed? When were the eyes and glasses last checked, and by whom? Does the patient wear the glasses as directed? Do the glasses improve the patient's vision?

9. NOSE: Difficulty breathing; sinus pain; epistaxis (nosebleeds); constant drainage.

10. MOUTH AND THROAT: Sores; problems in chewing and swallow-

ing; hoarseness; dental care; teeth grinding; pacifier, thumb, or finger sucking.

11. NECK: Stiffness; pain; masses.

12. BREASTS: Pain; discharge; infections; masses; nipple abnormalities. In the older girl: the early development of the breasts; asymmetry in size or shape during pubertal breast growth. In the adolescent boy: gynecomastia.

13. RESPIRATORY TRACT: Difficulty breathing; cough; sputum production, and color and consistency (thick or thin) of sputum; hemoptysis (coughing up blood); wheezing; asthma; history of pneumonia; chest pain.

14. CARDIOVASCULAR SYSTEM: History of heart murmurs; shortness of breath; endurance at vigorous physical play; squatting behavior; chest pain with exertion; sweating without exertion; cyanosis (especially with crying, feeding, or exertion); irritability; vomiting.

15. GASTROINTESTINAL TRACT: Vomiting (frequency, projectile or not, appearance); stool pattern (frequency, color, form, consistency, odor, greasiness, floating, mucous, blood, parasites). It is worth stressing here that clinicians frequently fail to learn about symptoms of diarrhea or constipation if they do not specifically ask about them. Exposure to intestinal parasites; abdominal pain; food intolerance and manifestation; unusual flatus; pica.

16. URINARY TRACT: Usual habits; color of urine; quality of urine stream; dribbling; urgency; frequency; dysuria; hematuria; polyuria; enuresis (nocturnal and daytime wetting). Edema, especially of forehead and hands.

17. GENITAL TRACT—MALE: Pain or discharge from penis; pain, swelling, or masses of testicles; other scrotal masses, including hernias; rash on scrotum. Changes in testicular and penile size, and appearance of pubic hair in early adolescence. In the sexually active adolescent, history of sexually transmitted diseases; use of contraception. Assess knowledge of sex.

18. GENITAL TRACT—FEMALE:

Prepubertal Patient: discharge, vaginal itching. If the patient is close to puberty (or approximately nine years old), the clinician should assess her knowledge about pubertal changes and menstruation.

Pubertal or Adolescent Patient: menarche date and age; frequency of menstrual cycles, how many days long, how heavy, regularity; pain with periods (dysmenorrhea); bleeding between periods; date of last period. Assess knowledge of sexuality; if patient is sexually active, contraception used; history of venereal disease. Vaginal discharge and itching. Obstetric history if not gathered in the past medical history. Attitude toward menstrual cycle; who told her about puberty; did she feel she was prepared for menarche?

19. MUSCULOSKELETAL SYSTEM: Muscle, bone, or joint pain; swell-

ing; tenderness; redness; limitation of motion or function; stiffness or deformity.

20. ENDOCRINE SYSTEM: Any general changes in weight (either gain or loss) and possible reasons for these changes, or changes in growth pattern.

Thyroid: masses in neck (goiter); exophthalmos; sweating; heat or cold intolerance; changes in activity level and energy; skin texture and excessive dryness or oiliness; changes in bowel habits; hoarseness.

Diabetes Mellitus: polyphagia; polydypsia; polyuria; enuresis; weight loss; change in temperament.

Pituitary: growth pattern changes. In the pediatric patient before growth is completed, the growth rate, especially in height, may inappropriately slow down or accelerate. If panhypopituitarism exists, signs of end organ hypofunction are also present related to the thyroid, adrenal glands, and gonads (postpubertal).

Adrenal: hypofunction may cause unusual pigmentation, weight-loss, weakness, anorexia, seizures (due to hypoglycemia). Hyperfunction may show changes in body contour (due to abnormal fat deposition), generalized obesity, unusual increase in facial hair, acne, deepening of the voice in females, poor growth in height, weakness, headache, and emotional lability.

Gonads: during childhood, gonadal tumors may cause lower abdominal pain or swelling in girls, testicular pain or scrotal enlargement in boys, and possible sexual precocity in either sex. Very small testes in tall boys often point to the presence of Klinefelter's syndrome. Hirsutism or virilization may develop in adolescent girls who have ovarian disorders, and the cause for delayed sexual maturation must be ascertained when an adolescent-aged patient remains prepubertal.

21. NERVOUS SYSTEM: Convulsions; weakness; headache; ataxia; paresthesia; fainting; speech problems; dizziness.

22. HEMATOPOIETIC SYSTEM: Anemia; pallor; unusual bleeding from cuts; epistaxis; blood in stools; spontaneous bleeding; easy bruising; enlarged lymph nodes; transfusions (with reactions, if any).

23. TRAVEL: Travel beyond the immediate vicinity, especially to areas where certain infectious diseases are known to be endemic—for example, histoplasmosis in the midwestern United States and intestinal parasites in tropical areas.

24. PETS: Include pets in and around the patient's home or school which may be significant in infectious and allergic disorders—for example, pet turtles which can carry salmonella and cats which can exacerbate respiratory allergies.

25. PSYCHOLOGICAL STATUS: This information is usually obtained during the developmental assessment and the patient profile. If the clinician has not yet completed the psychological data base, it should be done at this time, in the review of systems. The following symptoms are very

important and should be included in the evaluation of the psychological status: Unusual changes in mood or affect; memory lapses; difficulties in relationships with family, peers, or authority figures; depressions; "nervousness"; sleep disturbances; unusual eating behavior; phobias; hostility; destructive behavior; encopresis or enuresis in a previously continent (toilet trained) child; sharp changes in school performance.

CHAPTER 3

The Physical Examination: An Outline

Introduction
A. General Appearance
B. Vital Signs
C. Integument
D. Bones, Joints, and Muscles
E. Lymph Nodes
F. Head (general)
G. Skull
H. Eyes
I. Ears
J. Nose
K. Mouth
L. Throat
M. Neck
N. Breasts
O. Thorax and Lungs
P. Cardiovascular System
Q. Abdomen
R. Male Genitalia
S. Female Genitalia
T. Rectum and Anus
U. Extremities
V. Nervous System

INTRODUCTION

The *art* of the physical examination is to be flexible, not schematic, and to know what is important for each individual patient based on his or her age, the chief complaint, and the past medical and social history. Every clinical situation is unique, and its specific characteristics will dictate how complete the examination should be.

In an initial health evaluation, the physical examination should be quite thorough. The following outline covers such an extensive pediatric examination. The write-up of the examination is usually more abbreviated than we indicate here—but this will vary, of course, with the clinical setting and the experience of the clinician. (In Chapter 9 we shall discuss in detail how to skillfully make the physical examination a comfortable experience that produces the most data. At that time we shall review how crucial it is to establish rapport with the patient and gain his or her cooperation. Once again, here is where physical examination becomes an *art*.)

The following characteristics should be described whenever a mass or enlarged organ is noted during the physical examination.

1. Size: in centimeters
2. Shape: oval, round, tubular
3. Location: relate the mass to fixed structures, e.g., "5 cm below the right lower costal margin, at the midclavicular line"
4. Consistency: hard, firm, soft, fluctuant
5. Edge: sharp or round
6. Surface: smooth or nodular
7. Tenderness
8. Mobility
9. Attachment to other structures

A. GENERAL APPEARANCE

Here one records a synopsis of the patient's overall state of health on first inspection, the degree of cooperation, and any striking physical findings which the reader should know.

Example 1: Healthy, robust girl toddler who is shy with practitioner; cooperative on father's lap.

Example 2: Thin, pale boy; appears chronically ill; cooperative but obviously uncomfortable due to abdominal pain.

---

* This section is an extensive list of characteristics which may be included in the pediatric physical examination. It is intended to help the clinician be as thorough as necessary in this task. It is not intended to be a source of technical and methodological instruction. For this, turn to one of the texts on pediatric physical diagnosis.

Example 3: Hostile, uncooperative female adolescent; appears healthy and well-nourished.

Example 4: Pleasant, cooperative, comfortable teenage girl in wheelchair, with obvious arthritic deformities.

B. VITAL SIGNS

1. PULSE: indicate number per minute (note if irregular).

2. RESPIRATIONS: indicate number per minute (note if irregular).

3. TEMPERATURE: note location where obtained, i.e., oral (0) or rectal (R) or axillary (A).

4. BLOOD PRESSURE: routinely taken on an arm in cooperative children over three years of age. If the patient has a heart murmur or if there is a question of coarctation of the aorta, the blood pressure should be taken in both arms and a leg.

5. HEIGHT: in centimeters (and inches—to facilitate communication with most patients); state percentile according to growth chart.

6. WEIGHT: in kilograms and pounds; state percentile according to growth chart.

7. HEAD CIRCUMFERENCE: in centimeters; state percentile according to growth chart. Head circumference is usually not measured after about 18 months of age in an otherwise normal child.

C. INTEGUMENT

1. SKIN AND MUCOUS MEMBRANES: temperature, texture, moisture, color (including cyanosis), rashes, pigmented markings, turgor, bruises, scratches, scars.

2. NAILS: color, shape, clubbing, brittleness, pitting.

3. HAIR: color, texture, distribution, hirsutism, alopecia.

D. BONES, JOINTS, AND MUSCLES

1. SPINE: straight or abnormal shape (lordosis, kyphosis, scoliosis), malformations, limitation of movement, tenderness, pain with motion.

2. LIMBS: abnormal anatomy, limitations of movement, asymmetry in length and circumference.

3. JOINTS: deformities, loss of motion, swelling, heat, tenderness, redness, stability, crepitus, contractures.

4. MUSCLES: development, atrophy, hypertrophy, tenderness, strength, abnormal masses.

E. LYMPH NODES

1. LOCATION: cervical, occipital, posterior auricular, supraclavicular, axillary, epitrochlear, inguinal.

2. DESCRIPTION: size, mobility, consistency, tenderness, scars, sinuses, temperature, color.

F. HEAD (GENERAL)

1. SKIN: color, texture, sweating, lesions, telangiectasia, abnormal pigmentation.

2. SCALP: tenderness, masses, contusions, scars.

3. HAIR: texture and distribution.

G. SKULL

Shape, size, symmetry, tenderness, bruits, exostoses; fontanelle (size, open, flat or bulging when patient sitting and not crying); cracked-pot sound; transillumination (when indicated).

H. EYES

1. THE EYES AS A PAIR: asymmetry, setting-sun appearance, exophthalmos or endophthalmos, lid lag, strabismus, extraocular motion in six cardinal directions of gaze, convergence, nystagmus. Nystagmus is described as follows: if the quick component is to the left, then it is called nystagmus to the left. Reverse for the right. If there is no quick or slow

component, the nystagmus is called pendular. Note whether the nystagmus is vertical or rotary, or if it is present in only one direction of gaze.

2. EACH EYE SEPARATELY: lids, palpebral and bulbar conjunctivae, sclera, icterus, cornea, iris, lens; pupil size if unusually large or small; pupil shape; reaction to the light, both direct and consensual; accommodation.

3. OPHTHALMOSCOPIC EXAMINATION OF EACH EYE: clarity and location of lens, description of fundus, including cupping of the optic disc, appearance of retinal vessels, presence of hemorrhages or microaneurysms, exudates, macula. Frequently in infants only the red reflex can be obtained. Mydriatic eye drops are used if a more extensive eye examination is indicated.

4. VISION: if the child is cooperative, screening with the illiterate E test or a picture equivalent of the Snellen chart can be used, beginning around three years of age. Rough screening can be performed using toys or the examiner's fingers.

5. VISUAL FIELDS: this is performed as a gross screening test using the examiner's hands on a cooperative patient. If a precise evaluation of the visual field is needed to evaluate a central nervous system problem, the patient should be seen by an ophthalmologist.

I. EARS

1. EXTERNAL EARS: size, shape, configuration of the helix, tragus, antitragus; protuberance; low or unusual setting in relation to the eyes; tenderness, masses, deformity.

2. CANALS: presence of cerumen, discharge, odor, presence of a foreign body.

3. TYMPANIC MEMBRANES: color, presence or scattering of light reflex, ability to visualize bony landmarks, perforation, hemmorrhage, discharge, cholesteatoma, motion (with pneumatic otoscope).

4. HEARING: gross examination with tuning fork, ticking watch, whispered voice across the room. This can be supplemented by evaluation with an audiometer if there is any question of the patient's ability to hear well. Children should have hearing screening, using an audiometer, at regular intervals beginning at age three years.

J. NOSE

Gross external anatomy, obstruction, deviation of the septum, perforation of the septum, sinus tenderness, discharge, appearance of the nasal mucous membrane.

K. MOUTH

Examine all parts, including lips, buccal mucosa, tongue, teeth, and gums. Of particular interest are breath odor; lesions; lips for fissures, clefts; tongue for coating, abnormal movement; teeth for number present in relation to age, hygiene, repair, grossly abnormal bite; gums for hyperplasia.

L. THROAT

Appearance of tonsils, color of mucosa, exudate, lesions; palate for lesions and anatomy; uvula for position, movement with phonation, and configuration; posterior pharynx for mucosa and exudate; epiglottis and vocal cords should be described if seen on the routine examination of the throat.

M. NECK

Gross anatomy (webbing, asymmetry), movement, stiffness, pain, limitation of motion, masses, pulsations; trachea for central position and mobility; vessels for distention, pulsation, thrills, bruits, and radiating heart murmurs; thyroid gland.

N. BREASTS

In the prepubertal girl, the presence of an areola should be ascertained on each side of the chest. Between infancy and adolescence, discharge from the breast and masses in the breast are unusual; premature thelarche may occur in young girls without other signs of pubertal development. In the adolescent, the size, shape and symmetry of the breasts is noted, along with any discharge from the nipples or masses in the breasts.

During adolescent growth, the development of the breasts passes through the following five stages. These stages can be used for categorizing purposes in the medical record:

STAGE 1: This stage is the one found throughout childhood. The areolar surface conforms with the rest of the chest wall and the papilla may project from the areola. At this stage, a girl is considered prepubertal.

STAGE 2: This stage of breast development usually reflects the onset of puberty, but is also seen when premature thelarche occurs in prepubertal girls. A small mass of breast tissue can be palpated beneath the areola and often causes some projection of the areola from the chest wall as well.

STAGE 3: In this stage, the growth of the breast extends beyond the areolar border, and the outlines of the areola and the rest of the breast are confluent.

STAGE 4: Further growth of the breast occurs in this stage and, in addition, the areola projects from the underlying breast, in contrast with the outline shared in Stage 3. Many girls reach menarche during this stage.

STAGE 5: The breast is now mature, and the outlines of the breast and the areola are uniform again. The papilla may project slightly from the areola.

Breasts should be examined in both the male and female patient. In adolescent boys, gynecomastia is common and usually resembles Breast Stage 2; less frequently, gynecomastia reaches the size of Breast Stage 3.

O. THORAX AND LUNGS

(For clarity, the information is organized according to examination method and the usual order in which the examination is performed.)

1. INSPECTION: shape, symmetry, anterior to posterior diameter, deformities, expansion, depth and character of respiration, presence of nasal flare, use of abdominal and intercostal muscles, presence of end-expiratory grunt, position of comfort for respiration.

2. PALPATION: tenderness, tactile fremitus, thrills, symmetry of expansion.

3. PERCUSSION: tympany, hyperresonance, dullness, flatness, level and excursion of each side of diaphragm, position of mediastinum.

4. AUSCULTATION: breath sounds (description and location in chest if abnormal; for example, bronchovesicular breath sounds in all fields, ex-

cept for tubular sounds in right upper back); rales, rhonchi, wheezes (note whether inspiratory or expiratory); expiratory clicks (suggesting possible foreign bodies in the lung).

P. CARDIOVASCULAR SYSTEM

1. HEART: maximum apical impulse seen, felt "x" centimeters to the left of the midsternal line; presence of thrusts, heaves, pulsations, or thrills with location (e.g., faint thrill along left sternal border). Describe or draw a diagram of the area of cardiac dullness in relation to the midsternal and midclavicular lines (as determined by percussion). Heart sounds, whether clear, and their location. Murmurs with loudness, timing in the cardiac cycle, pitch, quality, location, transmission across the chest, change with different postures (e.g., Grade III/VI holosystolic low-pitched rumbling murmur heard best at the apex and radiating to the axilla). Venous hums, rubs.

2. PULSES: frequency, abnormal quality (e.g., water hammer), pulse deficit from arms to legs (usually brachial or radial compared with femoral); list or diagram of palpable pulses including carotid, brachial, radial, femoral, popliteal, posterior tibial, and dorsalis pedis.

3. VESSELS: usually describe with neck and extremities.

Q. ABDOMEN

1. INSPECTION: shape (flat, scaphoid, protuberant), scars, veins, peristalsis, obvious masses (see p. 51).

2. AUSCULTATION: peristalsis (listen for several minutes before concluding that the patient has an ileus), if normal, or if in rushes which coincide with painful sensations for the patient; bruits.

3. PALPATION: consistency (soft, hard), tenderness with location; spasm, guarding, pain (rebound, referred); straight leg raising (patient is supine; examiner raises the extended leg, thereby eliciting pain in the back and abdomen if there is irritation of the sciatic nerve). Masses and palpable organs (see p. 51). Organs to include are liver, gallbladder, spleen, kidneys, urinary bladder, uterus (pregnant or enlarged due to pathology).

4. PERCUSSION: shifting dullness, fluid wave, tympany; tympany can also be used to define the size and shape of masses and organs.

58   The Data Base: Foundation of Clinical Practice

   5. HERNIAS: location, such as inguinal, femoral, umbilical. Note whether the hernia is reducible. The presence of intestine in a hernia sac can often be determined by listening for peristalsis with the stethoscope on the sac.

R. MALE GENITALIA

   1. PENIS: tenderness, swelling, discharge, lesions, whether circumcized, location and shape of meatus, phimosis, urinary stream if noted.

   2. SCROTUM: wrinkling, swelling, tenderness.

   3. TESTES: size, consistency, position.

   4. EPIDIDYMIS: tenderness, induration.

   5. GENITAL STAGES: in adolescent boys, the genitalia develop through the following stages:
   GENITAL STAGE 1: At this stage, the genitalia are prepubertal: in addition to the penis being immature, the average value of the product of the length and breadth of the testis does not exceed 4 cm^2.
   GENITAL STAGE 2: This stage represents the first easily detected physical evidence for the onset of puberty. Though the appearance and size of the penis do not change from Stage 1, the testes become larger and the scrotum becomes somewhat more wrinkled.
   GENITAL STAGE 3: In this stage, the testes have grown larger than in Stage 2, and the androgen produced by them is sufficient to cause moderate penile growth as well.
   GENITAL STAGE 4: In this stage, the penis and testes continue to grow, and the glans develops.
   GENITAL STAGE 5: At this stage, the genitalia have reached mature development.

   6. PUBIC HAIR (this sequence applies to females as well as males): The appearance of pubic hair during adolescence can be assessed according to its amount, consistency, and distribution.
   PUBIC HAIR STAGE 1: At this stage, found throughout childhood, the vellus over the external genitalia does not differ from that elsewhere on the body.
   PUBIC HAIR STAGE 2: At this stage, a minimal amount of longer and somewhat darker stright public hair appears near the base of the penis or on the labia majora. This developmental stage may appear before, accompany, or follow Breast Stage 2 in girls; it follows Genital Stage 2, and sometimes Genital Stage 3, in boys.

PUBIC HAIR STAGE 3: The pubic hair is coarser, somewhat curled, and of moderate quantity at this stage, and has spread toward the inguinal areas.

PUBIC HAIR STAGE 4: At this stage, public hair has the full quantity and mature consistency of that found in the adult but has not developed on the medial surfaces of the thighs.

PUBIC HAIR STAGE 5: Similar to Stage 4, but including growth of hair on the medial surfaces of the thighs.

S. FEMALE GENITALIA

1. LABIA MAJORA AND MINORA: size, condition of surface, swelling.

2. CLITORIS: size, gross anatomy, urethral meatus.

3. VAGINAL OPENING (INTROITUS): appearance of mucosa, discharge, excoriation, scars, foreign body.

4. PUBIC HAIR: presence, developmental stage, distribution.

5. PELVIC EXAMINATION: vagina, cervix, uterine fundus, adnexa, ovaries, fallopian tubes, discharge, lesions, masses. Pelvic examinations are routinely performed only on sexually active adolescents. If the patient has a complaint which suggests pelvic pathology at any age, a pelvic examination is done.

T. RECTUM AND ANUS

External visual examination for fissures, prolapse, and cysts; digital examination for sphincter tone, masses, tenderness, uterus size; stool sample for color, consistency, hematest; prostate in the adolescent male. The digital examination is not done routinely in pediatric practice. It should be done if there are symptoms related to the rectum or abdomen.

U. EXTREMITIES

Color, edema, temperature, hair distribution, tremor, vessels for varicosities or phlebitis.

V. NERVOUS SYSTEM

1. MENTAL STATUS: level of awareness, orientation (time, person, place), ability to cooperate, quality of speech and language, memory, general knowledge, ability to perform simple calculations (per age); presence of delusions, illusions, hallucinations, affect; memory both recent and past; ability to think abstractly (per age); mannerisms, unusual conduct. Much of this information will be gathered and recorded under developmental assessment in the usual pediatric situation.

2. CRANIAL NERVES (NOTE: Roman numerals are the most common notation for the cranial nerves.):

   I. OLFACTORY: sense of smell and recognition of strong common odors such as coffee, vinegar, ammonia. This is tested only when indicated by complaints of particular symptoms which could be caused by a lesion in the frontal area of the brain.

   II. OPTIC: visual acuity, visual fields, and fundus with the ophthalmoscope.

   III. OCULOMOTOR: extraocular movements of the eye in all directions except lateral and downward-inward; pupillary constriction in reaction to light and accommodation; elevation of upper eyelid.

   IV. TROCHLEAR: downward-inward eye movement.

   V. TRIGEMINAL: muscles of mastication, jaw deviation; sensation to pinprick and touch on face; corneal reflex to touch with light cotton wisp. Note all three branches of the trigeminal nerve for sensation: opthalmic, maxillary, and mandibular.

   VI. ABDUCENS: lateral eye movement.

   VII. FACIAL: muscles of facial expression such as wrinkling of forehead, forceful closing of the eyes, smiling, puffing out cheeks, showing teeth; taste on the anterior two thirds of the tongue.

   VIII. AURICULAR (OTIC): hearing, air and bone conduction with tuning fork. Balance is tested later in the nervous system examination and reflects a combination of the function of the vestibular portion of the auricular nerve with the cerebellum.

   IX and X. GLOSSOPHARYNGEAL and VAGUS: swallowing, movement of the palate on vocalization and position of the uvula; gag reflex; taste on posterior one third of the tongue and sensation in the pharynx.

   XI. ACCESSORY: sternocleidomastoid and trapezius muscles,

tested by neck turning against resistance and shoulder shrugging.
XII. HYPOGLOSSAL: tongue for deviation, atrophy, fasciculations, and tremor.

3. MOTOR: handedness, voluntary movement of the extremities, muscular development, resistance to passive movement (tone), strength; atrophy; fasciculation; tremors; choreoathetotic movements; hemiballismus.

4. SENSORY: sensation to pinprick, light touch, temperature and vibration in all four extremities, trunk and face; position sense in toes and fingers; tactile localization; two-point discrimination, stereognosis.

5. COORDINATION: fine motor coordination; rapid alternating movements of hands and feet; finger-to-nose and heel-to-shin tests. Nystagmus noted when performing the cardinal directions of gaze may indicate a cerebellar lesion or malfunction.

6. POSTURE AND GAIT: posture—ability to retain standing posture with the heels together and eyes closed (Romberg test). Gait—if wide-based, unstable, presence of foot slapping, steadiness.

7. REFLEXES: deep tendon reflexes—compare both sides; describe, diagram, or put in table format and grade O to IV and note clonus; plantar reflex (Babinski); abdominal and cremasteric reflexes; primitive reflexes such as a jaw jerk, grasp, suck, Moro, tonic neck; anal sphincter reflex to touch.

8. SPINAL CORD IRRITATION:
   a. Kernig's sign: resistance to straightening knee, with hip and knee flexed and patient supine.
   b. Brudzinski's sign: neck flexion causes flexion at hips or knees; patient supine.
   c. Opisthotonus: arched back due to neck extensor muscles contracting pathologically.

CHAPTER 4

Screening

Introduction
Which Patients Should Be Screened?
Which Conditions Should Be Included in a Screening Program?
When Should the Screening Be Performed?
What Specific Methods or Tests Should Be Used?
What Factors are Important for a Successful Screening Program?
Example of One Schedule for Pediatric Screening Tests

INTRODUCTION

In the last decade Americans have begun to recognize the important role that preventive health care must play in their lives. Health care professionals are increasingly concerned about disseminating information to the lay public in order to promote early recognition of diseases or of circumstances which produce diseases. Such early recognition allows clinicians to treat a disease more efficiently and effectively and to ameliorate its course. It is also possible to prevent some diseases through eliminating etiologic factors, and (increasingly) to provide genetic counseling and prenatal diagnosis, and thus to prevent some diseases in future generations. Screening tools are adjuncts to the health history and physical examination;

all three are sources of information that are available to the clinician in making judgments about a patient's health. Screening tests may be administered as part of the history (as questionnaires), or as part of the physical examination, or they may be separate laboratory tests. The data they generate should be included in the health record.

Health care professionals are still grappling with the problem of conceptualizing screening and deciding what should be done. Lessler defines the term broadly:

> Screening is the acquiring of preliminary information about characteristics which may be significant to the health, education, or well-being of the individual and which are relevant to his life tasks. The means of data collection must be appropriate and reasonable with regard to the economics of time, money, and resources for dealing with large numbers of persons.*

A word of caution is needed here. Although screening tools can be very helpful, they can be misleading as well. Too often, clinicians will tend to ignore data from the history or physical examination and use screening tools as the only information on which to base their clinical judgments. This may lead to two kinds of erroneous conclusions: on the one hand, clinicians can develop a false sense of security and assume that a sick patient is well; or they can form the false impression that a healthy patient is ill. In situations of the first kind, a disease that might have been cured or ameliorated is left to progress to the point where a person's health may be threatened. Or possibly crucial genetic counseling is omitted. On the other hand, a clinician's false impression that illness is present can frequently lead to unnecessary and costly evaluation and possibly even treatment procedures, and will generate gratuitous anxiety for the patient and family. Both patients and examiners must remember that the use of screening tools is only one means by which the clinician assesses the patient's physical and mental health.

A number of issues regarding screening tests must be addressed to ensure that such tools are used appropriately. We present them here as questions:

1. Which patients should be screened for particular conditions or diseases?
2. Which conditions should be included in a screening program?
3. When should the screening be performed?
4. What specific methods or tests should be used?
5. What factors are important for a successful screening program?

Specific conditions and tests will be used to keep our discussion of these issues concrete. We shall also present a currently recommended screening schedule. However, screening procedures change rapidly with new technological and scientific advances, and clinicians will need to

---

* Lessler, K.: Health and educational screening of school-age children—definition and objectives. *Am. J. Public Health* 62: 191, 1972.

consult the most recent recommendations for particular clinical situations.

WHICH PATIENTS SHOULD BE SCREENED?

Certain personal and demographic characteristics are critical for choosing which patients to screen. These include a patient's age, family history, ethnic group, race, socioeconomic class, contact with a serious infectious disease, geographical region inhabited, and ethical and religious convictions.

AGE:
The neonatal period provides an opportunity to diagnose many congenital problems. Several convenient screening tests are now available for detection of inborn metabolic disorders such as phenylketonuria (PKU), congenital hypothyroidism, and galactosemia. Since these diseases occur in all segments of the American population, most newborn infants in this country are routinely screened for many of these conditions.

Lead ingestion is a very serious example of a problem in which the age of the patient (in combination with other factors) will determine the need for screening. Children normally have pica (ingestion of nonfood substances) from 9 to 24 months of age. However, the amount of pica and duration of the habit vary a great deal. There are a few children who have very little pica, but, then again, some as old as four or five years still ingest nonfood substances. Since lead ingestion is strongly associated with pica, all children between the ages of nine months and five years of age—or any others with pica—are theoretically at risk for lead poisoning and thus must be considered for lead screening. Of course, the decision about lead screening will also depend on the likelihood that a child was exposed to lead-containing substances (see Socioeconomic Class).

There are some conditions which are present throughout life, but for which special management or genetic counseling are only appropriate at certain ages. A good example of this is sickle hemoglobin. Children under two years of age with sickle cell disease are at high risk for life-threatening bacterial infection. In the past, clinicians frequently did not know when a very young child had sickle cell disease because the classical symptoms and signs had not yet become manifest and there was no test for the small amounts of sickle hemoglobin in a young infant. Now a method is available for doing hemoglobin electrophoresis on blood specimens for newborns (usually umbilical cord blood) to detect sickle hemoglobin. With the routine use of this as a screening procedure in all dark-skinned infants (especially those of Mediterranean, African, and

Arab ancestry), the primary clinician can institute early culture and treatment whenever infants with sickle cell disease show any signs of infection. This has been shown to decrease the rate of morbidity and mortality from infection in these patients.

Sickle cell disease usually becomes symptomatic in the young child, and there are no preventive measures which can be taken. Therefore, screening in childhood beyond the infant period is not useful.

When patients become old enough to enter reproductive activity, they should know whether or not they carry sickle hemoglobin, because its presence may affect their decisions about family planning. Adolescents can have a blood test to determine whether they are heterozygote carriers of sickle hemoglobin; presumably, patients with sickle cell disease (homozygous for sickle hemoglobin) or other variants would have been diagnosed during childhood. Research studies have shown that when high school students are screened and given a thorough program educating them about sickle cell anemia, they develop an understanding of the personal significance of the condition and become quite compliant with the entire screening program and follow-up. This approach has also been used with other genetic conditions such as Tay-Sachs disease.

FAMILY HISTORY:
In recent years, recognition of the number of conditions with a familial pattern of inheritance has risen dramatically. This has paralleled advances in technology which permit easier diagnosis of carrier states and detection of subclinical cases. In turn, alerting clinicians to carriers promotes earlier recognition of abnormalities and thus the possiblity for early intervention and amelioration of disease. Genetic counseling is also greatly facilitated.

One example of this is the group collectively termed disorders of lipid metabolism. A family history of coronary heart disease in close relatives under 50 years of age calls for the measurement of serum cholesterol and triglyceride levels at regular intervals; in certain cases it is useful to advise a special diet intended to keep the cholesterol level within the normal range. Another example is Duchenne's muscular dystrophy, a sex-linked disorder for which a screening test has been developed. A patient with a family history of this condition and who thus could be a carrier, might want to know if she in fact is one; she could, if test results are positive, obtain appropriate genetic counseling about future family planning. Even if she has an unaffected child, a mother with a positive family history will need to know if she is a carrier, in order to have the benefit of genetic counseling for future family planning. In the near future it will probably be possible to make a reliable prenatal diagnosis of this disorder.*

---

* Maurice J. Mahoney et al., Prenatal diagnosis of Duchenne's muscular dystrophy. *New Eng. J. Medicine*, 297: 968–973, 1977.

ETHNIC GROUP:
There are some inherited conditions which are more frequent among members of particular ethnic groups, mainly because of intermarriage within the group and the high number of individuals who are carriers of the genes which determine expression of the disease. One example of this is Tay-Sachs disease, for which the carrier rate is 1:300 in the general American population but 1:30 in the Ashkenazi Jewish population (of northern and middle rather than southern European ancestry). There is no way to prevent or cure the disease in a homozygous patient. However, screening for the heterozygous state in adolescents and young adults, genetic counseling, and elective abortion can help to prevent future cases of this fatal condition.

RACE:
The term "race" is not a scientifically precise or even useful term, but it is commonly used to designate people with arbitrarily selected physical characteristics, most frequently involving variations in skin color and facial features. For example, sickle cell hemoglobin is particularly common among dark-skinned people. Because of inadequate education on this subject, clinicians in the United States commonly think of sickle hemoglobin in association with the racial designation "black." But, in fact, Italians, Greeks, Turks, and certain Arab groups carry sickle hemoglobin with as great a frequency as many African populations. Thus, thinking only in racial terms can be dangerous or misleading, since children of *all* of these groups should be screened for the presence of hemoglobin S according to the guidelines listed above under age.

SOCIOECONOMIC CLASS:
Children who live in old and dilapidated housing or in neighborhoods where these conditions exist are at increased risk of having lead poisoning. Children of families in impoverished conditions generally live in poor housing (or their friends and relatives do); this increases the chance that, if they have pica, they may ingest paint chips which contain lead. Also, automotive exhaust fumes can so pollute inner-city air that very high lead levels have been found in children's blood and have been related to this source. Thus, children from one to five years of age who live in old housing or inner-city neighborhoods should be screened by blood tests for the presence of lead.

CONTACT WITH AN INFECTIOUS DISEASE:
Patients who are in ongoing contact with someone who has a serious infectious disease (such as tuberculosis) should be screened regularly. Early diagnosis permits early treatment, with less morbidity for the patient and less likelihood that the condition will be spread to other people. All pediatric patients should be routinely screened for tuberculosis at ap-

proximately 12 to 15 months of age, before receiving their measles immunization; at approximately 5 years of age at their preschool health evaluation; and again in early adolescence. Children living in areas with high incidence of tuberculosis should be screened more frequently, probably every year (see Rate of Conversion, p. 70).

GEOGRAPHICAL REGIONS:
Patients who currently live in, who recently have lived in, or who have recently traveled through an area with specific endemic diseases may need to be screened. Examples abound, including gastrointestinal parasites in subtropical and tropical regions and histoplasmosis in the midwestern United States.

ETHICAL AND RELIGIOUS BELIEFS:
Although the pediatric practitioner usually is not the professional responsible for the parents' health care, she or he is often in an excellent position to educate parents about genetic counseling and its availability in the community or within the larger geographic region. For example, it could happen that a 10-year-old boy might come for a routine health evaluation, accompanied by his 40-year-old mother who mentions that she is 8 weeks pregnant. She says that she is concerned about her chances of having a child with a chromosomal disorder related to her advanced age, such as Down's syndrome. Although the mother would have her own primary clinician for the pregnancy, the pediatric clinician in this case is in a position to answer many of her questions immediately, to discuss the situation with both her and her husband, and to make a referral for genetic counseling.

However, genetic counseling cannot be undertaken in a meaningful manner if the procedures which accompany it, such as effective birth control and elective abortion, are not broached as well. If the religious and ethical convictions of a patient or family do not allow them to consider such interventive actions based on test results, clinicians should withdraw gracefully from the discussion. Nevertheless, it is the clinicians' responsibility to attempt to educate patients about genetics and genetic counseling. They should also develop contacts with clergy and other community leaders who are sympathetic to birth control use and abortion, and who will help in counseling and reassuring patients facing these issues. But, we reiterate, clinicians should not attempt to coerce someone into genetic counseling who is morally opposed to it.

When a patient comes from a family with a history of a severe disease that is inherited, the clinician and parents should discuss the genetics involved, the implications for their future offspring, and the availability of tests to determine whether the parents are carriers or if a fetus has the disorder. Some parents will choose to have the tests and further counseling and to plan future pregnancies accordingly. Other parents do not believe that any form of birth control is acceptable to them, and so may decline to pursue the tests and counseling. However, even in cases of the latter sort, the primary clinician should be available to discuss their concerns and to give them emotional support during the decision-making process. We would add, further, that clinicians should provide such support no matter what decision the parents ultimately reach.

Fetal diagnosis using amniocentesis, ultrasound, and chemical and chromosomal analyses can provide valuable information about the health of the fetus. However, it is only appropriate to use these tests if the patient will seriously consider abortion, should the fetus be found to have a severe disorder. If the patient firmly believes that she could not contemplate having an abortion, then the risks involved in these procedures would not be acceptable (since no practical good would come of the tests).

WHICH CONDITIONS SHOULD BE INCLUDED IN A SCREENING PROGRAM?

The condition should be serious, prevalent, susceptible to detection before irreversible damage is done, and amenable to treatment or genetic counseling.

There is no simple way to evaluate the serious nature of a particular disease. Some diseases are life-threatening, some are extremely incapacitating, some have serious epidemiological consequences, and some have significance for genetic counseling alone. The clinician must evaluate the seriousness and consequences of each condition individually.

The *prevalence* of a condition is an important factor when one is considering the advisability of screening; so is *incidence*. The former refers to the frequency of a condition manifested in a population at any given point in time; the latter is the frequency with which new cases appear. A considerable amount of screening is done for rare (low prevalence) diseases with very serious consequences. This is especially true when treatment is available. An example of this kind of rare condition which can be treated is phenylketonuria (PKU), the incidence of which is 1 in 10,000 newborn infants. A special phenylalanine-restricted diet ameliorates the course dramatically.

It makes no sense to screen for conditions that have not been identified clearly and whose diagnostic criteria have not been specified. Without such criteria, it is difficult to know what, exactly, one is screening for—and whether the course of the disease can be altered by early intervention. Further, screening can only be justified if the patient will benefit from *early* treatment or counseling. If the results of treatment and counseling are not enhanced by early detection, and are equally effective if instituted after the disease has become clinically manifest, then screening is not beneficial and is not called for.

WHEN SHOULD THE SCREENING BE PERFORMED?

The examiner must decide when and how frequently the screening tests should be administered. Such decisions will depend on the age of the patient, lead time for the condition, and rate at which patients with previously normal results convert to abnormal test results.

AGE:
The age factor has been discussed above under the heading Which Patients Should Be Screened? If a condition has a particular age distribution, then the screening should be planned to intersect with those ages. Iron deficiency anemia, for example, occurs most frequently (in otherwise healthy children) at about 12 months of age and again in early adolescence; screening with hematocrit should be routinely performed at those ages.

LEAD TIME:
The term refers to the range of time between the moment a condition can be identified through screening and the point at which the disease causes severe or irreversible damage. A short lead time often means that screening is impractical. With childhood diabetes mellitus, for instance, the child has glucosuria only for a few weeks before presenting in ketoacidosis, with obvious symptoms. Therefore, testing the child's urine for sugar is not considered practical by most practitioners.

But a short lead time does not always rule out screening. Phenylketonuria (PKU), congenital hypothyroidism (cretinism), and galactosemia are examples of conditions which must be detected early in the neonatal period if they are to be treated successfully. Although the lead time is short in all of these conditions, the fact that the neonatal period is the correct time for diagnosis limits the screening period to a specific period which is the same for all individuals.

Long lead times make screening very useful. One example is iron deficiency anemia. Otherwise normal healthy children may use up their iron stores and exceed their daily iron intake very gradually. Mild anemia, which is common at one year of age, is not associated with significant morbidity, is not life-threatening, and is easily reversible. Even moderate anemia is not associated with very severe morbidity. So screening leads directly to successful treatment even after a delayed diagnosis. (This is in striking contrast to cretinism, where lack of treatment for even a few weeks leads to permanent mental retardation.)

RATE OF CONVERSION FROM NEGATIVE TO POSITIVE TEST RESULTS:
Tuberculosis is an example of a disease where the rate of conversion varies from one part of the population to another. High conversion rates, due to high exposure rates, are common in inner-city populations. Therefore screening schedules for tuberculosis will vary according to the place where the patient lives, goes to school, or works. Children from the inner city should be screened for TB every 1 or 2 years; children living in other, low-risk areas should have TB screening at about 1 year, 5 years, and 12 years of age.

WHAT SPECIFIC METHODS OR TESTS SHOULD BE USED?

The examiner should evaluate whether screening tests are acceptable, accurate, and reliable. Frequently, new tests are developed that are simpler to use but are too costly and thus not (generally) acceptable. Some may be inexpensive, but not accurate enough to be practical. A cautious, inquisitive attitude on the part of the health care practitioner is called for, and the patient's financial resources should be kept in mind.

ACCEPTABILITY:
People's attitudes may sometimes determine the acceptability of a test. Patients and parents are naturally concerned about physical discomfort, convenience, time required to perform a test, and cost. But clinicians' attitudes are equally important. Whoever administers the test must believe it is useful enough to warrant the trouble to administer it. Further, the clinician who sees a patient for follow-up will be likely to be conscientious about evaluation, diagnosis, and treatment only if he or she believes the screening tool is accurate and reliable.

ACCURACY:
Screening tools are not usually as accurate as diagnostic tools, but they are generally reasonably accurate. *Sensitivity* and *specificity* are the two parameters which determine accuracy. Sensitivity is the measure of how good the test is at detecting all true positives; it is defined as the percentage of the people who have the disorder who are actually detected by the test. As the sensitivity increases, fewer affected people are missed. Specificity refers to the percentage of people who do *not* have the disorder who are correctly identified as negatives by the test. As the specificity increases, fewer normal people are incorrectly labeled as positives. In an ideal situation, of course, the sensitivity and specificity would both be 100 percent. Naturally this is not possible in the vagaries of actual practice. However, we can work with less than 100 percent accuracy.

The predictive value of a screening test is defined as the percentage of those identified as positive who turn out actually to have the disorder. The predictive value of a test is obviously a consequence of its sensitivity and specificity, but it also partly depends on the prevalence of the condition for which one is screening. If the prevalence of the disease is low, statistical probability tells us to expect proportionately more false positive results, so that the predictive value will be less. False positive results have real consequences: they mean that people, inaccurately labeled as ill, will be subjected to the worry, cost, and inconvenience of returning for more definitive diagnostic evaluation. Mislabeling is an inevitable part of screening, but it should be clearly evaluated and minimized before screening is performed.*

RELIABILITY:
Screening tools must be consistent in measuring what they are designed to indicate. There are several measures of reliability. *Inter-observer* reliability means that two people observe and give the same findings. *Split-sample* reliability means that two tests on the same sample produce the same result. *Test-retest* reliability indicates that the same test on the same patient on two different occasions produces the same results.

A screening tool can be used clinically when it meets minimal requirements of acceptability, accuracy, and reliability. The skeptical clinician will remember that screening tools always have many limitations and that they are only one source out of many that provide the information necessary for making plans for patient care.

WHAT FACTORS ARE IMPORTANT FOR A SUCCESSFUL SCREENING PROGRAM?

Some of the most important factors of a successful screening program include: the amount of public education about the need for and availability of screening tests; efficient communication of records and data among health care professionals; resources for diagnosis and treatment; reasonable cost to the public; and awareness of the ethical implications of the program.

ADEQUATE EDUCATIONAL PROGRAM:
Public cooperation is essential for any large-scale screening program. Health care professionals should enlist the aid of local educators and media resources to disseminate information to the public about which

---

* Edward Bailey, et al. Screening in pediatric practice. *Pediatric Clinics of North America*, Feb. 1974, p. 123.

sections of the population should be screened, for what diseases they can be screened, and how this can benefit them concretely. Further, health care professionals should meet with each other and plan their educational activities in a coordinated manner.

EFFICIENT COMMUNICATION OF DATA:
Large-scale screening should be part of a program which can coordinate the performance of the tests, gather the results, and communicate them both to the patient and to appropriate health resources. Data that disappear into the twilight zone of stacked-up computer banks and never reappear are useless and wasteful. So are misplaced data or data delivered to clinicians long past the time of their usefulness. It is of utmost importance that the system for communicating screening data among health care professionals and to patients be carefully designed and well maintained.

RESOURCES:
The screening program is obliged to provide the people it screens with workable options for those who test positive. The program itself may have components that provide definitive diagnosis, counseling, treatment, and follow-up; or it may make arrangements with hospitals, clinics, or private clinicians to provide the necessary services. But, in all cases, both the patient who tests positive and/or a responsible clinician who has contact with the patient must be informed and a whole range of resources put at the patient's disposal. These include a primary care clinician, a secondary specialty care facility (where needed), or even regional and state-level facilities.

COST:
Costs to both society and each patient should be assessed. Monetary and nonmonetary costs to society must be evaluated. Public funds are frequently used for screening programs like tuberculosis surveillance, lead poisoning detection, and neonatal evaluation for inborn errors of metabolism. The cost of the program must be low enough so that it costs the public less for screening than for treatment of the previously unnoticed disease after it has progressed. For example, the cost of finding one case of PKU may be high, especially since it is so rare, but the long-term institutional care for the patient with untreated PKU is higher.

Monetary costs can be cut by centralizing both the training of technicians and the performance of tests (especially for highly technical laboratory tests). Other ways to cut costs include (1) having paraprofessional personnel perform office screening tests and (2) doing many tests for different diseases on one sample, as in metabolic tests on urine and blood.

The nonmonetary costs are difficult to estimate. Personal suffering and the quality of life for the patient and family cannot be calculated in dollars and cents. This factor always competes with monetary costs in administrative decisions about health care.

The monetary cost to the patient and family is also a serious issue. Health care professionals should try to arrange for third party payment for screening and follow-up. Where such payment is available, this should be mentioned prominently in educational materials about the program, since the public is already heavily burdened by health care costs. In areas of concentrated poverty it may be possible to get federal or state (or even private foundation) financing for all or part of the program.

ETHICAL IMPLICATIONS:
Large-scale screening programs sometimes misuse test results. Such programs frequently are designed primarily for research and thus lack any personal connection with the patient or family. Further, in many ways confidentiality is unthinkingly violated; this is especially true now that computers assimilate large quantities of data—and access to computer terminals is notoriously difficult to control.

In order to ensure the appropriate use of test results, the patient and parents must be fully informed about the test beforehand, and they should be told the kinds of results derived from the test and their possible significance. Also, they should be told the uses to which the results will be put. There have already been cases in which test results indicating sickle cell trait have been used unfairly against people seeking insurance. For decades, intelligence test results have been—and still are—used prejudicially in school and employment situations. Administrators of screening programs must be conscientious about maintaining confidentiality, so as to minimize possible misuse of the information from the program. This is more likely to be achieved if provision is made for consumer representation on policy-making bodies and open periodic review of the findings and achievements of the program with regard to patient service.

EXAMPLE OF ONE SCHEDULE FOR PEDIATRIC SCREENING TESTS

This is only one of many currently acceptable screening plans. Clinicians must formulate their own plans based upon the population from which a child comes and the latest available scientific knowledge about screening. The ages for initial testing and the frequency of repeat tests noted below are only for well children. Many of the procedures are also used for diagnostic evaluation. In that case, the ages indicated do not apply.
1. *Metabolic diseases:* These tests should be performed in the first few days of life. Examples include tests for PKU, hypothyroidism, and galactosemia. The test for PKU should be repeated at 2 weeks

of age to detect infants who had negative screening results because of inadequate milk intake prior to the time of the first test.
2. *VDRL:* This should be performed on umbilical cord blood to detect congenital syphilis.
3. *Blood type and Coombs' test:* These should be performed on umbilical cord blood to detect incompatibilities of blood type between mother and infant.
4. *Hemoglobin electrophoresis:* This should be performed on umbilical cord blood of all dark-skinned infants and those of relevant ancestry (see Ethnic Group and Race) to identify sickle hemoglobin. If screening is not done at birth or in early infancy, it should be performed in early adolescence for genetic counseling.
5. *Hemoglobin and hematocrit:* These tests for anemia are performed routinely at birth, 12 months of age, around 5 years of age, and in early adolescence.
6. *Height and weight:* These parameters should be measured and recorded on a growth chart from birth through 4 years of age on a regular basis, and then every three years in a child who is well. Some clinicians, however, believe these measurements should be repeated annually through adolescence.
7. *Head circumference:* This should be measured and recorded on a head circumference chart from birth through 24 months of age. Some sources recommend repeating the measurement every two years. In practice, the head is usually measured after 24 months of age only if there is reason to suspect excessive or inadequate head growth.
8. *Heart murmurs:* These should be evaluated as part of the routine physical examination from birth through adolescence.
9. *Hips:* The hips should be evaluated for congenital dislocation or excessive joint laxity from birth until the child walks. This examination is part of the regular physical examination.
10. *Hearing:* This should routinely be evaluated from birth through early childhood by gross hearing testing and by assessment of language development. Pure tone audiometry should be used as soon as the child can understand directions and cooperate, usually at 3 to 4 years of age. This test should be repeated every two or three years until adolescence in an otherwise asymptomatic child.
11. *Vision:* This should be evaluated from birth through early childhood by noting the child's ability to follow objects, to recognize familiar things by sight, and to coordinate eye-hand functions. The illiterate E test can be used at 3 years of age, and the standard Snellen test can be administered at 5 or 6 years of age. Vision should be retested every two or three years through adolescence.
12. *Lead:* Lead test should begin at 9 to 12 months of age if the child is at risk due to his or her life circumstances. Repeat testing every 6

to 12 months should be considered until 5 years of age, depending on housing conditions, the presence of pica, and the child's previous lead levels.
13. *Tuberculosis skin test:* There are many screening tests for tuberculosis, including the Monovac, Tine, and PPD tests. Every child *not* in a high-risk group should be tested before the measles immunization is given (around 15 months of age), before elementary school entrance (around 5 years of age), and in early adolescence (around 12 years of age). Children in high-exposure groups should be tested more frequently, probably every year.
14. *Urine culture:* It is now accepted practice that this should be performed on all toilet trained girls, beginning at 2 years of age if possible. The frequency with which the child should be retested is controversial, and so there is no established guideline for this.
15. *Urine protein:* It is now accepted practice that this should be evaluated at the preschool and preadolescent health evaluations in order to detect a wide range of renal diseases.
16. *Teeth:* Dental screening and cleaning by a dental hygienist or dentist should begin at 3 years of age, and should be repeated every six months, for life.

There are several tests which we have intentionally omitted because their value is controversial or pooly documented. Blood pressure, urine analysis, developmental tasks, and intelligence tests are some of these. Even some items which we have included—such as height and weight measurements—are rarely the earliest sign of disease. Nevertheless, they may occasionally be useful as screening tools. In general, however, the particular measurements which we have presented here are considered basic components of the pediatric health evaluation.

Suggested Readings
Unit II: Data Base

Chapter 2: History

Anyan, W. The adolescent's data base. Pp. 32–34 in *Adolescent Medicine in Primary Care*. New York, John Wiley and Sons, 1978.

Mahoney, E., Verdisco, L., and Shortridge, L. *How to Collect and Record a Health History*. Philadelphia, J.B. Lippincott, 1976.

Report of the Committee on Infectious Diseases, 18th ed. Evanston, Ill., American Academy of Pediatrics, 1977.

Chapter 4: Screening

Anyan, W. Possibilities in health screening in adolescence. Pp. 35–47, in *Adolescent Medicine in Primary Care*. New York, John Wiley and Sons, 1978.

Clow, C. and Scriver, C. Knowledge about and attitudes toward genetic screening among high-school students; the Tay-Sachs experience. *Pediatrics* 59: 86–91, 1977.

UNIT THREE

**Clinical Assessment:
Sources for the
Data Base**

CHAPTER 5

The Interview

Introduction
The Interview in Its Three Forms
    Initial Evaluation (and First Visit to Gather Complete Data Base)
    Follow-up Health Evaluation
    Visit for Episodic Care with Problem; Patient Known to Clinician
Components of the Interview: An Expanded Discussion
    Greeting and Introduction of the Clinician
    Discussion of the Clinician's Title and Role
    Introduction to the People Accompanying the Child
    Agenda
    Initial Questions for the Clinician from the Historian
Issues during the Interview
    Flexibility
    Confidentiality
    Technique of the Interview
    General Questions from the Historian
    Specific Questions from the Historian
    Third Party Questions
    "By-the-Way" Questions
    Challenges about the Clinician's Questions
    Questions about the Clinician
    Questions about Child Rearing
    Disagreements

>   Clinician's Feelings about the Parents and Child
>   Handling Strong Emotions of the Historian
>   Nonverbal Communication
> The Role of the Child during the Interview
>   Including the Child in the Parent Interview
>   Interviewing the Child
> Alternative Formats
>   Tense Historian
>   Unfocused Historian
>   Evasive, Withholding Historian
>   Historian with a Psychiatric Problem
>   Retarded Historian
>   Adolescent Historian
>   Foreign-Language Speaking Historian
>   Anxious Child
>   Concern about a Particular Physical Problem
>   Discomfort about the Sex of the Practitioner
>   Adolescent Parent

INTRODUCTION

The history is the most important part of the clinical evaluation. The interview with the parents and child provides the most essential part of the health history; it guides the clinician in performing the subsequent physical examination and suggests the choice of appropriate laboratory and screening procedures.

But the interview also serves important interpersonal functions. During the interview the child and parent begin (or reestablish) their relationships with the health professional. Those relationships will be affected profoundly by the quality of the interaction, which includes both verbal and nonverbal communication. In turn, of course, the success (or lack of it!) of those relationships will influence the accuracy of the history itself—and is therefore an important factor in the outcome of treatment. In light of these considerations the interview will fail if it consists merely of a series of questions designed simply to elicit factual data; rather, it must be a sensitive interchange that is led—but not dominated—by the practitioner. This chapter will discuss some of the techniques and problems of the interview; however, it will be limited to the context of nonemergency pediatric practice. The content of a complete health history is presented in the discussion of the total data base, Chapter 2.

In the normal course of events, the interview will take place at the beginning of the visit; naturally, the clinician should expect to gather additional information in the course of the physical examination. However, it is important to keep the interview and the physical examination separate—both conceptually and in practice. Examiners cannot do either an adequate interview or a thorough examination if they do them simultaneously. In addition, if the two are merged, the parent and child may get the impression that the examiner is rushed and disorganized.

Following the physical examination, clinicians should take the time to summarize their findings for the parent and child. In this summary they should share their impressions and present plans for screening and further evaluation or treatment. This summary is an extremely important element of the overall interchange. It provides child and parents with an opportunity to ask questions, to discuss their ideas about the child's health, and to pursue the significance of the clinician's statements. It also offers a vehicle through which clinicians can provide both child and parents with anticipatory guidance. A detailed discussion of the clinical summary is present in Unit 4.

THE INTERVIEW IN ITS THREE FORMS: A SUMMARY

The interview is a complex process during which examiners elicit the information that will compose the historical data base from the parents and child. It is a process that involves the interplay of people and their thoughts and feelings. This means that it should not be approached mechanically or too schematically. One does not use the outline of the data base: it is too lengthy and far more complete than the real interview needs to be, and its organization is based on the presentation of a complete written record of the history.

In this section we shall present a summary of the tasks to be completed in the interview, including their components and proper order. We shall differentiate between three separate clinical situations: the initial complete health evaluation, the follow-up health evaluation, and episodic care for known problems. Within the organization suggested, clinicians should use selected open-ended questions to determine whether there are any abnormalities or events that are likely to have a significant influence on the child's health and development, and should then proceed to the structured developmental observations and the physical examination.

COMPONENTS OF THE INTERVIEW: AN EXPANDED DISCUSSION

The three forms of interview have been summarized in terms of a series of components, most of which are common to all. In this section we shall discuss each of these components in some detail but as we do so, the

Summary of Three Forms of Health Care Visits

Initial Complete Health Evaluation (and first visit to gather complete data base)	Follow-up Health Evaluation	Visit for Episodic Care, with Problem (patient known to clinician)
1. Greeting and introduction of clinician	1. Greeting	1. Greeting
2. Identification of clinician's role and discussion of this information		
3. Introduction of people accompanying child	2. Introduction of people accompanying child (as needed)	2. Introduction of people accompanying child (as needed)
4. Presentation of agenda of visit		3. Presentation of problem
5. Questions to clinician from parent and child	3. Questions to clinician	
		4. Evaluation of problem
6. Dealing with questions— either answer them, or tell the parent/child how they will be answered	4. Dealing with questions	
	5. Interim health history	5. Interim health history
7. Current health—diet, habits, development	6. Current health	
8. Past developmental history		
9. Past medical history Perinatal Hospitalizations Serious illnesses and accidents Previous well child care		
10. Family social history	7. Update family social history	6. Update family social history
11. Family medical history	8. Update family medical history	7. Update family medical history
12. Review of systems	9. Review of systems	

components will be detached from their respective places in each of the interview forms. The reader might find it helpful to refer to the summary above in order to keep the order of the components within each of the interview forms in mind.

First, however, we wish to underline an important point: *At all stages in the interview, it is exceedingly important to address oneself directly to the child in a way that is appropriate for his or her developmental stage.* The patient, after all, should feel central to the interview and examination. Part of good health care practice is to assert, in one's dealings with patients, the validity of their feelings and perceptions—that is, to validate them as human beings. An alienated patient is not likely to derive maximum benefit from the health care that is offered.

Greeting and introduction of the clinician

The initial greeting and introduction of the clinician to the patient and parent are extremely important, especially if they are meeting for the first time. All too often, health care practitioners enter the examining room, nod, and proceed directly with medical questions. This aloof behavior can easily alienate the people involved, for it can communicate to them that the clinician is in a hurry, unfriendly, impersonal, or not interested in what the child or parent thinks. Clinicians will have much better rapport and will encourage more productive exchanges of information with patients if they take the time to make them comfortable initially, and if they make sure that all persons have opportunities to voice their own concerns about the health evaluation which will follow.

The initial greeting should include all of the people in the room, and the introduction should provide the name, title, and description of the role of the health practitioner. For example, "Hello, Mrs. Rivera. Hi, José. I am Ms. Smith, a nurse practitioner. I work with Dr. Jones and I will be doing many of José's checkups." On the other hand, with an adolescent or older child it is advisable to greet the patient first, since this establishes the patient's social significance and helps to gain his or her trust.

It is important to keep in mind that nonverbal communication has at least as much impact on people as what is said. Clinicians who enter the examination room and walk swiftly to a "sheltered" seat behind a desk, and who are stiff in deportment and formal in tone, will establish their "authority," but they do so at the price of lost trust, comfort, and intimacy on the part of the people whose needs they are supposed to be attending to. As a result, the clients may well be hesitant to share potentially vital information of a personal nature—which in turn may impair the quality of the health care they receive.

Discussion of the clinician's title and role

The clinician could say, "Are you familiar with the role of the nurse practitioner in our office?" Or: "Have you been to see a nurse practitioner before?" "Do you understand the way we work together?" If the parent or patient has questions about the function, training, or responsibilities of the health care practitioner—whether a nurse practitioner, nurse clinician, physician's assistant, physician, medical student, or intern—they should be answered as fully as possible at the outset. This helps them know what to expect from the clinician and often prevents unnecessary concern about the qualifications of the various members of the health care team.

Introduction to the people accompanying the child

Usually, a child is accompanied by a parent, older sibling, or other close relative (but sometimes the child is unaccompanied—see below). When the child is accompanied by someone other than a parent, the clinician should ask about the relationship of that person to the child, and should specifically request an explanation for the parent's absence. This usually takes place after the initial greeting and before one asks about initial concerns. If the child is accompanied by a parent who usually does not come with the child for health evaluations, the clinician should indicate awareness of this fact and inquire into the arrangement. Sometimes this will reveal important information about the family. For example, it may be the father's first visit because the mother has begun to work or is ill, or the parents have recently separated. When the child is unaccompanied, clinicians should use their judgment. It may be perfectly appropriate for a 16-year-old to come alone—but not for a 10-year-old. If the situation seems to be anomalous for any reason, one should inquire into the circumstances.

It is important to ascertain how well the accompanying person knows the child. As always, one should phrase the questions carefully, so as not to seem critical. If the adult and child do not live together, it might be wise to ask the adult how frequently she or he and the patient see each other, or how well they know each other. If the clinician believes the adult cannot give an adequate or reliable history, or if the adult expresses doubt that she or he can be an adequate historian, the clinician might say, "If there is information that I need after today's visit, I will call John's parents (or guardians, etc.). Whatever you can tell me now will be helpful." It is very important for the clinician to get in touch with an adult who knows the child well and obtain an interview. One needs an accurate and complete history—including past history and current daily habits—in order to assess accurately the physical and psychological well-being of the very young child. For instance, the health practitioner needs to know details about the range of the child's behavior with his or her caregivers, about eating habits and sleep patterns, and about recent developmental achievements.

When foster parents bring a child for a health evaluation soon after the child has been placed in their home, they usually have very little information about the child's past. Therefore, the examiner needs to have the legally responsible party sign a release of information form so that she or he can obtain data from medical and social agencies who knew the child. A social worker or case worker accompanying the child and foster parents should be interviewed.

Agenda

It is important to outline, briefly, the agenda for the visit. An example is, "I'll be asking you some questions, and then I'll examine José. Afterwards, I'll try to answer your questions." Of course, if the accompanying adult and child are quite familiar with the routine, it is unnecessary to do this.

Initial questions for the clinician from the historian

It is sound practice to give the parent and patient an explicit opportunity to ask questions early in the visit. The clinician can continue after the greeting with a statement such as, "Before I ask my questions, are there any questions you have for me, or anything you would like to remind me about?" If there are no questions, the examiner can say, "How have things been?" There are two important reasons for doing this. First, the clients' responses will tell the clinician what is foremost in their minds and frequently will provide crucial information to help the clinician decide how to proceed with the visit. Secondly, it is important for the patient and parents. If they do not have an opportunity to ask what they feel are important questions, their discomfort and tension will interfere with their ability to concentrate on the interview. It may also make them feel that the examiner is not attending to what they perceive to be most important, and may thus undermine their trust in the health care process. The opportunity to discuss their concerns early in the visit communicates to them that the clinician can be flexible in response to their particular needs.

The following example illustrates the kind of concern a parent may present when the question of interest is expressed in an open-ended fashion. A father brings his one-year-old daughter for a checkup. When asked if he has any particular concerns that he wants to discuss at this visit, he replies, "I am worried that Susie is too fat. I know she looks healthy, but I have always tended to be overweight, and I was a big baby. I've also read in the paper that big babies grow to be fat adults." At this point one can either pursue the question in depth or can indicate that one will discuss it later in the visit, after completing the history and performing the physical examination. In either case, the clinician should acknowledge that she or he shares an interest in or concern about the problem and will attend to it. This allows the parent to become involved in the health evaluation without feeling frustrated or insulted.

It is impossible to overstate how important are the clinician's responses to the parent's and patient's concerns. (A discussion of how to gather the specific data needed to answer given questions is presented in the section covering the evaluation of a concern.) Never accept evasive, monosyllabic answers. ("How have things been?" "Tough," or "OK," or "Can't complain.") Find something specific to ask about and use this opening to move outwards from the narrow issue to the patient as a person and then to the family situation: "How's the knee been? Any trouble walking? How about sports? You say you've kept away from sports because of headaches? How long have you had them? Are they connected to other problems? Any other problems? How are things at home? Dad still upset about his job? And Mom? She still getting headaches?" Clinicians should show involvement and concern because they *are* involved and concerned. Once the initial concerns have been discussed fully, the clinician can proceed with the health history.

ISSUES DURING THE INTERVIEW

Flexibility

The success of an interview depends on the flexibility and sensitivity of the interviewer. This is true for the health evaluation of the well child as well as for that of the sick child. The outline presented for the data base actually provides the underlying structure for the interview as well; however, one must be flexible and ready to alter the interview to suit the needs of the individual situation. Factors which determine the interview format include the number and variety of issues to be discussed, patient and parental attitudes, and the severity of illness. Further, historians vary: some patients and parents are quiet, passive, calm, shy, or taciturn; others are more nervous, angry, or dramatic. And clinical situations also vary, even in the non-urgent office visit. Although there is an overall plan for an interview, in actual practice clinicians must remain flexible and exercise their judgment.

Confidentiality

Confidentiality between the health care practitioner and the historian is an important implicit commitment which most people assume will be upheld. And it should be. However, there are a few limited situations when clinicians must not keep information confidential. For example: if it seems possible that a patient might harm himself or herself or someone else, health care professionals are morally obligated to report this to appropriate professional personnel or agencies—or to take measures themselves to prevent such a calamity from happening. In the case of child abuse or neglect, the obligation to break confidentiality is also a legal one; in the majority of states one is required to report the matter to the appropriate government agency.

But breaking confidentiality does *not* mean that the patient's or parent's rights can be overlooked. Whenever one must override the requirement of confidentiality, the clinician should explain this decision to the parties involved (the patient and/or parent) and should add that no information will be communicated without their being informed. In the case of child abuse, clinicians must not be afraid to report because they fear that a record of child abuse will prevent the family from being helped. Sometimes clinicians use such rationalizations to shield themselves from facing their own discomfort with a situation.

Technique of the interview

The ideal interview is complete, efficient, and yet flexible. This goal can be accomplished by using a modified open-ended approach, including both general and specific questions which are carefully chosen to elicit the necessary information. An open-ended interview is one in which the clinician asks questions which do not limit the answers implicitly or explicitly. Questions should be nonjudgmental and should foster honest replies which amplify, rather than restrict, the subject under discussion. The questions should lead to descriptions and explanations of events and feelings rather than to single word or yes/no answers. An effective interview is really a discussion—not just a list of questions aimed at learning facts.

It helps, of course, to ask questions that proceed in an orderly format from the general to the more specific, until all important details are noted and explained. The rationale is that the more general question will not bias the answer and will provide an opportunity for historians to bring up what they consider most important. The accuracy of recollections of events is greater when the respondents are encouraged to build a network of associations that are relevant, than when they are asked only to respond to direct questions. In addition, a flexible approach increases the motivation to report accurately and decreases irritation. The open-ended method is particularly useful if there is a complex diagnostic problem, if the historian is highly suggestible, or if the problem is emotionally charged. The child and parent may include information which the clinician did not anticipate and about which she or he would not have asked. After the historians describe the events in the order and with the emphasis they feel is important, then the clinician can gather a clear account of the actual chronological progression of the symptom and the surrounding events. It is unwise to attempt to impose chronological order on a history at the very beginning, since this will disrupt the flow of information.

Students or inexperienced clinicians are often too timid to ask parents and children about their feelings, especially about private and upsetting aspects of their lives. However, patients and parents are usually quite willing to discuss their personal problems with pediatric health practitioners if they feel that the clincan has been considerate of them from the out-set and if they perceive that the clinician's primary goal is to be supportive in helping them maintain good physical and mental health.

All questions, whether open-ended or more specific, should be phrased in a way that does not include an answer or suggest that a particular answer is "right" or "wrong." It is especially difficult to pose questions about child rearing, discipline, and sexual mores in a nonjudgmental way. Clinicians must choose their words carefully. They must also face and acknowledge their own attitudes, which will inevitably be revealed by nonverbal communication such as positive tone of voice and facial expression.

The words that clinicians choose in phrasing their questions are very important. It helps to select words that are familiar and easy for the individual historian to understand. Use of language that is too complicated for the historian (whether he or she is young or educationally disadvantaged) is inconsiderate and will make this person uncomfortable. People are frequently embarrassed to ask the meaning of words they do not understand, and this embarrassment may quickly turn to anger at the clinician whose lack of tact and sensitivity hurt them. Language that is too simple or childlike can also be insulting, especially to an adolescent or an insecure parent. Successful interviewing depends upon caring about people's feelings and acting upon one's perception of their emotional responses to the situation.

Really, all of this amounts to being tactful and using common sense. One can avoid questions that are very likely to irritate people and put them on the defensive. It is possible to avoid such unpleasant interchanges by choosing one's words carefully. For example, instead of asking, "Do you spank John?" it would probably be more productive to inquire, "How often do you have to discipline John?" "How do you do this?" Instead of "Do you hold Lisa when she takes her bottle?" (an aggressive, challenging question) try "How often during the day do you have a chance to hold Lisa?" "Is that during a feeding or at other times?"

Because the phrasing of questions is so important in the establishment and maintenance of rapport, we shall take the time to present a somewhat extended example of how to explore a serious topic. The approach taken is to ask a nonjudgmental open-ended question and to proceed to more specific questions:

Tony is visiting his clinician, Dr. Jane Silver, who needs to know about possible contact with tuberculosis (TB) in order to plan appropriate screening for Tony and his family and to initiate evaluation for the disease if it is present. In a low risk group, TB skin testing is usually performed only at the 1 year, 5 year, and early adolescent health evaluations. However, if a close friend of the family has been diagnosed as having TB, then Tony and his entire family will have to be evaluated. The question about TB contacts is very specific, but it should be asked in a way that allows for a non-defensive and honest, unbiased answer. One way Dr. Silver could ask this question would be to say, "As far as you know, have any of your family or friends had TB?" (A prejudicial way to elicit the same information is to say, "Of course, Tony hasn't been with anyone with TB, has he?")

If Tony has had contact with a person with TB, then Dr. Silver should proceed with a series of specific questions to elaborate the details, so that she can manage the case appropriately. Some or all of these questions would follow:

Who is the person with TB?
What is his or her relationship to Tony?
Has Tony been exposed to that person?
When did the contact occur?
How frequently did Tony and the person with TB have contact?
How close was the contact?
When was the diagnosis of tuberculosis made?
Was the tubercular person under treatment at the time of contact?
Do you know what kinds of medicine he or she was taking?
Who was treating this person?
Was the tubercular person ever hospitalized for TB?
Where was he or she hospitalized?
When did the hospitalization take place?
How long was the hospitalization?
Who else in your family or household was in contact with the TB patient?
Have you or the other household members been evaluated for TB since your contact with the tubercular person?
Has anyone in your family ever had a TB contact before?
(If the answer to this question is yes, Dr. Silver should ask for details.)

The answers to these questions about TB would provide the information needed to formulate a health management plan for Tony and his family. Although the proposed list of questions is neat and concise and the questions are quite specific, it is important to remain flexible throughout the interview. The clinician may have to explain some of the questions or may have to pursue issues raised by the historian's original answers.

General questions from the historian

At the beginning of this chapter we discussed the importance of giving patients and parents an opportunity to ask questions very early in the interview. Frequently, people will have no questions initially, perhaps because they are too uncomfortable to ask them or even to remember them. However, in the course of the interview or the physical examination they may be reminded of questions or may feel more comfortable about asking them. Sometimes parents are embarrassed to "bother" clinicians with a question. If the health care practitioner thinks this is the case, it is often helpful to say something like "Many parents ask about that. It's a natural concern." When a parent and patient feel accepted by the examiner, they will feel more comfortable asking difficult questions about medical, social, and emotional problems.

The clinician should be extremely cautious about giving advice or reassurance. Even superficially simple questions may have unforeseen significance, and the examiner should be careful to assess the particular situation. An offhand reassurance such as "Oh, she will grow out of it," may stop any further questions, although the parent is not really satisfied with the answer. This may interfere with communication for the rest of the interview, and a significant problem may go undetected. It is also important, although at times difficult, to remember that advice that is not synchronous with the family's cultural background and beliefs will not be helpful to them.

If health care practitioners answer a question without first gathering enough information from history, physical examination, or laboratory tests, they give the parent good reason to believe that they are careless, that they do not take the parent's concerns seriously, or that they do not want to think about the issue. Quick or "reflex" reassurance is often an attempt on the part of clinicians to reassure themselves. If one has the impulse to make such a gesture it should set off a warning signal to stop and ascertain what the source of discomfort is.

In the worst cases, inadequate evaluation of questions can often lead to erroneous clinical conclusions. This will not only seriously decrease the effectiveness of future guidance or counseling but also could result in the patient's suffering needless, and possibly severe, harm.

Specific questions from the historian

A number of factors go into the decision whether, and how, to answer questions at the time they are asked. These include: whether one has sufficient data to answer the questions accurately; how simple the answer is; who is in the room at the time; and how much time all parties involved (clinician, child, parent) have for the visit.

A few general principles apply to answering questions. The first, and most important, is to answer the child's questions promptly and straightforwardly. The answer may be brief, but it should address the child's concerns and fears, and it should reduce the possibilities of needless agonized fantasizing on the child's part. Second, the clinician should answer promptly simple questions that are not especially emotionally charged and which have straightforward factual answers. Many questions about procedures, immunizations, and health maintenance routines can be completely and simply answered in language that the parent and older child can understand. Some of these questions will cover methods or amount of payment; roles of members of the health care team (especially newer members such as physicians' assistants and nurse practitioners); why a particular procedure is being performed (such as the PKU test at birth and at two weeks of age); and why a procedure is not performed (such as the smallpox vaccination). Third, it is wise to postpone elaborating on detailed issues and managing people's concerns until late in the interview, when further data from the developmental assessment and physical examination will be available for formulating an answer.

When the questions are not simple, clinicians should acknowledge their complexity and should tell the child and parent how and when these questions will be addressed. For example, clinicians should explicitly state that they need to gather more data from the interview, physical examination, or laboratory tests before they can give a good answer on a complicated matter. Occasionally, health care practitioners may need to say that they will discuss the situation later, with the parent alone and not with the child, but in such cases they should explain the reasons for this arrangement to the child.

However, if a parent wants to discuss a concern immediately, and insists on it, the examiner may consider the issue of maintaining rapport sufficient reason to make an exception and will decide to respond, as will be discussed later in Evaluation of a Complaint or Concern.

Third party questions

Parents frequently want to know the clinician's opinion about statements made by family and friends, and they may want advice about how to handle other people's criticisms. Toilet training is a topic that frequently draws a lot of gratuitous advice on the "right way" to toilet train a child from intrusive friends and relatives. (Mostly, this advice does little more than make parents feel insecure or defensive.) Or the parents may have read and talked about how to manage this developmental task. Most often, the health care practitioner should try to reinforce the parents' own well-founded ideas and to give them the confidence to proceed with less conflict. The clinician might say, "This is a complicated problem to solve. You will find that other people may disagree with what you and I have decided together. I am confident that we can find the right way for your family."

"By-the-way" questions

Parents sometimes ask a question as an aside—in the middle of a discussion, during the developmental assessment or the physical examination, or at the end of the visit. Frequently they introduce their question with the phrase "by the way." Clinicians should note the phrase, and should remember that the question or topic it precedes frequently is not as casual and simple as it seems at first.

Usually, questions introduced in this offhand manner are about issues which have concerned the parent for some time, and which may be controversial within the family. These questions should be handled like any other concern that has been introduced without the "by-the-way" phrase; they require thorough evaluation with the open-ended technique before they are answered. Clinicians should be aware that adolescents frequently use "by-the-way" questions to lead into a discussion of a current problem. The adolescent often will not inform either the clinician or the parent about the problem before or at the beginning of a visit. Then, as the visit progresses, and as the adolescent feels more relaxed about opening up the issue with the clinician, she or he will slide into a casual-sounding "by the way."

In sum, "by-the-way" questions should never be ignored. It is important not to allow the pressure of scarce time at the end of the visit or other matters to lead to a haphazard or inattentive response. Clinicians should sensitize themselves to the "by-the-way" manner of asking and should answer such a question or issue fully—either when it is asked, or at a clearly designated time in the near future.

Challenges about the clinician's questions

Occasionally, a parent or patient asks why the interviewer has asked a particular question. This may be a straightforward attempt to understand the reason behind the question; but it may also indicate that the person is particularly wary or that the question touched a sensitive area. This question, like other reactions to questions, should be noted; they may form patterns which illuminate the way a patient or parent is feeling.

If the historian seems annoyed by a question, examiners can usually alleviate the tension by explaining their reasons for asking. One might say, "I need to ask these questions so that I get all the information necessary to help you and your family decide what the problem is and what needs to be done for treatment." Or one may also choose to acknowledge and empathize with the historian's annoyance: "I know it can be irritating to have to answer so many questions." Of course, if the irritation is a pattern which interferes, it must be evaluated and managed as a problem.

Questions about the clinician

Parents sometimes ask personal questions of clinicians. In pediatrics, these most often concern whether he or she is married and has children. One should answer such questions accurately; but it is not necessary—or even advisable—to discuss one's own personal life beyond giving a few simple facts. If clinicians become friends to their patients it may paradoxically make them less able to be helpful. Of course, strict formality and reserve are not required. One aims for a comfortable but clearly professional relationship. Occasionally, patients and parents are hostile because they worry that the clinician, who has not experienced the same stress that they are suffering, will be unsympathetic or even inattentive to details of management. Clinicians in this situation should not try to defend themselves or describe what they have suffered. Instead, one should address the underlying fears nondefensively by explaining that one empathizes and understands, even though one has not had the particular experience: "Of course I can't understand your situation as well as you do, since

I never really went through it, but I am really concerned and will try very hard to understand you. And I think we will be able to work together well enough to help you."

Questions about child rearing

EVALUATING THE SITUATION:
Questions about child rearing practices often reflect very complex problems in family relationships, although at first glance they may appear to be simple questions about the best way for parents to behave. It is not unusual for discussion of a relatively minor inquiry to lead into a discussion of a major family problem. Health care practitioners should be alert to questions such as: "What should I feed the baby?" "How should I teach her to use the toilet?" "Should she have a pacifier?" "At what age should I take the pacifier away?" "What is the best way to discipline my child at this age?" "How should I handle his sister's jealousy?" "Is it OK to spank Alphonse?" "Should I let Mary Lou use birth control pills?" and "Should I allow Heidi to smoke?"

When a question about child rearing is raised, the examiner should ask several open-ended questions to learn about the parent's ideas as well as to explore the complexities of a situation. However, it is important for clinicians to explain the process of exploration they are undertaking; otherwise they may give the patient or parent the impression that they are evading the question. Thus, it helps to say something like, "Before I try to answer your question, it will be helpful if I understand a little more about it." One can gather information about the parent's views and experience by asking such questions as:

>   What have you tried, or thought about trying?
>   How did things work out when you tried it that way?
>   How did you feel doing it that way?
>   Why do you think that did (or did not) work out well?
>   What did you do in that situation when your other children (if there are siblings) were that age?
>   What does your spouse think about this issue?
>   Do you agree with his (her) ideas?
>   Have you received opinions from other family members and friends?
>   What did they suggest?
>   What do you think about those ideas?
>   Why do you think those suggestions aren't good? (if the parent has a negative reaction to those suggestions)
>   Are there specific ways in which you think I might be able to help?

In some situations a question that appears straightforward on the surface, may reflect considerable family controversy and even heated argument. For example, Mr. Jardin has brought his three-year-old daughter Mimi, for a checkup. He asks Dr. Silver, "What do you think about children sleeping in their parents' bed?" Dr. Silver should first ask about the circumstances which prompted the question. Then, with the questions listed above, she should ask about Mr. Jardin's ideas and feelings about the present way of handling the situation, and the alternatives which have been considered. She might add "How would you like to change that arrangement?" and "What other circumstances in your family would have to be different in order to alter the sleeping arrangements?" The answers to such questions will help Dr. Silver and Mr. Jardin to decide whether the problem is inadequate space, inadequate financial resources, or the fact that Mimi does not want to sleep alone. In addition, it is quite possible that the parents have different opinions about whether it is best for Mimi to sleep with them (assuming that she has somewhere else to sleep); or one parent may really feel like having Mimi in bed, although he or she thinks it would be best not to.

After all the circumstances and possible options for change have been identified, and after it is clear what each parent really wants, Dr. Silver can talk with the Jardins (mother and father) and to Mimi as well; together, it should be possible to come up with a plan which is realistic for their family. This approach makes it more likely that whatever plan is agreed upon will, in the end, actually be carried out. This point is not something to be taken for granted when one is trying to effect changes in family patterns and dynamics.

Health care professionals should keep in mind that even uncommunicative parents usually have their thoughts and feelings about child rearing. Occasionally, they do not want to tell the clinician their ideas—either because they fear the clinician will be harsh and judgmental about their thoughts or because they feel hostile toward the clinician, and so withhold information.

PRESENTATION OF THE CLINICIAN'S OPINION:
It is important to give one's opinion to parents who wish a professional assessment of their decision about child rearing practices. In a simple matter it is often sufficient to indicate agreement, approval, or support. For example, a parent may be trying to foster a sense of responsibility in a six-year-old child by having her put away her clothes and do simple chores in the care of a pet. On being told of this plan, it would be supportive for the clinician to give a friendly nod with a few words of approval. If the situation presented by the parent is more complex, the clinician can agree, emphasize what she or he thinks are important parts of the plan, amplify and add ideas, and answer specific questions about the plan.

The *manner* in which the health care practitioner presents an opinion will be a critical factor in the ability of a family to accept and implement it. Clinicians should present their opinions in clear language that the family can understand, and at the same time should not be condescending toward them. Health care practitioners should make it a point not to use jargon, because it creates an unnecessary communication barrier, is intimidating, and does not clarify the issues (in fact it may fail to communicate any information at all). The clinician's use of jargon and language that is more sophisticated than a family can comprehend puts the family in the position of needing to ask more questions, feeling more dependent on experts, and feeling more uncomfortable—hardly factors that contribute to good health care management.

When presenting ideas about child rearing, clinicians should take the trouble to organize what they have to say so that the family will have something clear to respond to. Occasionally health care practitioners become defensive when parents question their recommendations. Needless to say this is not desirable, especially if it leads to a quarrel with the family. It is much better for patient care if clinicians are prepared to be open, to explain their positions, and to refer to the goals of the parents and the considerations that prompted the recommendations. They may also refer to sound clinical experience and scientific evidence as needed. If the family members do not state any questions, but still seem unsatisfied or puzzled, the practitioner should probe a bit—ask if they have a particular situation in mind, or if they are concerned about an area that was not discussed. Sometimes it may help to comment "You seem puzzled (dissatisfied, confused) by what I just said. What puzzles you?"

There are some parents who will follow the clinician's advice even though they disagree with it. Even people who pride themselves on being mature and independent will frequently follow advice from an expert professional, although they do not understand the rationale for the plan and may even disagree with it. Sometimes parents will *try* to follow such advice when they are really not persuaded that it is correct. These parents may confuse the child by their inconsistent or halfhearted attempts at following instructions, or they may fail to carry out the plan and then feel guilty or angry about it. Occasionally, parents are afraid the clinician will reject or belittle them, and so they do not mention their disagreement and the subsequent failures. All of this discussion amounts simply to this: insensitivity on the part of a clinician in communicating with the family members may severely reduce the likelihood of being helpful with child rearing.

Some parents are particularly insecure and want the clinician to tell them what is correct. Health care practitioners should support the insecure parent, but their long-range goal should be to teach parents to evaluate situations, make their own decisions and plans, and gain confidence in their ability to be competent parents.

Often the child rearing issue is discussed with only one parent. The practitioner must indicate, however, that it will be necessary to involve the spouse, other significant family members, or even other people taking care of the child (such as teachers, day-care workers, or sitters) in the decision. And of course the child should also be included as soon as he or she is old enough to comprehend even a simple explanation of the situation.

Disagreements

It sometimes happens that disagreements arise between the clinician and the patient or parent. If a disagreement occurs, the clinician must keep in mind that it should be resolved in the best interest of the child. For example, information about sleeping arrangements is part of the pediatric data base. If the sleeping arrangements do not conform to the health care practitioner's values or standards, she or he might say, "How does that work out?" or "How do you feel about that?" If the child or parent indicates that the arrangements are satisfactory, the clinician must give careful thought to whether his or her concerns are irrational, arbitrary, ethnocentric, or exaggerated.

Child rearing practices, even within the same culture, are diverse. Clinicians, parents, and patients often believe that their own opinions are the only correct ones (or at least the very best), and they may stubbornly refuse to consider other equally effective approaches. When there is disagreement, rather than impose their own prejudices, practitioners should aim to support the family's approach to child rearing, as long as this approach is based on good intentions, comfortable feelings, and a sound grasp of the pertinent facts.

Although there may be many ways to approach a particular aspect of child rearing, it is important that the parents and other people taking care of the child have a fairly consistent approach to the child. In addition, the parents should be prepared to evaluate the child's progress and to alter the plan if necessary. A flexible, individualized approach to child rearing is much more important than almost any particular decision. The practitioners should always try to communicate their opinions in the context of support for a general approach to child rearing which is thoughtful and empathic.

When clinicians disagree with the parents' ideas about and their past solutions to problems, they should express their reservations tactfully and indicate whether and how they intend to pursue the topic further. In their discussions with the family, clinicians must convey the idea that they are committed to maintaining the physical and emotional health of the child. They should not be intimidated (by implicit threats that the family will leave treatment) into avoiding disagreement; and at the same time they should try not to become unsympathetic to the parents. Parental compliance with the position taken by a clinician—whether it be advice about medication for a seizure disorder or encouraging independence in a passive adolescent—depends on the trust and understanding that exist between the health care practitioner and the family.

Clinicians must acknowledge that there is great diversity in child rearing patterns. Some of the diversity represents small differences in style which do not significantly affect consequences. However, some practices are detrimental to the child's physical or emotional health—at least according to our cultural standards—and need to be changed. If the issue is very important, then the clinician must pursue the discussion, whether or not the parent is interested in his or her opinion at first. Occasionally, the parent or child will become annoyed and may even threaten not to return. However, if the clinician is to be an effective advocate for the child, he or she is obligated to tell the parents (and possibly the child) that there is cause for concern. Naturally, it is important to do this tactfully, though firmly.

Clinicians should express their disagreement in a way that does not belittle, intimidate, or antagonize the family, and at the same time is honest. They should allow the parents ample opportunity to ask questions without becoming defensive, and should try to understand the parents' objections to suggestions. It is important to organize and present whatever evidence, including clinical experience and scientific data, will help convince the family to give serious thought to one's professional opinions and suggestions. Parents are more likely to listen to, and seriously consider, the opinion of a practitioner who can calmly explain the rationale for his or her recommendations.

There will be some situations in which the clinician cannot persuade the family to try the recommended plan. In such instances, it is appropriate for the health practitioner to acknowledge the disagreement but to make it explicitly clear that this is not necessarily the end of their dialogue. It may be helpful to say, "This is a difficult problem to solve. You need to try different solutions until you find one that is best for your family. I would like to hear from you in a few weeks to find out how things are going." The clinician should follow these words with an active effort to contact the family if they do not touch base in a few weeks' time.

Even when the family disagrees with the health care practitioner, if they can view the clinician as an ally of the family who is committed to working with them until the problem is solved, they will not be reluctant to return and ask for reevaluation and help with further management.

Clinician's feelings about the parents and child

It is very important for clinicians to identify and reflect on the strong feelings they often have toward patients and parents. Historians may be angry, suspicious and accusatory, unappreciative, withholding, uncooperative, undependable, seductive, or demanding toward practitioners. In response, clinicians often feel irritation, anger, hurt, embarrassment, frustration, sexual stimulation, identification, fear, or pity. They can also feel judgmental, rejecting, critical, or disgusted with patients and their families. It is destructive to ignore these feelings, because even a well disciplined clinician will express them in a way which, although not obvious, will be perceived by patients and parents. Usually this perpetuates a cycle of negative feelings and behavior. However, thoughtful analysis of the feelings can provide a greater understanding of the relationship between the clinician and family. Such analysis can then be used to deal constructively with the person who provokes the feelings.

Often, just understanding the relationship changes the practitioner's behavior enough to stop a destructive cycle; but sometimes clinicians have to talk openly about the problem in the interaction. If the parent or child does not find it easy to talk about feelings, or if it does not seem necessary, the clinician should mention the behaviors which are contributing to the problem. This may lead to a discussion of the feelings; or the discussion of the behavior may be helpful by itself. For example, withholding parents need to know that the clinician notices their behavior and that it is impossible to make any sound clinical judgments without sufficient information. Demanding patients need to have their inappropriate demands identified and need to be reminded of the limits of the services offered. However, this should be done sympathetically as well as firmly: "I know how hard it is to get here, but we do not do home visits in these situations."

When it is necessary to discuss the feelings behind the behavior, practitioners may begin the discussion by talking about their own feelings and restating their commitment to help the parents and child. Sometimes an impression of criticism can result, if the historians' feelings are discussed first. A comment about how feelings can interfere with the work is appropriate, and then the clinician can ask the historians how they have been feeling about the realtionship.

The ability to use the information about feelings is a valuable skill in building and sustaining a professional relationship with families. Like other skills which the clinician learns, it requires thoughtful practice and grows with clinical experience. However, practitioners can never be helpful to patients in these discussions if they are unable to accept their own feelings. It is a common mistake to regard as unprofessional and to feel ashamed of the many strong feelings which are stirred up in all of us who work with children and families.

Handling strong emotions of the historian

Sometimes a parent or a child will begin to cry, or may express intense rage or extreme anxiety, either when a serious problem is the focus of the discussion or when the respondent is reminded of an idea or feelings during the course of an interview. Most clinicians have to learn to resist the urge to make things right quickly by reassuring the person that things are not so bad or that they will get better. It is also an error to communicate that there is no need to talk more about it because the clinician really understands how they feel. The practitioner has to find a way to demonstrate empathy and support without foreclosing the discussion.

It is usually most supportive and informative if the interviewer allows the parent or child time to experience the feeling by remaining silent for a short while. A gesture or a phrase to indicate empathy, such as touching a shoulder, offering a tissue, saying "I can see it is hard," or "I can see you're upset," will usually communicate support and allow the conversation to go on. Sometimes a parent seems ashamed or inhibited and needs to be told that it is all right to cry or to be very upset in the clinician's presence. The decision about whether or not to include the child in this part of the interview may need to be discussed (see p. 102). Clinicians should ask questions about the feelings and thoughts if the conversation seems to stop, when it is not clear what prompted the strong feelings. They may use questions such as "What were you thinking about then?" or "What is it that made you upset?" However, when a serious problem is being discussed, the practitioner is not surprised that the historian shows strong feelings, and therefore it is necessary to use different questions, such as, "Of course thinking about your father's death is hard. What has been the hardest thing about it for you?"

Sometimes a parent or child will become irritated with the clinician for asking more about a painful experience: "How do you *think* it feels when your mother calls you a slut?!" Practitioners should never insist on the continuation of the conversation, nor should they counterattack. They can comment that they know it is hard to talk about painful things; or they can explain that of course they know in general that a situation would be hard for any person, but that every human being is different and the differences are very important to understand. Finally, they should always make it clear that they are available, that they think it is often helpful to talk about strong feelings with a professional person, that they feel capable of being helpful but that they know it is up to the child or the parent to decide when, where, and with whom to talk about these private and difficult issues.

On rare occasions, practitioners may have to ask distraught historians to control their emotions so that their work can proceed. This is actually very unusual, but it may be appropriate when there is a pressing acute problem to solve, and after some attention has been paid to the upsetting feelings. The clinician could say, "Please try to pull yourself together. I know it is difficult, but we should try to get on with the evaluation of Kenneth's cough and fever. I will make sure to talk further about the situation with your husband at another time."

Nonverbal communication

Nonverbal communication—although largely unintentional—is as important an element of an interchange as what is said verbally. Using facial and bodily gestures, as well as positioning relative to one another, people constantly amend, amplify, negate, deny, mitigate, satirize, undercut, render ironic, or emphasize what they say to each other. For the most part, such nonverbal communication expresses how they *feel*: about themselves, the situation, and others present. Sensitive clinicians will constantly monitor the nonverbal communication between themselves and the parent(s) and patient, and that which occurs between parent(s) and child as well.

Health care practitioners should think about their location in relation to the parent and child. When all present are at a physically equal level, for instance, when they are all seated, there is less opportunity for parents to feel that a clinician thinks he or she is superior. Children, too, are less likely to be afraid of clinicians who are seated at their level. Clinicians who sit rigidly back in their chairs, and perhaps even fold their arms in front of them, put both the parent and child at a distance and appear stern and judgmental.

It is important to be aware of posture. For instance, slumping may communicate fatigue, depression, or unhappiness in the clinician, and the parent or child may assume that this relates to them. The clinician who is unkempt or sprawled out may appear sloppy and too casual, and this in turn can be "read" by the parent or child to mean that the clinician is incompetent, sloppy in method or thought, or not respectful of the parent and child.

It is very important to monitor the reactions of children or parents whom one touches, perhaps on the arm or shoulder. Although perhaps intended to convey concern or emotional support, these gestures may be perceived (consciously or unconsciously) as a sexual intrusion or as patronizing by members of either sex. Naturally, such physical contact can be very reassuring if the clinician and parent are comfortable with each other and if a sound professional relationship exists between them.

Eye contact between the clinician and the parents and child is an important way to indicate interest, concern, and attention. However, this too can have negative as well as positive content.

This discussion of nonverbal communication has concentrated on the interchanges between family members and the health care practitioner since the clinician's sensitivity to these issues will improve his or her ability to provide good health care to the family. However, it is important not to overlook the issue of how family members are communicating nonverbally among themselves. The alert clinician will find that monitoring nonverbal communication between the parents and the child, and between the parents themselves, will yield a wealth of important information that may contribute significantly to the clinician's determination of the family situation and consequently of the best way to proceed in health care management.

For example, the way in which a parent holds a young child may reveal many things. If the child is held stiffly, in an uncomfortable position, or with minimal body contact, there is sufficient reason for the clinician to suspect that the parent may be experiencing conflicting feelings toward the child. Conversely, a parent who is relatively free of conflict and feels love and affection for a child will hold the child closely, cuddle it, and perhaps kiss it or "coo" at it on occasion. Similarly—through such things as how close or distant from one another they sit, the amount of eye contact they make, the degree to which they interrupt one another, the extent to which they do or do not touch each other on the arm or shoulder on occasion, and the stiffness of their bearing—parents will reveal how they are getting along with each other (or with an older child who is no longer receiving the intensive body contact that occurs with infants).

A great deal has been written about nonverbal communication in the last few years, and there are numerous popular books on "body language" that are available on almost any book rack. Although we would encourage young health care practitioners to expose themselves to these materials in order to develop their sensitivity to such issues, we would caution them not to take too literally the "definitions" of specific gestures and body positions that are sometimes proffered. Like language, nonverbal communication is extremely malleable and, even more than language, it is intelligible only in the context of the culture of the people who are communicating. Moving close may be a reassuring gesture to members of Spanish-speaking ethnic groups—but may be perceived as intrusive and possibly even mobilize resentment among white Anglo-Saxon Protestants. Similarly, whereas middle-class American whites tend to need eye contact in order to be reassured that they are being listened to, this is not the case with the lower-class American blacks. (Incidently, white clinicians sometimes feel rejected by lower-class blacks who seem to be "avoiding" eye contact with them. Although the possibilities for hostility and rejection in such a situation are real, nevertheless it is likely that in quite a few instances the clinicians' "reading" of the nonverbal behavior of their black client or patient is culturally biased and hence based on wrong assumptions.) It would be wise for health care practitioners who work primarily among people whose ethnic background differs from their own to make some effort to get informal "coaching" on the conventions of nonverbal communication as practiced among members of these groups.

THE ROLE OF THE CHILD DURING THE INTERVIEW

Including the child in the parent interview

The main concern of the examiner throughout the interview should be to gather as accurate and complete a history as possible without making the parent or child unnecessarily uncomfortable. It is inevitable that family members will experience some emotional discomfort when the discussion turns to social, psychological, and serious health problems. However, if the clinician is sensitive to the patient's and parents' needs, he or she can minimize the discomfort and manage it constructively.

One problem that needs careful thought on the part of the clinicians is how and when to include the child in discussions about sensitive issues. Some parents are quite willing to discuss psychological and social problems privately with a health care practitioner, but they do not want the child to hear the discussion. Often this is appropriate, but in other cases it will be apparent that it is best to include the child. However, even in such cases it is best initially to honor the parents' preference about excluding the child. Later, during that visit or on a subsequent one, the child can be brought into the discussion after the parents and clinician have shared some precise information about the problem and have discussed the issue of including the child. (It may be necessary to work out ground rules for doing so.)

Sometimes it is necessary to exclude a child from the interview even though the parent does not think so. Parents may forget that certain information they give the clinician may be extremely upsetting to the child. Children may be upset when the parent is very angry or sad, or when he or she is describing violent, sexual, or criminal behavior, or other frightening events. With regard to this issue, often the emotional tone of a report is more important than the content of what is said.

It is also advisable to have the child out of the room when the parent is very critical, shaming, or hostile toward the child. A parent may begin to say things like "Alex has been bad since the day he was born!" and then begin to list his many faults. It is embarrassing and upsetting to a child to listen to a very negative public account of his behavior. In such circumstances the examiner should tactfully interrupt the parent, indicate that this particular issue should be discussed when the child is not present, and proceed with the less emotionally charged material for the time being. This can be accomplished quite directly, by saying, "I think you and I could discuss this better at another time because it may be upsetting and confusing for Alex." Children two years of age and even younger can become very distressed by what they hear a parent saying. The clinician must guard against underestimating the impact of the interview on the child.

Interviewing the child

Deciding on an appropriate role for the child in the interview is quite difficult. Children vary tremendously in their capacity to converse with an examiner in a health evaluation. The child's age, stage of development, cognitive abilities, language skills, and level of anxiety all influence this capacity. The content of the conversation and the behavior of the parents toward the child during the interview are also important. Therefore, the clinician must carefully consider all of these factors before deciding what degree of participation is appropriate for the child. However, it is always advisable for the clinician to enter into some verbal interchange with the child before proceeding with the physical examination.

If the child and examiner are familiar with each other from past visits, and if the child is not too shy, the clinician can initiate the interview with the child in a direct manner. If they do not know each other, or if the child is particularly shy, it is better to greet the child along with the parents, but to interview the latter first. Most children will observe the examiner's manner with the parent. If the clinician is calm, friendly, and approving, the child will sometimes enter the conversation spontaneously. More often, however, the child will be a quiet listener; at an opportune point the clinician can include the patient in the conversation by directing a comment or question toward the child. It is usually best to begin the conversation with neutral comments, before any questions are attempted. Showing the young child a toy or a book may be very helpful. For the older child a discussion of favorite activities or hobbies can be a good opener.

The interchange between the clinician and the patient may remain limited, or it may become a full interview. For example, a four-year-old child may be comfortable and may enjoy chatting with the health care practitioner about his or her home, school, family, and favorite toys. Another child of the same age may be very anxious about the possibility of having an injection, and so may be unable to converse easily with the clinician, even though she or he has quite adequate verbal skills.

If the child seems particularly afraid or shy, the clinician should ask the parent about the child's discomfort. If the problem hinges on something specific like a fear of injections, it is best to discuss this and try to alleviate some of the anxiety. However, in doing so, it is most important for the parent and clinician not to deceive the child into thinking that there will be no injection or other intrusive or frightening procedures when, in fact, there probably will be some.

It is important to be careful to frame and word one's questions to suit the child's age, cognitive and verbal abilities, and style of communication. Experienced clinicians will inquire about the whole world of the child's experiences: family, home, school, playmates, pets, favorite toys, and activities. Only gradually will they focus their questions directly on the child's health. All of this information is of great potential value and even a child as young as three years of age can give the clinicians some helpful information about a current complaint.

As the child grows older, remembers more, and becomes more competent in verbal skills, the examiner can inquire about past as well as current body functions. Whenever possible, questions about the current complaint should be addressed to the child before the adult is interviewed, so that the child's answers are not biased by what she or he has heard the adult tell the clinician. This is particularly true if there is a physical, psychological, or behavior problem; it is less important for the routine questions about the child's daily life.

Questions about causation or reason (i.e., using terms such as "how?" or "why?") are usually quite difficult for young children to answer and may frighten them from further conversation. These questions make many children think the interviewer expects a particular response (as in fact is true of their teachers in school), and the child is afraid to give the wrong answer. Playing it safe, the child says, "I don't know." Therefore it is wise for examiners to avoid such questions until they know a child quite well.

Although every child is different, some generalizations can be made about children's abilities to participate in the interview. These principles differ according to the child's stage of development.

INFANT AND TODDLER:
Of course, the preverbal child is not, strictly speaking, interviewed; but observations of the child and of the patterns of interaction between the child and the parents during the interview are very important (see the section of this chapter on nonverbal communication, and also Chapter 7 on Developmental Assessment).

PRESCHOOL CHILD (approximately three to five years of age):
As children approach three and four years of age, their verbal skills increase to a level where they should be able to tell the health care practitioner about their daily life (if they can be made to feel comfortable enough). Children at this age may even be able to relate some of the characteristics of a symptom, such as a stomachache or leg pain, although usually they can only describe their current experiences; recollections about past events tend to be incomplete, or at least not readily communicated in a clinical setting. It is usually appropriate that a parent be present during the entire visit, including the interview and the physical exam-

ination, since children at this age feel more secure with a parent in the room.

SCHOOL-AGE CHILD (approximately five to ten years of age):
Children in this age group should be able to answer most of the questions about their current life, including descriptions of family, home, school, and daily habits. At the older end of this age range, children may be able to answer more complex questions about events in the recent past and about their health history, as well as questions from the review of systems. Clinicians often underestimate the ability of the school-age child to participate in the interview.

It is important for clinicians to interview children of school age; not only are they a source of valuable data, but health care management of such a child will be greatly facilitated if the child is made to feel a part of the decision-making process. Interviewing the child suggests that the clinician thinks of the child as a competent individual who can share the responsibility for his or her own health care. Also, as the patient reaches adolescence, he or she will make better use of the relationship with the clinician if the two of them have established a good relationship over the years.

Generally, it is advisable for the parent to be present during much of the visit. However, it is also important for the health care practitioner to have some time to talk with the child alone, even if there are no problems. This gives the child an opportunity to say things he or she might feel uncomfortable saying in front of the parents. It also gives real meaning to the idea that the clinician builds a relationship with the child as a separate, responsible person. Whether or not the parent is present during the physical examination will depend on the age of the child, whether the parent is the same sex as the preadolescent child, and cues from the child indicating whether or not he or she prefers the parent to be present.

ADOLESCENT:
In general, the adolescent patient should be allowed considerable independence and privacy in the clinical relationship. This means that the clinician should invite the adolescent to discuss the history and any present problem alone, perform the physical examination alone, and discuss the clinical summary with the adolescent. Together, the clinician and the adolescent can also decide what aspects of the clinical problem and its management should be discussed with the parents and what additional useful information they can supply. Depending on the nature of the problem and the additional history which is sought, the discussion with the parents can take place in either the presence or the absence of the adolescent. What is important is that the adolescent be aware of the process, and be as active a participant in it as possible.

Naturally, it takes time to develop the kind of clinical relationship with an adolescent that has been described. This is most easily achieved by progressive transitions in the relationship as the child matures and the parents learn to trust the clinician. In the absence of such a long-standing relationship, the clinician will need to devote some time during the first health promotion visit to establishing the necessary rapport with the family.

Since adolescence covers a wide developmental spectrum, the care of very early adolescents must be based on the clinician's careful assessment of the patient's maturity and the parents' willingness to allow the child to be more independent. Naturally, the more mature adolescent will play a greater role in arranging health care, will often arrive for care unaccompanied by a parent (perhaps accompanied by a friend), and will assume nearly full responsibility for managing care between visits. If, in relation to age or grade level in school, the adolescent appears more immature or dependent than expected, or if the parents appear not to want to allow the adolescent to be more involved in the process of care, these findings should be noted as important and problematic clinical data.

ALTERNATIVE FORMATS

Some unusual circumstances which may demand that the examiner alter the usual order of the visit should be mentioned at this point.

Tense historian

If the adult or child historian is very tense, the clinician can frequently only surmise the cause. Sometimes the examiner will decide that it is appropriate to ask a historian why he or she is acting tense, even though they have just met. However, in most cases, it is advisable to delay doing this until a follow-up visit. If the problem still exists, the clinician might say, "As we talk about your child's health, I find the conversation very tense. Do you have any idea why it is that way?" A terse "No" may be the only response. In that instance, one can acknowledge the discomfort and express the hope that things will improve. On the other hand, the questions may prompt the historian to talk about the tension, and the clinician can obtain some insight into the discomfort and may possibly help to reduce it.

At the very least, such a question lets the historian know that the interviewer has noticed that something is amiss, is concerned, and feels that it is appropriate to discuss the problem. It is important to make it clear that one is not accusing the historian of a lack of cooperation; rather, one is trying to be helpful. For example, in a case where the parents did not like the previous clinician and consequently changed to the current one, the clinician might say, "I know that you asked to see me because you had some disagreements with Dr. Barlow who used to take care of Jonathan. Is that related to the difficulty we are having now?" Of course, the historian may opt to simply accept the proffered explanation as a way of avoiding further discussion—even if it is not accurate. However, it is usually possible for the clinician to tell whether a historian is being truthful or is evading an honest discussion.

In very rare cases, a historian (either parent or child) is so upset that it is necessary to make the interview as brief as possible. This may occur in the presence of distressing social or emotional problems. In this situation it is advisable to do a brief structured interview and physical examination quickly, and then to decide on a format for addressing the problem. Quite possibly it may be easier to proceed separately with the parent and child, or it may be necessary to set aside a subsequent visit for exploration of the issue.

Unfocused historian

It may be impractical to use an open-ended interview format if the historian is very talkative or preoccupied with his or her own concerns. Open-ended questions allow great latitude and may suggest that the interviewer has unlimited time to listen to answers.

It is often productive to be somewhat lax and to allow verbose or tangential answers for a short time during the first interview with a parent or patient. However, if this pattern of response is more than merely a symptom of anxiety early in the interview, and persists, then the clinician must intervene and limit the answers. Of course, this must be done tactfully, to avoid insulting the historian. One way to accomplish this is to ask increasingly specific questions; often the answers will become more concise. One can even be more explicit and say, "I need to ask you some specific questions so that we can cover the necessary information for today's visit."

However, we do not wish to suggest that tangential answers be forgotten. Even answers that seem unrelated to the clinician's questions should be explored at some later time. They may actually contain very valuable information, or, rarely, they may point to serious problems—for instance, when disorganization is a result of psychiatric disorders such as psychosis, mania, or delirium.

Frequently, parents have concerns of their own about their own health, their marriage, or problems of other family members. If these problems are very urgent, they can easily become the focus of the history, even though it may not be appropriate to discuss such concerns at that point in the interview or in front of the child. The clinician should take control of the interchange in this situation and should direct the conversation back to the original focus from which the historian wandered.

After the practitioner has listened long enough to clearly communicate interest, a supportive but directive comment is called for, such as "I can understand why you are concerned about John's difficulties in school. I would like to discuss it further with you, either at the end of today's visit or at another time. Right now, we need to get back to Ann's checkup. Can you tell me what Ann's usual diet includes? Tell me about her meals on an average day."

Evasive, withholding historian

Occasionally, the opposite problem arises. The historian is very terse, answers with single words or short phrases, gives evasive answers, or says "I don't know" very often or when it obviously is not true. As in the case of the unfocused historian, the clinician confronting such a situation must attempt to accomplish two things at once: try to understand why the historian is acting this way, and get the interview rolling. Frequently, success in the former results in accomplishing the latter. Does the behavior reflect the historian's anger at the clinician or institution? Were there prior situations when the historian had an unpleasant experience which now interferes with a fresh and open start with the clinician? In a teaching institution parents sometimes fear that they are receiving inferior care, or that they will be the subjects of experiments. Is this a factor here? Perhaps something the clinician did or did not do has upset the historian. Then again, a parent may feel guilty for having caused the child's illness (perhaps due to negligence—real or supposed) and fears that the health care practitioner will expose his or her mistakes. Or the unresponsiveness could also be the result of a psychiatric problem, such as depression or psychosis. If there is any clue to a possible problem, the subject should be broached and discussed openly and honestly.

If the historian is extremely terse and negative, and it is not possible to discover the cause of the problem, the clinician is still obligated to gather as much information as possible in order to formulate an adequate plan. In this situation, it becomes necessary to use a more direct, specific approach than usual. One may have to be very explicit and open, perhaps saying something like "I know that you do not want to talk with me today, but I need to have certain information in order to take care of your child. I will make the questions as brief as possible." Then the clinician should proceed in an efficient but friendly manner with a list of direct, specific questions. Straightforward questions about diet, sleep, elimination, and physical health are less threatening than those involving social relationships, behavior, and feelings. The more threatening questions should be asked later, after the clinician has had an opportunity to build a more positive relationship with the family. It is important not to become intimidated by the historian, but it is usually best to avoid forcing an angry person to a confrontation.

If the parent or patient has a particularly difficult time working with a specific health care practitioner or institution, this fact should be taken seriously and noted as significant data. Occasionally, such difficulties reach the magnitude of a separate problem and must be handled with special attention, consultation, or the invitation to change to a new primary clinician.

Historian with a psychiatric problem

On rare occasions, in the course of a visit the examiner realizes that a historian has a significant psychiatric problem. The historian may exhibit bizarre behavior, hallucinate, be extremely suspicious, be confused about past and recent historical information, or be very depressed. The differential diagnosis of these symptoms will not be discussed here; however, we shall consider what the clinician should do upon finding that a historian is significantly disturbed.

The clinician has two goals: (1) to obtain help for the disturbed person, and (2) to assess the home situation for the child. To attain both goals it is necessary to speak with a responsible friend or another family member and also to consult a mental health professional. If the clinician is adequately trained or is the only professional available, it may be appropriate to do some of the social and psychiatric assessment on the spot. However, consultants will have to be called eventually and it is usually best if they are involved as early as possible.

The examiner must make an immediate decision on how to proceed. If the historian is extremely depressed, the clinician might say, "I am very concerned about how unhappy you look, and I would like to have a doctor talk with you who knows about these problems." If the disturbed person is acting very suspicious, the clinician should be cautious about acting too forcefully, but it is crucial to be completely honest and straightforward. If a psychiatrist is available, as in a hospital clinic, it may be possible to arrange for the consultant to see the person immediately. When this is not feasible, the clinician must assess the need for hospitalization to protect the person from harming himself, herself, or others, make a referral (see Unit 4) and proceed to assess the family support system. It is of the utmost importance not to "give up" if a parent refuses professional help. In such an event, the clinician can and should initiate ongoing work with the family to achieve a means of coping with the problem.

In order to assess the home situation in relation to the child's needs, the practitioner must speak with other family members. Frequently this is done in collaboration with a social worker. If the parent is not competent to care for the children, it is necessary to make alternative arrangements, either for care with other family members, or with the aid of a public agency.

Retarded historian

On rare occasions, the historian—either the parent or the adolescent patient—is retarded. If a clinician encounters a retarded parent, it is necessary to try to learn whether the parent can manage his or her everyday family responsibilities. Also, one should ascertain what support systems exist for the parent. It may be necessary to consult with a social worker to evaluate the parent's ability to raise the child and to assess the available family and agency supports. The retarded patient is almost always accompanied by a competent adult. If a retarded child is alone, the clinician must gather as much information as is possible from the patient, and then contact the family.

A word of caution: frequently, a parent is labeled "retarded" because of slow or halting speech, a very quiet manner, or an inability to ask questions or answer them quickly. People who are poor and educationally disadvantaged are frequently erroneously miscategorized, based on a judgmental and ethnocentric evaluation of their skills and some superficial clinical impressions. Their planning and decision-making abilities may be quite adequate, even though they appear "slow" because of their verbal liabilities. The clinician should always be suspicious of labels applied to a parent's intellectual abilities. One should assess each situation personally and proceed only after obtaining adequate current data.

Adolescent historian

Adolescent patients frequently have special concerns related to their stage of development. High on their list of concerns are those which bear on the extent of their physical growth and sexual maturation, their physical and personal attractiveness, sexual activity, peer relations, and their increasing drive for independence from parents and other authority figures (including clinicians). Most often, adolescents form good relationships with clinicians, especially when the clinician actively attempts to prevent the adolescent's role in the relationship from becoming any more dependent than absolutely necessary.

At times, some adolescents may view the clinician as another adult who is an adversary. If the clinician treats the adolescent with respect and interest, and provides the young person with privacy and appropriate information, such problems can be kept to a minimum. However, there are other factors that may precipitate this kind of reaction. For example, the adolescent who appears for care at the insistence of a parent or a "third party" such as a school guidance counselor or law enforcement officer may feel coerced and may behave indifferently or uncooperatively during the interview. It is important to distinguish these adolescents from others who in fact are concerned about health matters but find it very difficult to acknowledge their concerns and consequently attribute all of these concerns to a parent.

As was suggested previously, adolescent patients deserve and require time alone with the clinician, and usually the parent interview can be deferred until after the adolescent has proceeded through the full evaluation. Adolescents are more actively concerned about the confidential nature of the clinical relationship than are younger patients, and the health care practitioner should be prepared to discuss this aspect with the adolescent patient and his or her parents. This does not mean, however, that most adolescents expect their parents to be excluded. The opposite is true; most adolescents are uncomfortable if their parents are not included in their care.

Foreign-language-speaking historian

When the child's family speaks a foreign language, the clinician must assess how skilled they are in the locally spoken language. Occasionally, the practitioner assumes that the parent speaks no English and immediately asks for an interpreter to help during the visit. However, first appearances may be deceiving: the parent may be able to communicate adequately, and thus may be insulted by the request for an interpreter. If there is any doubt about the parent's language abilities, the examiner should say something like "I do not speak Spanish. Do you speak English?" If the parent answers with anything less than a very firm yes, the clinician can offer the services of an interpreter, but should allow the parent to decide whether one is needed.

Sometimes a friend or relative who does speak English accompanies the family and can serve as interpreter. In many clinics and hospitals, there are pediatric clinicians or other health workers who can interpret. However, the choice of interpreter is important and deserves careful consideration. A relative or friend may be a very adequate interpreter for the discussion of fairly routine matters; but the parent may be reluctant to have the friend involved in a discussion of family social problems or even of certain medical problems. In such cases an "anonymous" interpreter is called for. However, there are many cases where a friend is more helpful —especially if the child is ill or if the parent is disorganized or upset. Clearly, the choice of an interpreter is a clinical decision.

Examiners often feel unnecessarily hurried. This may induce them to "skip over" important information when they work with interpreters. Typically, they will neglect to introduce themselves properly and fail to greet the family members. It is also essential to take the trouble to explain one's title and role, especially if these are not traditional ones in the medical context.

Working with an interpreter is not easy. It is best to speak to the interpreter exactly as if talking to the family, and to carefully observe the family as they answer, in order to reduce the likelihood of misunderstandings. When an employed health center interpreter and parent first meet, they will probably exchange socially important comments very early in the visit, which will not be translated. The clinician, although left out, should accept this, particularly in the Hispanic culture, as a routine and even necessary way to begin an interview.

Interpreters who work for health care institutions vary in ability and style. A competent interpreter will often take the initiative in asking a series of open-ended questions and will then give the translated version to the clinician quickly. One should be careful, however, not to accept the interpreter's assessment of the situation; and even the translation of "factual" materials may be shaded by the interpreter's assumptions. An obvious example of this problem would be an interpreter's reporting that a child has a urinary tract infection, whereas the specific complaint is burning on urination. There is, of course, a great deal of information to gather, and there are many decisions to make before the diagnosis of a urinary tract infection can be made. The interpreter may be correct, but the diagnosis can only be made after the appropriate diagnostic steps have been taken, including a full history, physical examination, and laboratory tests. Interpreters are also frequently tempted to impose on the clinician their judgments about the character of a parent or the parent's ability to care for the child properly. These examples by no means exhaust the matter, and in practice these problems are much more subtle than the examples perhaps indicate. It should be stressed that these problems can be very serious and require the clinician's alert attention.

The examiner can faciliate work with the interpreter by asking only one question at a time, especially if the questions are open-ended. If one asks a series of questions, the interpreter may forget them or, the parent may fail to answer one, and the interpreter will not go back for the missing information. It may be necessary for the health care practitioner to reiterate a complex chronology—just as he or she would for a parent who did speak English—and have the interpreter corroborate its accuracy.

Anxious child

Occasionally the child is very anxious about the physical examination and is disruptive during the interview. This is especially true of three- or four-year olds. If the child cannot stay in a playroom or waiting room, and cannot play quietly in the room where the interview is being conducted, then it may be necessary to proceed with the physcial examination with only a minimum of history. Frequently the child will be more calm after the dreaded physical examination is finished, and the history can be completed at the end of the visit.

There are occasions when it is better to yield to the imperatives of the situation and omit the physical examination. The child should be told to play for a while, and the clinician can then proceed with the complete history. Unless there is a current complaint or a previously existing medical problem, the physical examination can usually be omitted without missing important new data. Also, informal observations of the child during the interview can be very informative, and frequently a physical examination may be more successful at a later visit.

Occasionally a child may be upset by the specter of such intrusive procedures as immunization injections or painful laboratory tests such as finger-stick blood tests. The distraught child may refuse to cooperate with the history or physical examination, which forces the examiner to adopt some strategy to deal with the problem. One choice in this situation is for the clinician explicitly to postpone the injections and laboratory tests to a separate visit, and only to do the history and physical examination at the current visit. On the other hand, if it is very difficult to have the child return, or if it seems unlikely that the parents would bring the child back for painful procedures, then it is best to get the injections and laboratory tests over with right away, early in the visit. The child might calm down afterwards and be willing to play while the complete history is obtained from the parent. Later, it is even likely that the child will cooperate with the physical examination. However, this format should only be used as a last resort and if the clinician is sure the procedure is appropriate.

If a child over three years of age shows a great deal of anxiety or cannot be comforted, the examiner is obliged to do a very careful interview to assess the reason. Is this child unusually fearful in other situations? If so, is this a symptom of a serious emotional problem? Excessive fear during the health assessment is significant at any age, even if there are no other reported fears, and should be treated as important clinical data by the examiner.

Concern about a particular physical problem

It is sometimes neccessary to proceed rather directly to the physical examination early in the visit, if concern about a particular physical problem warrants this. The remainder of the history can be completed subsequently. For example, such a situation would exist if a patient had a rash and the parent and patient were very concerned about the diagnosis, etiology, and treatment. The health care practitioner may proceed from the history of the rash directly to the examination of it, and then to a brief discussion of its diagnosis and treatment. Afterwards, the clinician can return to the data base. Sometimes, after a question about a rash has been asked, it is adequate to say "I will check that carefully when I do the physical examination, and then I will discuss whatever treatment is indicated." This approach is less disruptive to the interview, and most parents and patients can be comfortable with it. If, however, the child or parents seem very concerned, it is better to relieve their tension and alter the sequence of the interview and physical examination.

Discomfort about the sex of the practitioner

During the adolescent and preadolescent years, the child may not feel comfortable with a clinician because of the clinician's sex. Most frequently, the patient will be uncomfortable with a clinician of the opposite sex. More infrequently, the patient is concerned about homosexual feelings and may be very anxious, especially during a physical examination, if the clinician is of the same sex. If the patient expresses such concerns, one should be prepared to discuss them openly. Occasionally a patient cannot verbalize his or her concerns. It is possible, however, that the examiner will recognize them intuitively, and it will then be up to the examiner to initiate the conversation. In some rare instances, it will not prove possible to resolve the discomfort associated with this issue; then the practitioner should arrange for someone else to examine the patient, and it may be necessary to switch clinicians.

Adolescent parent

Not infrequently, the patient is an infant or very young child, and the parent of the patient is still an adolescent. A grandparent often accompanies the infant-adolescent pair to the health care setting; this is potentially one of the most delicate clinical situations. The clinician must ascertain, sometimes help the family to clarify, these important factors: who is the primary caregiver for the child; who makes the major decisions about the patient's care; and who wants to be the responsible caregiver. Sometimes the grandparent functions as the infant's parent, and the adolescent resumes her usual work, school career, and social life. This may be what the grandparent wants, but it is not necessarily what the adolescent wants. The adolescent mother may want to be the primary caregiver, but the grandparent cannot allow her such a responsiblity (there may or may not be good reasons for this). Alternatively, there are situations in which the adolescent functions as the parent but if given a choice would prefer to relinquish the responsibility to the grandparent. It is rare for an adolescent father to be as involved as the mother in the child's health care (especially if unwed), but this discussion would also apply to him if he were involved.

In such cases clinicians should identify themselves clearly as the health care practitioner and advocate for the infant. Their efforts should be bent on assisting the family in making decisions which are best for the infant. In addition, clinicians should be supportive of the adolescent. The challenge to the health care practitioner is to assess the situation in a nonjudgmental way, to avoid being caught in any controversy between the grandparent and the adolescent parent, to evaluate the adolescent's capacities for parenting, and to help promote her maturation into a responsible adult.

Usually, it is easier for everyone if the adolescent parent has her own clinician for her health care and does not have to share the same health care practitioner with the infant. If she does have the same clinician, she may feel jealous of the attention given to the infant by the clinician. Further, she may also feel infantilized because her clinician takes care of babies. In instances where the health care practitioner is young or a student, it is advisable for the clinician not to care for both the mother and the child. A student may identify over-closely with the mother and find it difficult to maintain the emotional distance necessary for competent clinical work.

A possible solution for providing health care for the parent-child couple is for one health care team to have the responsibility for the entire family, but for the infant and parent each to have different health care practitioners. This combines the advantages of separate clinicians with the increased communication and better planning possible on a team.

CHAPTER 6

Evaluation of a Complaint or Concern

Introduction
Location
Character or quality
Intensity or quantity
Chronology
    Onset
    Duration
    Periodicity and frequency
    Course
    Context
Factors affecting symptoms
    Aggravating factors
    Alleviating factors
Associated phenomena
Scope of inquiry
Psychological and organic complaints
The interview as a complex interpersonal exchange
    Three examples:
        Three-month-old with rash
        Six-month-old with diarrhea
        Eight-year-old with enuresis

INTRODUCTION

In order to completely evaluate any complaint, whether it be organic or psychological in nature, health care practitioners should ascertain the following: where the symptom is located; what it is like (including a detailed description of the somatic and psychological components); how intense it is; when it began and what course it followed; circumstances under which it takes place, including factors which are associated with the complaint and especially those elements which aggravate or alleviate it; and associated symptoms.*

This section will describe these categories of data in detail and will provide illustrative examples from pediatric practice. Clinicians should use these categories as a guide in conducting the open-ended interview, but of course should adapt them to the needs of the individual clinical situation.

LOCATION

Knowing the bodily location of a symptom is of great help in determining its etiology. Pain is the most common "marker" of the location of a problem. To evaluate a complaint of pain, the clinician must help the child describe both its exact location and any movement of the pain from one area to another during the illness. It is important to know if the pain is felt superficially or deep in the body. Pain is often felt right at the site of the problem, and remains there, as in the case of ankle pain following a localized injury like a sprain. However, the pain pattern may also be quite complicated. Appendicitis is first felt in the periumbilical area and then moves laterally and downward to settle in the right lower quadrant (at McBurney's point). Sometimes pain radiates or shoots from a primary focus to an adjacent part of the body. An example of this is the pain of renal colic, which is first felt in the flank or the anterior lateral abdomen, and which "shoots" down to the groin. Referred pain is felt in one place but has its source in another part of the body. For example, hip pathology may cause only knee pain, and irritation of the diaphragm from peritoneal disease in the abdomen may cause only shoulder pain.

There are some standard questions that clinicians ask to elicit information about pain. Parents may be asked "Where does Joan say the pain is?" "Does Robert point to the place that hurts?" "Do you know if the pain is always in the same place?" Questions addressed to a younger child will usually ask for a demonstration: "John, show me where your tummy

---

* William L. Morgan, Jr., M.D., and George L. Engel, M.D., *The Clinical Approach to the Patient*, Philadelphia, W.B. Saunders, 1969, p. 35.

hurts. Point with one finger (here the examiner may hold up a finger) right to the place that hurts." Older children might be queried further: "Does the pain move to other places?"

Knowing the depth of pain—that is, how superficial it is or how deep it seems to be located in a body cavity, now how severe it is—is sometimes helpful in determining where the pathology is located. If a patient says the pain is on the chest wall and is superficial, the clinician will need to examine the skin, muscles, and bones. If the patient complains of pain deep in the chest, one must consider the heart, lungs, esophagus, and stomach as possible sites of origin. However, it is crucial to keep in mind that pain felt on the surface may be the result of pathology in internal organs.

CHARACTER OR QUALITY

It is particularly important to help the child explain or describe the quality or nature of a complaint in his or her own words *before* the parents and examiner begin to suggest possible terms. The clinician can initiate this part of the interview by saying "Tell me what it feels like." This should be followed with questions which encourage the patient to refine the description, such as "What do you mean by an ache?" Sometimes a patient will offer a subjective image of what the symptom feels like, such as "squeezing" or "twisting." After the patient has tried several times to describe the symptom, the examiner can suggest other descriptive terms such as "dull," "sharp," "burning," or "knifelike." (Note: A child as young as four or five years of age sometimes can accurately describe a symptom she or he is currently experiencing but may need assistance from parents in describing the chronology and other elements of the problem.)

INTENSITY AND QUANTITY

The intensity and extent of the symptom refer to the patient's experience of it as well as to the amount of functional impairment involved. The terms also refer to the size and shape of an observed abnormal physical finding. Examiners should ask specific questions directed at these parameters: for example, "How bad is the pain? Would you say it is very bad, moderate, or mild?" The language used in the question may have to be modified for the pediatric patient, so that the child can understand the question. An example would be asking a six-year-old child if the pain were "very bad, medium, or not very bad," or if it "hurts a lot or just a little bit."

People have a variety of ways of expressing their subjective experience of discomfort. Some underestimate and some overestimate severity. Judgments about severity of pain involve assessment of the characteristic reaction to painful situations and the nonverbal aspects of communication; the response to a direct question about severity is not sufficient. Sometimes, the *degree of impairment* is a more helpful indication of the severity of the symptom than is a patient's description. For example, a child who has only a mild stomachache frequently will play well and maintain his or her usual activities—even though complaining bitterly. A child with severe abdominal pain, however, is usually quite limited in activity during the episodes of pain and cannot be lured to play even by the most pleasant offers. Then, when the pain lessens, the child will resume more typical activities.

When there is a physical abnormality like a rash or other lesion on the body surface, the extent and exact location of the lesion are very important. A mass felt inside the body should be described as accurately as possible and the description should be supplemented with measurements in the physical examination, so that current size can be recorded and changing size can be evaluated.

CHRONOLOGY

The chronology of a symptom refers to the onset, duration, periodicity, frequency, and course of a symptom. It is particularly important to obtain an accurate account of a symptom's chronology, because such information is often most helpful in determining the severity of a problem, the need for immediate intervention, and even the etiology of a problem. Each of the elements of chronology will be considered in some detail.

Onset

The clinician should try to obtain an exact time of onset. Naturally, patients tend to remember the details of timing more easily if the complaint began recently, and they can usually be helped to remember the approximate time of day and the day of the week when a symptom began. It is unusual for a child to remember the exact time of day (such as 11:05 A.M.) when a complaint was first noticed, unless it was associated with some other event such as leaving for school or going to sleep. If the complaint began more than one or two weeks prior to the interview, the patient can be expected to be more vague about the time of onset. But no matter how recent the onset, the best way to get accurate information is by the open-ended method. And, occasionally, medical records will contain data from previous histories which give details surrounding the onset of the condition.

Other facts about the onset which are also important include the setting where the complaint began and whether the onset was sudden or gradual. If several symptoms or events occurred in close succession, the exact order of events should be carefully determined, because they may suggest important causal relationships.

Duration

The examiner should ask about the duration of each symptom. Duration is closely related to severity and thus is helpful in assessing the urgency and importance of a complaint. A severe headache that lasts 30 minutes is much less worrisome than one that lasts 3 days—at least from a diagnostic point of view.

In pediatric practice, parents are usually not concerned when mild symptoms have a short duration. Often, a mild symptom may persist or recur over many weeks or months before the parent seeks a clinical opinion. In this situation, it is very informative to ask, "What made you come (for health care) at this time?" The answers vary a great deal. Sometimes the reason is that the length of time that the symptom has persisted has itself become worrisome; sometimes the symptom has become more severe. Frequently the clinician learns what the parent thinks the diagnosis is, what an important relative or friend thinks, or about concurrent significant family problems which made the parent anxious. An example of the concern about a specific diagnosis is the parent who brings in a little girl because of bruises. These bruises may not differ significantly from those which her siblings have nor be any different from bruises that this same very active girl has had for much of her childhood. However, the clinician eventually learns that a cousin recently became ill and was diagnosed as having leukemia. Thus the parent is really asking whether the girl's bruises could be a symptom of leukemia. An explicit answer is needed in order to allay the parent's fears.

Periodicity and frequency

These parameters are grouped together because the data about them are often intertwined in the history. Some symptoms are continuous, but many occur periodically. The time interval between recurrent episodes may be regular or irregular. Knowledge of these parameters is often very helpful in determining the etiology of a symptom, especially when they are correlated with other factors which occur in the same patterns. One example is unilateral flank pain in an adolescent female which is alternately on the right and left sides, and which recurs regularly every four weeks, halfway between menstrual cycles. The accurate description of this pain and its periodicity will lead directly to a diagnosis of *mittelschmerz*, which is a pain caused by the mature ovum's rupturing out of the ovary. Another example of periodicity is abdominal pain associated with peristaltic waves. These waves, or movements, of the intestine can often be observed by looking at the patient's abdomen and can be heard by auscultation. They may appear during the examination while the patient is reporting the pain or exhibiting the facial expressions of someone in pain. The correlation of these periodic phenomena will point to the critical diagnosis of intestinal obstruction; the pain results from intestinal dilatation with each peristaltic movement.

Other periodic relationships to note are symptoms related to circadian rhythms of sleep and wakefulness, and morning vomiting with brain tumors.

Frequency is also helpful in determining the seriousness of an underlying pathology. A stomachache which occurs three times a year is much less worrisome than one which recurs three times a week. They both deserve evaluation, but the more frequent symptom is consistent with potentially more serious pathology, either structural or functional.

Most patients and their parents can approximate the frequency of a symptom. If they cannot, the clinician may have to help by saying, "Would you say the headaches occur every day, once a week, or once a month?" Another way to approach the question is to ask, "How many times has Ann had a headache in the past two months? Do you think the headache was the same as before that time, or do you think it has changed?" If the frequency in the last two months is different from what it was before, the clinician should ascertain whether the headaches are becoming more or less frequent.

Course

The history should include a detailed description of the nature of any symptoms since their onset. This information is best collected after the historian has presented a complete current description of the symptom. As the clinician gathers information about the onset, duration, frequency, and periodicity of the symptom, the historian will usually volunteer descriptions of how the character of the symptom changed over time. However, it may be necessary to make a specific request like "Please go back to the beginning and tell me what happened to the headaches since they first began." Some historians need even more specific questions such as "Do you think the headaches have become more severe since the beginning?" "Have they stayed the same, or have they become worse in some way?"

The course of a symptom will naturally be intertwined with associated factors, and the course of these factors must also be ascertained in order to evaluate these interrelationships. The significance of the course and relationship of symptoms is illustrated in the following example:

A father relates that his child has a "cold." One possible description would indicate an upper respiratory infection which began two days ago.

The symptoms began with clear rhinnorhea, were followed on the second day by an occasional wet cough, and were accompanied throughout by a slightly decreased appetite and temperature varying from 98°F. (36.7°C.) to 100.8°F. (38.2°C.), without any medication. Another description of a "cold" indicates a different situation. In this case the symptoms began eight days ago with clear rhinnorhea and wet cough. These symptoms persisted for three days and then became more severe. Temperature elevations to 104°F. (40°C.) were noted, along with a deep cough with copious mucous, grunting respirations, and an exhausted appearance. It is obvious from the descriptions of these two "colds" that the second represents a much more serious illness. Thus the depth of evaluation, and the treatment, will be very different in each case.

Context

It is important to know where the patient was when the symptom began, and in what context(s) it continued and recurred; all of these data may be helpful in evaluating the etiology of a problem. Specific information—such as what the patient was doing and even whom the patient was with when the symptom first occurred or recurred—often are valuable clues to the nature of the problem. A child who develops abdominal pain only at breakfast time on school days is more likely to have a psychogenic school problem than a child who has abdominal pain which wakes him from sleep at night. A teenager who becomes lightheaded and has tingling sensations only in stressful or tense situations may be hyperventilating. A child with a papular vesicular rash may have been visiting two weeks earlier with a child who had chickenpox. The specifics of the setting need to be discussed in relation to the individual clinical problem.

FACTORS AFFECTING SYMPTOMS

The clinician should always ask two basic questions: "What makes the symptom better?" and "What makes the symptom worse?" *Aggravating factors* often stress the system involved, so that symptoms are produced. For example, a child's knees might hurt after he plays ice hockey for long periods of time. Inquiry into other weight-bearing activities would probably corroborate the impression that the pain is directly related to stress on the knees. Often, the patient cannot think of other factors, but clinicians can "play detective" a bit, asking about likely possibilities to gather support for their ideas or intuitions about etiology. In the case of our hockey player, it might well emerge that walking up stairs or bicycling may produce the same symptoms.

Alleviating factors can include treatment or avoidance of a noxious agent. By treatment we mean both the home remedies and professionally advised treatment recommended on previous occasions, which the patient tried before the current visit. It may include medication, exercise, and diet. One very helpful source of information is a list of treatments which failed to alleviate the symptom. Heat and rest used to treat a sore knee will alleviate mild pathology caused by trauma but will not alter the pain related to severe, progressive destruction from neoplastic disease. Another example is the patient who has been taking appropriate doses of penicillin for seven days without improvement in her sore throat. The clinician can deduce that the patient does not have a streptococcal sore throat, and must look for a different etiology for the symptom.

Avoidance of a noxious agent is a common mode of treatment. One example is the disappearance of abdominal pain in a patient who has a lactose intolerance and eliminates milk products from his or her diet. Another example is the teenage girl whose difficulty with puffy, itching eyes comes to an end after she stops using a particular eye makeup. Often, patients or parents do not have accurate ideas about the physiology of their symptom, but they do notice important information which leads to a diagnosis.

ASSOCIATED PHENOMENA

Data about associated factors are crucial for the accurate evaluation of a problem. Proceeding from the open-ended format, the clinician then has to address the problems posed by differential diagnosis and formulate incisive and specific questions that will provide the information needed to make a diagnosis. In the case of a child with purulent drainage from the eye, for example, the clinician must ascertain whether the drainage is an isolated symptom, whether there are other associated symptoms related to an upper respiratory infection, or whether data recorded in the history suggest that the symptom is part of an illness such as measles. When the symptom—as presented—is vague (such as "trouble breathing") the clinician must learn more about it: Is the child breathing rapidly, coughing, producing sputum, having trouble catching his or her breath or getting enough air? In addition, it is advisable to ask about fever, vomiting, fluid intake, lethargy, irritability, and past history of asthma or other respiratory illnesses.

SCOPE OF INQUIRY

It is important to keep in mind that the complaint may reflect disease in a system of the body completely different from the obvious one that appears to be troubling the patient. Therefore, the examiner's questions must cover a broad enough scope to evaluate this possibility. A common example is the child who presents with vomiting and fever, but who, further evaluation reveals, has had rhinorrhea and a significant productive cough for several days. Physical examination and laboratory tests confirm that she has pneumonia. The initial complaint of vomiting did not represent primary gastrointestinal disease but rather respiratory pathology. There are many examples in pediatric practice in which the above principle applies. Fever, abdominal pain, headaches, poor growth, and rashes are all problems with diverse etiologies.

The clinician must appreciate the complexity of the diagnostic process and must maintain flexible opinions throughout the process and even beyond, into the treatment phase (mistakes in diagnosis are not uncommon). The outline provided for the review of systems can be helpful to the beginning clinician, but good diagnostic skills are only developed through a great deal of experience with a variety of sick children.

PSYCHOLOGICAL AND ORGANIC COMPLAINTS

Clinicians sometimes err by attempting to separate symptoms artificially into two discrete groups: psychological or organic. For example, an adolescent female patient may complain of feeling "washed out," vomiting, fatigue, and poor appetite; she could have hepatitis, be pregnant, or be depressed. Or a patient with diabetes mellitus may be having enuresis; the etiology of the enuresis may include a variety of possible causes such as a urinary tract infection, poor control of the diabetes with high blood sugar and increased urine formation, or psychological and family problems. Thus it is clear that the clinician will be able to begin to delineate the pathology causing a specific symptom only after a careful, complete interview, a physical examination, and laboratory tests. At all times the complex interrelationship of body and mind should be remembered and taken into account in the gathering and assessment of data.

THE INTERVIEW AS A COMPLEX INTERPERSONAL EXCHANGE

The art of interviewing and examining is complex indeed. All the factors we have just discussed must be integrated into a form which allows a thorough but comfortable exchange within the limits of the visit. Clinicians must use their knowledge of interpersonal skills, of pathophysiology of symptoms, and of differential diagnosis to guide them in conducting the interview. The examples presented below illustrate how to evaluate three common pediatric complaints using a modified open-ended approach. The questions are clearly directed toward gathering specific data, but they are phrased as much as possible in a way that will prompt accurate, unbiased information from the historian.

EXAMPLE 1: Mr. Johnson comes to the office with his three-month-old son, Harry. He says, "Ms. Hutchins, I really need help with this terrible rash that Harry has. We just don't seem to know how to get rid of it." The clinician might answer, "I'd be glad to see what I can do for Harry. I'd like to ask you some questions in order to learn more about the rash and then see what we can do." She should ask the following questions, in approximately this order: (Questions 1–9 elaborate the symptom as described in the Introduction to this chapter, which deals with the evaluation of a complaint or concern.)

1. When did the rash first appear?
2. Where is it?
3. What does it look like? (More specific questions about the appearance of the rash will be suggested by Mr. Johnson's answer. Ms. Hutchins may have to ask if the rash is red, fine, bumpy, raised, looks like hives, looks like pimples, etc.)
4. Has the rash improved, remained the same, or become worse since it began?
5. Is it constant, or does it appear and fade away?
6. What makes it better?
7. What makes it worse?
8. Have you used any medicines or other treatments?
9. What were the results?
10. Does Harry have any other symptoms? (The answer to this may suggest that the rash is one symptom of a condition that is not limited to the skin, or it may suggest that the rash itself is associated with other symptoms. An example of the second case would be oral moniliasis, or "thrush," which can cause discomfort, difficulty in eating and drinking, and irritability.)
11. How is Harry eating, drinking, sleeping?
12. Is he urinating normally?
13. What are his stools like? (It is important to ask specifically about color, consistency, and frequency.)
14. Are the stools any different now compared with the way they were before the rash appeared?
15. Has Harry vomited, been unusually irritable or lethargic, or had a fever recently?
16. Have any new foods been added to his diet? (Rashes are frequently manifestations of allergy, and foods are often the basic cause of the problem.)

17. If so, which ones and when were they added?
18. Has Harry been in contact with anyone who is ill or who has a rash? If so, when? What were the person's illness and/or rash like? (Rashes may be infectious in origin.)
19. Has Harry had this type of rash previously? If so, what was it from and what did you do for it?

    If the rash is on the perineum or buttocks and the child is not toilet trained, it would be wise to ask:
20. What kind of diapers are you using? If cloth diapers are used, are they washed by machine or by hand? Are the detergent or bleach or other washing agents different from products used before the rash appeared? (Contact dermatitis in the diaper area is not an infrequent diagnosis. It can be caused by detergent used to wash underpants as well. These questions illustrate how to pursue a possible etiology if the particular clinical situation suggests a certain cause.)

EXAMPLE 2: Mrs. Stone comes to the clinic with her six-month-old daughter, Susan. She says, "I am very glad you could see us today, Mr. Russell. Susan has had diarrhea for days, and it is really awful." The clinician might say, "There are several questions I need to ask, and then I will examine Susan. I am sure we can find out how to make her feel better." He should then proceed to ask the following questions:

1. When did the loose stools begin? (The symptom should be evaluated according to the format elaborated earlier.)
2. What do the stools look like? (The clinician may have to ask specifically about color, consistency, odor, presence of blood or mucus.)
3. How frequent are the bowel movements now?
4. How does this differ from Susan's usual bowel habits?
5. Have the bowel movements become more or less frequent since this illness began?
6. What seems to make it worse or better?
7. Have any medications been tried?
8. What were their effects?
9. Did Susan begin to eat any new foods around the time the diarrhea began?
10. If so, when, and what, and what was the relationship to the onset of the diarrhea?
11. Has Susan's diet been changed since the diarrhea began? If so, what has been the effect of this? (The main treatment for uncomplicated, acute diarrhea is dietary. The regimen of clear liquids gradually progressing to easily tolerated solids to the full diet usually alleviates diarrhea. As with any treatment, if the clinician knows what a family has already tried, she or he can better assess

both the severity of the symptom and the ability of the family to manage a problem.)
12. Has Susan vomited? If so, elaborate, as for any other symptom.
13. How much food has she eaten in the last week?
14. How much fluid intake has she had since the diarrhea began? (If the diarrhea is of more than a few days' duration, it is adequate to know the food and fluid intake of the last few days.) (Questions 12, 13 and 14 are included because the examiner needs to know if the child's output has exceeded her intake; these data permit a gross estimate of how dehydrated she might be.)
15. Has Susan had a fever?
16. If so, how high has it been, and when did it occur?
17. How is Susan acting? Is she more irritable or more lethargic than previously? How is she sleeping and playing?
18. Has Susan had diarrhea before? If so, when was that episode, and what were the cause and treatment?
19. Does she have any other symptoms, such as cough, runny nose, or abdominal pain? (Diarrhea may be "parenteral" in origin, which means there is no primary gastrointestinal disease, but the diarrhea, like fever, is nonspecific. Young children with ear infections and respiratory infections will frequently have mild diarrhea.)
20. Has Susan been in contact with anyone who is ill? In particular, do any of those people have diarrhea? (The diarrhea may have an infectious origin.)

The foregoing list of questions represents a fairly thorough initial interview about a common symptom. If some questions produced answers that needed further amplification, then of course the clinician would pursue them systematically. An example would be the presence of blood and mucus in the stools; the possibility of a bacterial infection of the gastrointestinal tract or of parasitic infestation would then be more likely, making it more appropriate to ask about water source, sewage system, problems with plumbing, travel to a place where water sources might have been contaminated or where the child may have become infested with gastrointestinal parasites.

The above questions illustrate how a clinician must use his or her knowledge of pathophysiology and differential diagnosis as a guide to constructing the interview.

EXAMPLE 3: Enuresis is an example of the many symptoms in pediatrics which may have an organic or psychological basis. The data (as reflected in the example below) must be gathered using questions intended to clearly rule in or rule out the psychological and the physical causes for enuresis. If the clinician attends only to organic or psychological information, she or he risks making a diagnostic error, with serious consequences for the child's mental or physical health. However, enuresis is most frequently the result of a failure to control the body during sleep. Therefore, when it is not associated with serious family pathology, and does not have an organic basis the symptom can be alleviated by the practitioner's talking with the child.

Mrs. Thomas brings her son to the office and says, "Ms. White, I need your help because Jack—who is eight years old—is wetting the bed again. What can we do about it?" The health care practitioner might say, "Before I can answer your question, we will have to talk about the bed-wetting. After that, I'll examine Jack, and we will make a plan about how to solve the problem."

It is crucial, in such a case, to interview both the parent and the child. If the child knows the clinician quite well, and is comfortable enough to discuss the problem with her, she can begin the interview with the child right away. If the child is not so comfortable, Ms. White should begin the interview with the parent and later include the child. The questions to the child may be interspersed throughout the discussion, or they may be grouped together. In the following example "CHILD" indicates questions particularly suited for the interview with the child.

1. When did the bed-wetting begin? (Questions 1–6 elaborate the symptom and its course.)
2. How often does it occur?
3. What, do you recall, happened around the time the bed-wetting began?
4. Were there any new or stressful events at that time?
5. Does Jack only wet at night?
6. How well does he control his urine during the day? (CHILD)
7. Is there any difficulty with bowel control? (CHILD) (Difficulties in bowel control occur more often when there is an organic basis for poor urinary control, such as a neurologic lesion. Severe psychological problems may also be indicated if the enuresis is functional.)
8. What do you do when Jack wets the bed?
9. What do you say?
10. Do you punish Jack? If so, what kind of punishment is used?
11. What does Jack say or think about the bed-wetting and punishment? (CHILD)
12. Does Jack have urinary frequency, pain or discomfort on urination, increased amounts of urine, or urgency? (CHILD)
13. What does the urine look like? (CHILD) (The answers to questions 12 and 13 may support the diagnosis of urinary tract infection. Polyuria suggests diabetes mellitus and diabetes insipidus as possible origins of the enuresis.)
14. What is the urinary stream like? (CHILD) (Urinary stream becomes unusually splayed if there is distal meatal stenosis. The

stream may be dribbling if there is outflow obstruction or if the bladder cannot contract properly.)
15. Does Jack have a greater fluid intake than he used to have? (CHILD)
16. Has he had any fevers? If so, when did they occur? Were they associated with any symptoms? (Fever, if *not* associated with symptoms such as cough, rhinorrhea, etc. [suggesting an upper respiratory infection] may be due to recurrent or chronic urinary tract infection.)
17. How has Jack's health been in general, both recently and previously?
18. Has he been growing in height and weight as you would expect? (Poor growth is consistent with chronic renal disease.)
19. Have there been other changes in behavior or development that you or his teacher have noted?
20. Does he seem happy?
21. Has Jack told you about any new concerns lately?
22. How does he get along with other people, including his parents, siblings, peers, and authority figures such as teachers? (CHILD) (Questions 19–22 help in assessing the psychological profile of the patient. Enuresis may be only one symptom of psychological difficulty. It is important for clinicians to treat the entire patient, not only the enuresis.)
23. What have you tried so far to treat the enuresis? (The examiner will not only learn what therapy to try again—and what to avoid—but also about the opinions of the parents and something about their problem-solving abilities.)
24. What were the results?
25. What do you think is the reason for the bed-wetting? (CHILD) (Again, the clinician learns how the parents have analyzed the problem. This is helpful when the clinician presents a management plan to the family.)
26. At what age was Jack toilet trained? (Enuresis has a relationship to difficult toilet training in some patients. It is another piece of information which may be helpful in evaluating the cause and planning treatment.)
27. How was the training done?
28. Was the training successful for both urinary and bowel control?
29. Was any one aspect particularly difficult?
30. Were there any difficulties with the toilet training?
31. Is there a family history of bed-wetting? If so, in whom? What do you know about the course of that person's bed-wetting? (If the family has had a particularly upsetting experience in the past, they may be exceptionally fearful of the course for the child. An exam-

ple of this is the case of a patient who was told he would "outgrow" the enuresis, but who really had urinary tract disease which remained undiagnosed. After many years, the diagnosis of chronic urinary tract infection and severe renal damage was made. This was probably avoidable early in the course, but the damage was irreversible many years later when it was finally discovered.)
32. Is there a family history of urinary problems? (Elaborate as indicated.)
33. With whom does Jack sleep?
34. Do they share a bed or a room?
35. Does that person also wet his or her bed? (Occasionally, enuresis is associated with certain sleeping arrangements. They may be directly related to the enuresis, or may be one example of many things which upset the child.)

The above questions illustrate how a clinician can evaluate both the functional and the organic basis for a problem. The answers will provide the basis for further evaluation, including history, physical examination, and laboratory tests to determine the etiology of the symptom.

CHAPTER 7

Developmental Assessment

Introduction
The Developmental History
    Outline of an Approach to Developmental Assessment
    Discussion of the Outline: General Issues
    The Components of the Outline Expanded
        General Personality Characteristics
        Relationships of the Child
            Parents and/or other primary care-givers
            Siblings
            Peers
            Authority figures
            Family and social (nurturing) environment
        Achievements and Their Use
            Child under five years of age
            Child over five years of age
        Past Development
    Observations: Some General Comments
        Unstructured Observations: General Comments
            At the Office
                Infant, six months old
                Preschool child, four years old
                School-age child, nine years old

        Adolescent
        Home Visit
        School Visit
    Structured Tasks: General Comments
        An Approach to the Child and Parents
        The Setting
        Representative Tasks
            Six-month-old infant
            Four-year-old child

INTRODUCTION

Health maintenance includes the prevention and amelioration of abnormal conditions, both physical and mental. In both spheres, the early identification of problems can lead to intervention which decreases morbidity and prevents or diminishes detrimental sequelae. Thus, the detection and management of developmental and psychological problems are essential components of comprehensive pediatric care. This chapter describes the process of gathering the data needed for developmental evaluation and presents an organization of this information which is especially useful for primary pediatric care. We must stress, however, that it is not meant to be a manual of normal child development or a discussion of developmental problems; hence the more complete developmental evaluation, which is usually performed by a subspecialist, is not presented here.

Every child needs periodic developmental assessments, but there is no single right way to do them. Each clinician must decide the frequency and extent of the assessments, who should perform them, and how they should be done. Factors affecting these decisions include the particular patient population, the clinical setting, and the clinician's skills.

A developmental assessment begins with the prenatal visit, and even if a patient enters one's practice when she or he is older, information about the pregnancy and the child's early development—especially that of the infant period—is an important foundation for the organization of subsequent data. The developmental or psychological assessment retains its importance throughout the patient's childhood.

Some developmental assessment should be part of every well-child visit. However, the extent of the evaluation will vary a great deal; it will vary among patients and even for the same patient at different times. Frequently, a health care practitioner who has a good ongoing relationship with a competent family will only update the developmental history briefly and make appropriate observations during the course of a visit. But even in the most abbreviated assessment, if the identification of developmental problems is left entirely to intuition without some systematic data collection and formulation, even experienced clinicians will miss many children who could benefit from timely assistance. Periodically a more thorough evaluation should be undertaken for all children, to be sure that less obvious problems are not being overlooked.

A brief assessment during the pediatric follow-up visit is usually adequate for identifying developmental problems if the clinician has already gathered a rather complete data base, either over years of primary care or at the point of intake into the practice. As a result of ongoing interest on the part of the clinician, the parents have been helped to understand that she or he is interested in their child's development. Thus they are likely to bring up their concerns if they are given a chance to do so; the interval history, although brief, provides just such an opportunity.

At this point we must digress a bit to discuss the importance of the relationship between the practitioner and the parents in terms of its effect on developmental assessment. The brief follow-up assessment relies heavily on the parents' report of the child's behavior. Therefore, the parents' inclination and ability to communicate their thoughts and observations are crucial. If a clinician and a family have not known each other for a significant length of time, or if the parents have difficulty in communicating with the clinician about their child (either because they are not competent in describing the child or because there is a problem in the clinician-parent relationship), the examiner is obligated to take the time to do an expanded assessment, including intensive direct observations.

There are a variety of circumstances which require that extra attention be paid to developmental assessment. If a child is at high risk for developmental or psychological problems, a thorough assessment should be done frequently. The child's risk may be related to any number of factors, including his or her own physical illness, birth history, sensitivities, or the fact that the child is difficult to care for. Further, the child may be at risk because members of the family have physical or emotional problems, or there may be social or financial difficulties which can lead to problems of parenting. If a health care practitioner learns that a family is undergoing acute stress, or if a clinician becomes concerned about a child's development or the parent-child relationships in a family, a more thorough assessment naturally is indicated right away (see Chapter 6 on the evaluation of problems or concerns and Chapters 12 and 13 on assessment of psychological problems).

An adequate but brief developmental assessment relies mainly on the history and careful informal observations made during the office visit. It is also important for the examiner to interview the patient, and it may prove fruitful to present a few specific tasks to a young child. However, testing the child's skills really is only a small part of the developmental assessment in pediatrics, and it does not require elaborate equipment or a great deal of time. In fact, the ability to successfully complete certain tasks can be misleading: many children with normal skills and developmental landmarks have serious psychological problems.

When parents are unable to give an accurate history, the examiner must rely more on his or her own observations of the child and of the parent-child interaction. In addition, when the parent is not an accurate historian the clinician should not depend on the parent's ability to report concerns; rather, one should proceed in a careful manner to obtain detailed reports of behaviors and supplement these with data from other sources, such as a teacher's report. It is particularly hard to assess problem-solving (adaptive) skills and language development in the young child without a good history. Examiners should be prepared to evaluate problem-solving abilities, especially in the preschool child, by using specific task-directed toys such as puzzles, color-matching games, and drawing materials (see pages 157, 158, and 169–171 for more details).

Sometimes a clinician may have difficulty in making firsthand observations of expressive language because a child is too shy to talk. If the reports about the child's language are insufficient, it is important to be particularly conscientious about helping the child to become comfortable enough to engage in some conversation during the evaluation, possibly with a parent. Sometimes it will be necessary to make a home visit in order to assess a patient's speech as well as other aspects of the child's development. Home visits will be discussed later in this chapter.

Many children spend a significant amount of time away from their parents, in day care or in school. Usually, one can rely on the parents' and the older patient's reports of adjustment, achievements, and activities in settings away from the home. However, if the interview is incomplete or seems unreliable, it is advisable to communicate directly with the appropriate person in the school or day-care setting. This should be done with the knowledge and permission of the parents. Sometimes it is helpful to visit such institutions, because it is difficult to interpret the reports of unfamiliar people working in a setting which the clinician has never seen.

It is best if the primary clinician, whether nurse practitioner, physician, nurse clinician, or physician's assistant, is as competent in developmental assessment as in other aspects of pediatric evaluation, such as gathering a medical data base, performing a physical examination, and choosing appropriate laboratory tests. Developmental screening should not be delegated to a peripheral paraprofessional, because an accurate developmental assessment requires familiarity with the family and their cultural background and depends on a trusting relationship between the examiner and patient. It is relatively easy for an assessor merely to score a failure when a child does not do a particular task properly; but it is often very difficult to know why a child failed the task at that particular time and to deduce the clinical importance of that failure. Only someone who knows the child and the family is likely to be able to interpret the child's behavior during a structured evaluation. Also, it is much easier to gather the personal information necessary to assess the quality of the life of a child and his or her parents if the developmental and psychological information is gathered within the context of a continuing clinician-patient relationship.

Some pediatric health care practitioners might argue that a clinician could take the quantitative information about someone else's screening test and synthesize it with her or his own qualitative information. Although this is one option, it gives a less comprehensive picture than that obtained when the ongoing clinician gathers the data, because the clinician will have missed a valuable opportunity of observing both the child and the parent, and their interactions, during the more formal tasks. Indeed, very important characteristics of the child may be observed as the structured tasks are administered: some children have a shortened attention span when they become anxious; some are not motivated to approach a challenge; some are terribly shattered by a failure; and some do not know how to ask for help. The ability to tolerate frustration varies, as does the degree of satisfaction and pride with success. Some children are impulsive and possibly also rigid, but may be bright as well; others are more thoughtful, more reflective and flexible. These important features would probably not be included in a report done by a person who is not a skilled *clinical* observer. Nor would the clinician have a chance to assess the parents' responses during the structured tasks, which may be very valuable. In addition, most young children will be more comfortable and therefore present a more accurate picture of their best performance, if their own familiar health care practitioner integrates developmental assessment tasks into a routine health visit. Finally (and by no means least importantly), the interactions among clinician, parents, and child which occur naturally during the observations of the child's behavior and the subsequent discussion of the child's developmental status are very important elements which strengthen the relationships among all the parties.

Structured interviews, questionnaires about symptoms, behavioral check lists, and various abbreviated psychological tests (such as the Denver Developmental Screening Test, Draw-A-Person, and reading readiness tests) can be useful in specific practice settings and may be somewhat helpful guides for students. However, it is important to note that they have many limitations, just as do other diagnostic tools. Too often, abbreviated psychological tests are not used properly, and they can be detrimental if they are not administered sensitively and skillfully. Unfortunately, scores are very concrete and may induce a false sense of their validity. The scores of screening tests, at their best, are useful as warning signals. I especially wish to stress that these tools are not effective when used alone, because they lack the historical data that a clinician needs in order to recognize many psychological problems. If screening tools are used, the clinician should recognize their limitations, gather an adequate history, and use them in combination with data from many different sources in the formulation of problems and plans for management. If this broad perspective is maintained, then psychological screening tools can be useful adjuncts to the clinical assessment of developmental problems.

Students and young clinicians are liable to become excessively concerned with a low (or high!) score on a particular test. It is important to become comfortable with variability as the commonplace of human existence. The "normal" is always to be thought of as a range of variation; over time, a clinician will encounter patients at all points within the normal spectrum of child development. This is really no different from the normal spectrum of somatic medical problems and the tremendous variety of detail a clinician encounters when performing physical examinations. Thus, whenever a particular part of the history or developmental observation is assessed, it must be viewed in the context of the full range of what is normal rather than as an isolated score or pass/fail rating. Once again we stress that this ability to assess the significance of behavior or achievements is not terribly elusive and is gained through clinical experience.

Many practitioners avoid developmental assessment because they feel incompetent. In truth, many are not sufficiently trained to interview and observe young children or to evaluate psychological data. Also, good developmental assessment takes more time than many clinicians feel they can afford to provide. One must be convinced that psychological work is worthwhile in order to charge adequately for it. Then again, some pediatric clinicians do not like the developmental and psychological aspects of pediatrics. Many such clinicians are well trained and can afford the time, but find this aspect of pediatric work very frustrating, or view it as unscientific and thus not worthy of their time. However, the developmental assessment is a critical aspect of primary care. It involves skills which can be learned, just as the medical history and physical examination are learned. And it is bad practice to avoid it.

THE DEVELOPMENTAL HISTORY

The developmental history should be a description of the child viewed within the contexts of family and social environment. It is a profile of the child's developing personality, including his or her important relationships, accomplishments, and ability to use skills effectively. This information constitutes a major part of the patient profile contained in the data base.

In addition to the developmental history itself, there are always important data in the medical history, the social history, and the clinician's observations made through the course of a visit. Interactions between the parents and child that occur during the history and physical examination should be noted. Also, valuable data are provided by the (positive and negative) exchanges between parents and between parents and clinician about the child and his or her behavior. Parents will often reveal how they feel about their child through expressions of affect with regard to the child's body—such as pleasure in the child's physical growth or repulsion at bowel movements, vomitus, or genitals.

All of the historical information and observations should be organized in a way that helps the clinician to make an accurate formulation at the conclusion of the visit. Although there are many ways to organize this information, the student practitioner should learn to use one system consistently. Whatever the system, its organization should be practical and complete. The following outline is a guide for developmental assessment. Each listed component will subsequently be elaborated on and discussed, and clinical examples for representative children at different ages will be provided.

Outline of an approach to developmental assessment

    A. General personality characteristics: especially mood, affect, feelings about self
    B. Relationships of the child
        1. Parents and/or other primary caregivers
        2. Siblings
        3. Peers
        4. Authority figures
        5. Family and social (nurturing) environment
    C. Achievements and their use
    D. Past development

Discussion of the outline: general issues

Too often, clinicians rely solely on a survey of the child's achievements. However, in actuality many children with significant emotional problems are able to perform all of the age-appropriate tasks. Also, many clinicians rely on much too general statements by parents or other historians. It is critical for a practitioner to gather details about any activity or relationship, including the feelings associated with them. General statements without details are not very useful and are often incorrect. For example, labels such as "colicky baby," "hyperactive," and "bad" are virtually useless alone, and thus need further elaboration. Through an assemblage of details about behaviors and especially about the emotional atmosphere of the home, it is possible to render a substantial picture of the child's life. Similarly, if one gathers only a superficial account of the child's environment, it is likely that one will miss crucial information. If problems are present, the clinician may want to supplement the history with the History of One Day (see Chapter 8).

Information about the past can be discussed as it pertains to each area of current functioning (i.e., gross motor: current skills, past landmarks) or it can be discussed separately. Generally, however, the interview flows more smoothly if the clinician asks about current abilities in all categories first, and follows with questions about the past. Parents often become confused if asked to mix descriptions of the current situation with past events.

The technique of gathering the developmental history essentially amounts to that of an open-ended interview. Beginning with the most open-ended, nonthreatening questions, the examiner then follows up with specific questions. One way to begin is to say, "Are there any questions you want to ask about Ann's development?" Usually parents will not have any questions at first, but as the clinician proceeds with the interview, they may be reminded of something that has worried them. Often, parents think that the clinician is most interested in the child's physical health, and they do not expect the practitioner to be interested in, or to have the time to ask about, psychological issues. It is important to be careful to communicate that one is interested not solely in problems but in any questions the parents have, even if they are questions about variations of "normal" development.

The first developmental history is part of the prenatal interview. The parent-child relationships begin with the fears and dreams of the parents long before the infant is born. Problems in the relationship with the unborn child may be detected during pregnancy. When the clinician first meets the family into which the patient will be born, he should begin to learn about each parent's background, their marriage, other children, and the circumstances surrounding the conception (including whether it was planned) and pregnancy. When there are unusual stresses, they are explored. It is also important to know the supporting resources available to the family, such as extended family, friends, and trusted professional people.

The clinician should learn whether there are any organic factors which put the infant at risk, such as toxemia, a history of previous Rh incompatibility, or a family history of metabolic disease. Factors which put the mother and father at risk for defects in parenthood, such as depression, past history of poor parenting when they were children, and prenatal complications of pregnancy, should be elicited.

In the delivery room, the first words to the nurses and doctors about the baby, and the parents' report of their first impressions of the infant are important data. (This may not be available to the pediatric clinician.) During the postnatal hospital stay, observations of the parents and infant together and discussions with the parents provide valuable information for later developmental assessment. The clinician begins to learn whether the parents' perceptions coincide with observed behaviors of the child and whether the parents have appropriate expectations for the child at that age.

Beginning with the health evaluation at two weeks of age, the developmental interview follows the outline presented above, but the details vary for each age. If the family is new to the clinician, the history should be quite thorough, with at least one broad question for each category of the developmental history. These might be phrased as follows: "How would you describe Jason?" "How does Jason get along in school with other children and his teachers?" "How are his grades?" "What does he do in his spare time?" If the clinician knows the family well and there are no overt concerns, an open-ended question to cover the major categories of the developmental assessment will suffice. Questions about personality, extended family, and the parents' marriage are not required at each visit —if the previous visit was within the last few months. One can always ask more specific questions whenever the parent or child suggests that all is not well.

Whenever there is any clear problem or concern, or whenever the clinician notes nonverbal cues or inconsistencies in the history that suggest a problem, the topic should be pursued with more specific questions: "Tell me more about his school work." "In what situations is Jason fearful?" "Do you know why he is afraid then?" "What do you do?"

The components of the outline expanded

We shall now consider in greater detail the four major elements that must be explored in the course of the developmental assessment: the child's general personality characteristics, relationships, achievements, and past development. Guidelines for observation and evaluation and methods of eliciting information are illustrated with specific notes on what to look for and what questions to ask.

GENERAL PERSONALITY CHARACTERISTICS

This section includes information about the child's mood, affect, energy level, fears, and feelings about self. Clinicians frequently omit anxiety and depression, which can be masked and thus difficult to ascertain in the preverbal and young child.

The interviewer may begin to learn about these characteristics with an open-ended question such as: "How would you describe Naomi to someone who did not know her?" The answer usually reveals which characteristics the parents feel are particularly prominent. It can tell as much about what the child means to the parents as it tells about the child. Discrepancies between the parents' report and the clinician's observations are very important to note because they reveal problems with the parents' experience of the child, which may in turn indicate significant problems in parenting.

In order to help the parents elaborate on this description, the clinician may need to continue with further questions such as:

How does she feel about herself?
What does she do when she is upset, unhappy, or angry?
What things make her cry?
Is it easy or difficult to end her crying?
How do you do it?
How does Naomi handle situations when she is physically hurt?
What kinds of comforting make her feel better?

If the open-ended questions are not adequate, then more specific probes may be necessary: "Would any of these terms be helpful in describing Naomi—even-tempered; moody; independent; clinging; resilient; active; calm; happy; unhappy; serious; carefree?"

Although the open-ended technique is used, the clinician should direct the questions toward certain general personality characteristics. For instance, most children will seek assistance from adults when needed. If the child never turns to others for help, or is very fragile and seems unable to deal with even small incidents like minor falls without help, the practitioner should gather more data.

It is important for the clinician to make an attempt to learn whether a child has any remarkable or unusual characteristics or sensitivities. "Unusual" does not necessarily have a negative connotation, of course, but if the question is put too abruptly a parent may easily leap to the assumption that the clinician is worried about the child's development. One way to introduce this section is to say: "Each child has his or her own individual style, and I am interested in learning about Naomi in that way. Are there characteristics of hers which you think are distinctive? I am interested in things that you feel are positive attributes, as well as those characteristics you do not like or are concerned about."

One important set of data concerns the child's activity level and attention span. Here are some questions that are frequently useful in helping parents to report this information:

How would you describe Naomi's activity level?
Are there times when she does quiet things?
What does she do when she is busy and active?
When she gets overexcited, are there ways you can help her to be calmer?
What are they?
Can Naomi pay attention to things?
What are some examples of toys or activities to which she pays close attention?
Is she generally interested in *things*?
Is she interested in *people*?

It is often difficult to determine whether the child is normally active and has a reasonable and age-appropriate attention span. However, the parents' report of their own perceptions and also of the teacher's view can be helpful data, especially if there are items reported that seem to be extreme in any direction, or if such a report contradicts the clinician's own observations. Naturally, a detailed description should be obtained if the history suggests unusual activity on the part of the child or marked contradictions in observers' perceptions.

Another area to evaluate is whether the child has any unusual or exaggerated fears. Frequently, a straightforward approach is adequate: "Does Naomi have any special fears?" If such fears do exist, it is important to gather enough details about them to be able to evaluate whether or not they are age-appropriate and also whether they are unusually severe. Some infants startle in reaction to loud sounds. Many toddlers are fearful of barking dogs and loud trucks. These would be considered within the range of normal if the child's reactions to noise are not too severe, if the child can be easily comforted, and if they do not interfere with his or her regular activities. However, a ten-year-old child who is extremely afraid of dogs, who cannot be reassured about the friendly intent of the pet dogs of friends, and who is limited in his or her social activities by this fear does have a significant psychological problem that should be addressed clinically.

Times of transition, breaks in routine, or unusual occurrences during the average day are especially difficult for some children. It is helpful to learn how a child responds to some commonplace stresses, because unusual or severe reactions may be signs of abnormal psychological adjustment. Transitions—including separation, sleep, and even changes from one activity to another—are significant events for a child and inevitably stressful to some degree. Illness is another stress which can alter a child's behavior and interfere with his or her relationships.

For the apparently well child, the clinician should ask a few open-ended questions such as:

Does John have any difficulties related to going to sleep?

How does John react when the family's daily routines change?

What are the things he objects to most strongly?

It is very important that the clinician also try to learn whether a child's responses to stresses such as illness and transitions are age-appropriate or unusually severe—as well as how the parents handle such difficult situations and to what degree they do or do not support the child. Part of a child's maturation involves developing ways to cope with stress. For example, with separation an infant may cry in great protest and then be distracted by a toy; a toddler may clutch an object left by a parent as a reminder or may hold his or her favorite stuffed animal or blanket tightly. School-age children may frequently ask when the parent is returning and follow the time on a clock. Adolescents and adults will frequently think about the person from whom they are separated, and they may use the telephone or write letters in order to maintain contact during a long separation. This subject can be broached by asking some specific questions about common situations involving separation from parents:

How does John react when you go to work?
With whom does he stay if you go out in the evening?
How does he react to being with the sitter?
How have you and your wife been handling John's feeling about being left with the sitter?
Do you think he has a problem in this area?

Other potentially difficult transitions include waking up from sleep, going to school, visiting a friend's house, returning home, changing from one play activity to another, and even changing from winter clothing to spring clothing. These areas may be discussed during the routine developmental history, during the 24-hour history (see Chapter 8), or in the context of evaluating a problem.

RELATIONSHIPS OF THE CHILD

An examiner should specifically ask about important people in a child's life, since it is necessary to have information about these relationships in order to assess whether the child has problems in the area of social adjustment. These data should include not only interactive behavior but also the emotional tone and feelings the child attaches to them, and the meaning these people have for the child—and the child for these people.

Parents and/or Other Primary Caregivers: An assessment of child-parent relationships requires the clinician to obtain complex information about how the child and parents experience one another, the meanings they have for each other, and the feelings they generate in each other. Throughout the visit, the clinician should observe nonverbal communication for clues about these issues. It especially pays to note how the parents feel about and respond to the child's behavior, and how they behave toward each other when dealing with issues such as discipline and child rearing practices.

However, a clinician should also pursue information about these social relationships directly, by asking about them:

How does Naomi get along with you?
How do you and your daughter get along?
What things do you like the most about Naomi?
What things that you do together are fun for you?
Are there quiet times when you relax together? Would you describe a few?
What things about Naomi give you the most pleasure?
What about your daughter are you proudest of?
What about her do you enjoy the most?
What things make you happy?

What is the most difficult thing about living with Naomi at this stage?

What things make you angry with her?

Does Naomi get along better with one of you than with the other? Can you elaborate on this?

The answers to these questions are very helpful in determining whether the parents see their child as an individual with a separate personality or whether they tend to see the child as an object of their dreams. For example, a young teenage mother may like her infant son mainly because he is like a doll to play with, or because he represents her own accomplishment in life. Therefore, she may expect the child to be well behaved and cute all the time. She is disappointed when he is fussy because she does not enjoy being a responsible caregiver to a real person with complicated needs and potentials that vary from her preconceptions. The mother of a three-year-old daughter, on the other hand, may experience her child as inconsiderate to her because she does not sit still through an adult movie; or the father of a competent seven-year-old boy may be ashamed because his son does not excel in the areas in which the father wishes he himself had been successful.

It is important for clinicians to come to terms with the fact that parents' feelings toward their children are frequently far from what one might wish them to be. And a clinician must be able to face such problematic relationships clearly and see them for what they are: a parent may have an especially tense relationship with a particular child, or a parent may seem to hold a grudge against a child or just not like him or her very much. If a parent does begin to make strongly negative and hostile remarks about a child over two years of age during the interview, then the examiner should move quickly to stop the discussion and postpone this aspect of the history to a time in the near future when the child is not present to hear the parent's remarks.

Sometimes it is necessary to do some sleuthing. If the parents' answers suggest that their family is not troubled by *any* of the conflicts such as sibling rivalry, separation anxiety, or oppositional behavior, an astute clinician will be skeptical and will inquire about the home life in more detail. Likewise, if the parent or child casually mentions an area which the clinician feels is potentially serious, then a more detailed discussion of the issue is appropriate. Indeed, especially those topics that are introduced with the common offhand phrase "By the way . . ." usually merit active investigation.

It is important to ask about the child's relationship with both parents, even when one parent is not present at the visit. These questions can be quite direct:

Tell me more about Ann's relationship with her father (or mother, if the father is present at the visit).

What kinds of things do they do together?

How much time does he spend with the children?
Are there things that he particularly likes to do with the children?
How much was he involved with the children when they were younger?
What things make him most angry with the children?

If the mother is not a full-time homemaker, she should be asked these questions with regard to herself; also, if the father is the historian, he should be asked these questions about the mother.

In instances where the parents are not living together or where there is marital conflict, it is especially important to learn whether the historian is satisfied with the relationship the child has with the spouse and other caregivers. However, it is important to keep in mind that disagreement between caregivers is an important issue in most families, even where there are no major marital problems.

Discipline, including limit-setting and punishments, can often be discussed conveniently in the context of any difficult situation mentioned in the history. Parents will often bring up a toddler's difficulty in sharing toys, an older child's willfulness and wish to be in control of his parents, or an adolescent's rebelliousness toward rules and responsibilities. After the problem is broached by the parents, the practitioner should be prepared to follow up:

How do you and your husband handle that situation?
Do you both agree on that method of discipline?
How do you manage your disagreements?

Even when discipline is not mentioned directly, it is advisable to ask about it specifically: "Tell me about the way you and your husband discipline Henry."

Patterns of child rearing, including discipline, are deeply ingrained, and most parents raise their children much as they were raised. Although a clinician may have a rational argument for using a different method to discipline a child, it is very difficult for parents to change their habits, and rarely will they change their opinions on rational grounds. Also, in formulating the significance of a particular disciplinary method, one should keep in mind the fact that there are a great many perfectly adequate ways of raising children—even though a lot of these patterns will differ from what the clinician has been socialized into thinking is best. The crucial factor in how parents raise children is the emotional atmosphere in the family. A parent who spanks a child may communicate dissatisfaction with a particular behavior, which is quite natural; but the same act may also communicate hatred and a desire to hurt the child physically. Only a careful interview will tell the clinician about such qualitative differences between parents. (See Chapter 5 on child rearing.)

If a child is older than four or five years of age, one can ask direct questions to evaluate the feelings he or she has toward the parents:

What can you do to please your parents?
What can you do to make your parents happy or proud of you?
What can you do to make them mad or disappointed?
What things that they do are hardest for you to bear?
What things are best for you?
If you had some free wishes, how would you change things in your family?

The examiner can also learn about family relationships through a child's play with dolls or from drawings the child is asked to make during the visit.

Siblings: It is important to inquire about a child's relationships with siblings. A parent and an older child can be asked directly how the child gets along with his or her siblings. One should ask specifically if there is sibling rivalry or if the older children are competitive about school work or their accomplishments. Questions for the child include:

How do you get along with your brothers and sisters? (If there are several siblings, the clinician should try to learn with which siblings the child has the closest relationship and with which he or she has the most difficulties.)
What kinds of things do you do with them?
What things are the most fun for you?
What do you do to make them happy?
Which one is your closet friend?
What things make you angry about your brothers and sisters?
What things do you do that make them angry?
What do you do to solve the problem when you are not getting along?

Peers: Both the parents and an older patient can provide the examiner with information about the opportunities the patient has for peer relationships and about what they think of their qualities. A parent should be able to tell the clinician about the child's contact with peers. For the younger child these will be limited to children encountered in the neighborhood, play group, nursery school, or day-care center; for the older child they will include children encountered in school and after school. The practitioner should ask the child of five years of age and older specifically who his or her friends are and what they like to do together. Is there a special friend? What kind of person is this friend? What is the most fun about this friend? Social activities such as church and scout groups are important areas for peer contact. Exploring this area provides an opportunity for the clinician to learn about the child's life from the child directly and, through this conversation, to assess the child's language skills in a natural context. If the child is interviewed alone, it might be a good idea to use these questions early in the conversation since they are not so threatening.

Authority Figures: The examiner should interview the parent and older child about adults other than parents with whom the child has significant relationships. For a young child these frequently include baby-sitters and nursery school or day-care center teachers. The older child's authority figures will be school teachers, guidance counselors, coaches, and groups leaders (scout, religious). The older child, especially an adolescent, may also be working, and the quality of his or her relationship to employers or fellow workers is significant. Both the pleasurable and the difficult aspects of each relationship should be explored if there are developmental problems.

Family and Social (Nurturing) Environment: This category of information includes data about all members of the patient's household (including those other than the nuclear family), extended family, close friends of the family, and the diverse relationships between these people. Also of interest are the neighborhood, the various community groups to which the family belongs, and socioeconomic factors.

It is important to bring up questions about relationships even if they seem to be intrusive and embarrassing to ask. Do not, for example, omit to inquire: "How are things between you and your husband?" or "Are there any areas which are particularly difficult for you and your husband?" Most parents will not think it is too personal, if they have had an opportunity to talk with you for a while; they will frequently appreciate the interest and concern and will usually answer such questions honestly.

If the household includes persons from outside the nuclear family, the examiner should be sure to ask about their relationships to the child and to the rest of the family as well. A frequently encountered example is the family where the maternal grandmother lives in the home with the nuclear family of the patient. Some useful questions are:

How does the arrangement with your mother work out?

Are there any problems with having her in your home?

Sometimes grandparents have difficulty accepting the life style of today's children. Have you noticed that in your family?

There may also be grandparents who do not live in the household but are near enough to visit and know the grandchildren well. In many cases, friends who are contemporaries of the parents are available to help out in a crisis. Other important factors include the type of neighborhood in which they live, the church or synagogue and other social groups to which they belong, and agencies with which the family is involved; these should be noted. One may ask:

How long have you lived in this area?

Do you have family who live in this part of the country?

Do you see them often?

Do they help you with the children at all?

Do you have friends who can help when you need it?

To whom else would you turn for help if your family needed it?

Have you ever needed help f...   re-
    spond?
Do you have someone to talk...   ...her
    about the children or any...
Are you members of a church...
What kinds of activities is your...
Do you have any contact with a...   ...o-
    ciation or with social worke...

Every family can benefit from the...
of stress. It is valuable for the clinician t...
the support which is available to a famil... ...ion may have
been obtained as part of the family social history. However, if it was not
gathered earlier, the developmental history provides a convenient opportunity to fill that gap.

ACHIEVEMENTS AND THEIR USE

In this section of the developmental history the clinician should ask about a child's current achievements and interests. It is helpful to use different approaches for the younger and older child; therefore, we provide the following two separate outlines. Naturally there will be some overlap between five and seven years of age.

Child under Five Years of Age: *Large Muscle Skills (Gross Motor):* Specific questions will vary with the age of the child. For the toddler, the clinician should find out, for example, if the child climbs stairs, alternates feet when climbing the stairs; can use a walking toddler bike; can use a small slide, can climb into an adult chair. For the older preschool patient, the examiner should ask whether the child can ride a tricycle and has the opportunity to ride one; whether or not the child uses a jungle gym and slide; and how well he or she climbs.

Small Muscle Control and Manipulative Skills: The parents' history is a helpful supplement to the clinician's observations. Questions about toys with small parts, ability to use buttons and zippers successfully, and interest in small toy figures are helpful in obtaining information about the child's development and skills in this area.

Problem-Solving (Adaptive) Skills: This is one area in which the history is of secondary importance to clinical observations as a source of data. The history is somewhat helpful, however, when parents tell about a child's play, use of puzzles, drawing, use of blocks, and interest in other manipulative toys. As the child reaches the preschool years of three and four, his or her increasing knowledge about shapes and number concepts becomes a useful part of the history.

Language and Communications: Both expressive language and comprehension should be discussed. For the very young toddler one can ask what kinds of things the child says; for somewhat older preschoolers one can inquire about the extent to which the child tells the parents about what she or he does and observes and whether the child can express needs verbally. It is important to ask if the patient seems to understand when he or she is spoken to, and whether people outside the immediate family can understand the child's speech. Toddlers and young preschool children very often use jargon or very immature speech, so that it is difficult for strangers to understand them. If this pattern persists, it may be a sign of abnormal language development.

Usually, the clinician has the opportunity to hear a child speak during a visit, if only to a parent. However, a young child may be so shy that she or he will not talk at all. If the child does talk, the examiner should listen and assess the level of language used. If a patient refrains from any speech during the examination, one may want to visit the child at home where she or he is likely to be more comfortable and consequently more willing to interact with a stranger. With some extra effort, then, it should be possible to assess the language of even a very shy child.

Personal-Social: This category can be subdivided into social skills, self-awareness, self-help abilities, and fantasy play. Of course, expectations vary with the age and developmental stage of the child.

1. *Social skills* include a complex array of abilities. One important element to consider is the usual progression of an infant's awareness of other people through the following stages: Initially, infants respond to voices and become quiet when someone picks them up. Later they develop a social smile; this progresses to reaching out and grasping at a person's face or other parts of the body, such as hands.

Another important skill is a child's ability to discriminate among people. Already in infancy, a normal child can tell strangers from familiar people. Around six months of age many children begin to protest when strangers come near or try to hold them. Toddlers develop this further and protest about separation from familiar people.

Play also is an important social skill for a young child. Infants learn to initiate play with adults, often by giving a toy or otherwise engaging the person. Later, children learn to ask an adult or child to play with them. In the preschool group, beginning as early as 30 months of age, children begin learning to share and take turns. This ability is not usually mastered fully until four or five years of age.

2. *Self-awareness* includes knowing one's own body parts. Infants from about 10 to 12 months learn to show this by pointing to and/or naming parts on their own body, or on another person or a doll. Older infants learn to identify themselves in a mirror, and preschoolers later learn to use pronouns appropriately (I, me, them) and to know their own sex.

3. *Self-help skills* include being able to feed oneself and use eating utensils as one grows older; undressing and, later, dressing are important self-help skills as well.

4. *Fantasy play* begins with domestic mimicry; toddlers imitate the

household chores which adults perform around them in their daily lives. Toddlers will sweep the floor and "help" to make a bed. Soon after, they will treat a doll the way adults treat children, including feeding, hugging, spanking, and reprimanding it. Later they engage in more complex fantasy play with assigned roles, dress-up, and conversations with imaginary figures.

Child over Five Years of Age: It is assumed that any deficits in large muscle control, small muscle control, and problem-solving skills will have been discovered by the time a child reaches school age. The assessment of the child between five and seven years of age overlaps the assessment of the child under five years of age because there is naturally a range of variability in what children are exposed to, what is expected of them, and what they are able to do; and because some of the characteristics, such as being too shy to talk to the clinician, may persist. Therefore, it is useful to be flexible in one's approach in this transitional period. From age seven years through adolescence the history about the child's achievements and their use can be organized according to the categories discussed below.

If the child has not received adequate health care or has not attended a school, the clinician should take nothing for granted. For practical purposes it is wise to assume that no one has performed an adequate developmental assessment and, therefore, to "start from scratch." This, of course, involves doing a thorough developmental history and careful clinical observations, especially of problem solving and language development. This is because parents are more likely to miss or deny delays in these areas than in others, and because evaluating them involves quite a bit of direct observation.

It is helpful to divide the school-age child's achievements into the following groups: school performance, extracurricular activities, hobbies, and athletics. Also, it is useful to simultaneously explore the activities in detail and discover how the child feels about them.

School Performance: The examiner should inquire into a child's school performance, including the quality of grades achieved. Also, specific information on a child's reading, mathematical, and writing abilities should be recorded. This can be followed with some questions of a more subjective nature:

What do you like the best about school? Why?
What is your favorite subject?
What do you like the least about school?
What is your least favored subject?
Are there any subjects that are particularly difficult for you? (This has often already been mentioned as the least favored subject.)

These questions will sometimes yield answers that indicate problematic areas. They can be followed up with more searching questions. Also, it is advisable to ask the parents what they think about the patient's school adjustment, what the child is learning, and how, if at all, they are involved in the school.

Extracurricular Activities: This includes a variety of activities, often school-based, in which the child learns a wide range of skills and socializes with peers. It may include sports, stamp collecting, music, and other interests.

Hobbies: These may have already been mentioned in extracurricular activities, but they may be overlooked if they are not school-associated. Hobbies generally include those activities outside of school or a job that a child pursues somewhat seriously, such as music, art, dancing, animal raising with a 4-H group, or hiking. Frequently, hobbies are social activities as well, since they are pursued in a group.

Athletics: The clinician should ask if the older school-age child participates in athletics. Not infrequently, children who avoid athletic activities feel inadequate; also, their lack of participation may deprive them of easy access to socially significant peer groups.

PAST DEVELOPMENT

The practitioner can gather information to determine whether the child's gross motor or language development was significantly delayed by asking parents questions about their child's developmental landmarks:

> Can you tell me approximately how old Leon was when he first sat alone?
> When did he walk without support?
> How old was Leon when he spoke his first words?
> How old was he when he combined words to make sentences?
> Has he had any problems with speech?

However, one should keep in mind that information about developmental landmarks has limited usefulness because parents have great difficulty in remembering the ages of these accomplishments. In addition, if the child has had any significant delay, there is almost always some manifestation of it in current functioning, and thus it is likely to be noted in the course of the physical examination. Also, information about it usually is to be found elsewhere in the history.

OBSERVATIONS: SOME GENERAL COMMENTS

This portion of the developmental assessment includes both unstructured or naturalistic observations and those made during the presentation of structured tasks. The child and family can be observed in many different settings, including the clinician's office, the child's home, a day-care center, or a school. In the office, it is important to remember that one's observations should begin with what takes place in the waiting room, and then continue in the examining room.

Unstructured observations are made by watching and listening to a child and parent (or teacher) in a more or less natural setting. *Structured observations*, which include psychological tests and some screening procedures, such as the Denver Developmental Screening Test, are made with the aid of special equipment or special techniques used in a prearranged format.

Direct observation of the interactive behavior of the child and his or her parents is an extremely important aspect of any pediatric developmental assessment. Observation supplements and validates the picture of both patient and parents which initially was presented in the developmental history. Sometimes these observations yield information that contradicts the history. Also, parents are often unable to tell the clinician that they are disappointed or worried about their child, or that he or she produces negative feelings in them. They may feel guilty or ashamed about these feelings and therefore may be afraid of criticism. Parents may become used to their child's unusual characteristics; they may deny problems, and sometimes they are not aware that a particular behavior or skill represents a problem. Therefore, direct observation is an invaluable supplementary method for detecting problems both in the child's development and in the relationship she or he has built with other family members (particularly the parents).

A clinician's intuitive impressions are important; one should not prematurely dismiss—or accept—such hunches or impressions. They should be kept in mind as one gathers the developmental history and as one makes observations. Their critical assessment may later lead to important formulations. An example of such a development is the case of a practitioner who notices that a child is unusually unhappy and anxious early in the office visit. This observation should not automatically be dismissed as an acceptable expression of fear of the clinical situation, nor should it be interpreted as an a priori sign that the child has significant psychological problems. The child's behavior must be evaluated along with other information about his or her response to stress and observation of the progress of resolution of the anxiety as the visit proceeds.

Student clinicians often find it difficult to be disciplined about making developmental observations, especially unstructured ones. It is hard to notice both the child's and the parents' affect and behavior when one's own anxiety is prominent. However, students should work at being as observant as possible during an entire visit. Then, at the end, the case should be formulated using all the information that has been gathered. Frequently, observations that are not made deliberately during the visit are still available to clinicians when they consult an outline at the end of the visit.

A formulation of the case should take into consideration the normal range of developmental variables, and it should be articulated within a consistent and practical format. Following an outline usually helps to direct a clinician's attention to many areas simultaneously, and it promotes a sensible and balanced formulation. The following outline describes detailed examples of developmental observations in four different age groups:

1. General personality characteristics
2. Parent-child interactions
3. Large muscle skills
4. Small muscle skills (especially hand)
5. Problem-solving (adaptive) behavior
6. Language and communication skills (both receptive and expressive language)
7. Personal-social skills

The age groups discussed are: infant, preschool, school-age, and adolescent. These descriptions are not intended to be a manual of child development, nor are all possible observations mentioned. Instead, this section is intended to present suggestive and heuristically useful examples of "typical" observations a clinician should make. The practitioner should extrapolate from these situations to the actual children evaluated in his or her clinical practice.

Unstructured observations: general comments

The unstructured observations described below are most frequently made during a well-child health evaluation in a clinic or private office. However, they can also be made during a visit to a patient in a newborn nursery, home, day-care center, school, or hospital.

The clinician should keep the outline in mind and simply remain alert and observant throughout the visit. If any observations need more data, it is fine to ask about specific behaviors at the time they occur. After the visit it is important to rethink the entire visit, make note of significant observations, and put them into the context of the history and structured developmental observations in preparing a final formulation.

AT THE OFFICE

Infant (six months old): *General Personality Characteristics:* The examiner should note the predominant characteristics exhibited by the infant during the visit. The child may be passive or active, content or fussy, relaxed or tense, engaging or unfocused, sleepy or alert, cuddly or rigid, easy or difficult to comfort. Most infants go through two or more behavioral states during the average visit. (*State* is a commonly accepted term which denotes a person's state of consciousness, mood, degree of comfort, and behavioral organization.) For instance, the infant may arrive content, alert, and sociable. During the visit she or he may become hungry and may cry. In most cases the parent will be able to tell what is wrong and try to comfort the infant, for instance, by feeding the child if that is what is called for. If the visit occurs during the patient's usual naptime, the parent may not be able to comfort the child until the visit is over and the infant can go to sleep. A clinician's opinion about a child's personality should take into account the various states noted during the observation period, the stresses on the child, and the child's responses to parents' care. All of these data must be interpreted, of course, together with the parents' description of the child at home.

Parent-Child Relationship: The examiner has to assess whether the parents are aware of their child's needs and whether they are able to meet these needs appropriately. Indicators of parents' competence in this area are: their being prepared with diapers, appropriate clothing for the weather, and bottles (if the child is not breast-fed). The emotional tone of the interactions between parents and child is the main indicator of whether an appropriate mutuality has been achieved. Also, observations of how the parents hold and carry the infant, whether they talk to the child, and how they diaper and feed the baby are very valuable in this part of the assessment.

It is important to note how the parents respond when the child becomes upset, whether the ways they try to comfort the child are appropriate, and whether they in fact are able to comfort the child. Also significant is how the parents feel when their child is upset. This can be ascertained through observation of the tone of the interaction, spontaneous comments, and even by direct questions, such as "How do you feel when the baby cries?" Parents vary greatly in this regard; they can be concerned, irritated, ashamed, or even indifferent. A parent may even be angry at or upset with the child, declaring that the child "is crying on purpose, to get back at me." Such a response probably indicates serious difficulties between the parent and child. A parent may also be overly concerned or identified with a child—unable to leave the child at all or excessively upset when the child cries.

The parents' responses to their infant's body is another valuable area to observe. Their verbal—and especially nonverbal—responses to the child's body in general, and their responses to the child's mouth, genitals, stool, and vomitus in particular, often tell an alert clinician about feelings which parents might not describe straightforwardly during the history. Parents who feel good about their child are usually able to tolerate with equanimity, and even a good-natured joke, such unpleasant experiences as soiled diapers or spitting up. When parents do express or act out strong negative feelings or inhibitions about their child's body or bodily functions, it may mean that they have a serious problem in their emotional ties to the child.

It is also advisable to note whether the parents take pleasure in the infant's accomplishments and whether they express affection toward the child. Most parents, even if they are having difficulties, will be enthusiastic about the positive aspects of their relationship with their infant. If these positive feelings are lacking, it is a very important indication that a problem exists.

Large Muscle Skills: As they mature and develop, infants have a predictable progression of resting postures when they are placed in different positions. Therefore it is important to observe the infant's postures in various positions in order to assess this development. (This is also true for reflexes, and is discussed on page 221.) The six-month-old infant in the supine position should have symmetrical posture, with the head in the midline or moving to follow objects with the eyes. When prone, the legs should be extended. The infant should be able to sit, although he or she may need support to remain balanced. The head should be centered over the trunk without any bobbing. The quality of body movements (e.g., smooth or jerky), muscle tone, and the infant's ability to move should also be noted, as should the presence of any abnormal movements.

Small Muscle Skills (Especially Hand): It is very important to observe the infant's fine motor skills—both when the child is supine and when she or he is sitting either alone or supported on a parent's lap. The clinician should note how the child uses his or her hands and fingers: each hand individually, each hand in relation to the others, and the hands in relation to the body, eyes, and mouth. A contented and relaxed six-month-old child will move his or her hands together and apart, and will grasp things such as a rattle or the tubing of a stethoscope. The child will not be able voluntarily to release the grasp, however, although he or she may well lose interest in and inadvertently drop the object.

There is a well-known progression of grasping behavior. It is presented here as a practical note to the reader. As always, dates are approximate, but they do serve as guidelines in developmental assessment.

The neonate has fisted hands much of the time. As the infant matures, the fists are held open more of the time, and by 12 weeks of age the fists remain open. By 16 weeks of age the infant can hold things in a purposeful way (unlike reflex holding in the younger infant). At about 20 weeks of age the child can grasp a one-inch cube precariously, but cannot release it voluntarily. Subsequently (around 24 weeks) the infant learns to grasp a cube by using the palm and all fingers and to hold the cube reliably. By 28 weeks the child has a radial-palmar grasp of a cube (uses the thumb side of the hand and the palm) as well as the ability to gather in a small pellet with a raking motion of the whole hand. Around 32 weeks the child uses a radial raking motion to get the pellet and tries the scissors grasp, but usually is unsuccessful. Thirty-six weeks marks a great hurdle:

the child has a radial-digital grasp of a cube and a successful scissors or other grasp of a pellet, and further learns to release the cube. By 48 weeks the child learns to pick up objects, even pellets, with a neat pincer grasp. From then on the child masters many complicated tasks such as building towers and continually improving visual motor coordination.

Problem-Solving (Adaptive) Behavior: The clinician should think about which small muscle skills the child has and how those skills are used. What problems does an object present, and how does the infant use hands, eyes, and the entire body to solve these problems?

The six-month-old child should be able to transfer small objects (rattle size) from one hand to the other and to put things in his or her mouth. Frequently, such an infant will assist a parent in holding the feeding bottle, or will put one or more fingers in the mouth.

Looking behavior should be well coordinated by this age. The child should follow an object or a face over the entire visual field and should be interested in and use the eyes to examine his or her own hands. The coordination between seeing and motor behavior is also developing; the child can reach for a seen object which arouses interest.

Language and Communication Skills (Both Receptive and Expressive Language): A six-month-old infant will make many soft vowel sounds and will repeat sound patterns. He or she will be just beginning to make consonant sounds like "da." These sounds may be made while the child is alone, in response to someone talking to the child, or in response to an interesting object. The infant can communicate discomfort clearly, using a wide variety of sounds that range from complaining or whimpering to a brief protest and loud continuous crying. A child of this age does not comprehend any specific words but will be interested in speech, especially from familiar adults. Most six-month-old infants can be comforted or stimulated by being talked to.

Even deaf infants have normal vocalization until this age. However, they do not respond normally to sounds like the ringing of a bell, crinkling cellophane, or voice sounds. Subsequently, their spontaneous vocalizations become much less frequent, and these do not progress to the repeated consonants and jargon typical of the older infant and toddler.

Personal-Social Skills: The six-month-old infant initiates smiling in a social way. The child knows his or her own parents or other significant caregivers and may respond differently to strangers. Frequently, the parents do not notice the difference between the child's response to them and to strangers, and many prefer to think that their child is friendly to everyone. In fact, from the neonatal period on, most children do show subtle differences in behavior with different people. Parents sometimes need to be reassured that the discrimination which may be manifested as differential responses to strangers is an important sign of normal development. Each individual child responds selectively to different familiar and unfamiliar people throughout his or her development. The neonate may be comforted most easily by a primary caregiver. At six months of age children begin to develop a negative or anxious reaction to strangers. At 13 months many children are at their peak of separation anxiety. In fact, fear of separation reappears later in normal development.

Children at this age also begin to learn games such as peek-a-boo. Initially, playing games is a social response with gurgles of pleasure and anticipation. Later it develops into more complex play that prominently features imitation.

Six-month-old infants frequently are beginning to act on their own behalf. They often will resist when someone tries to pull a toy out of a hand. They will also be putting things (including food) into their mouths; and they will be starting to "assist" their parents by grabbing a spoon or cracker and feeding themselves.

Preschool Child (four years old): It is both informative and helpful for a preschool child to have some play materials, such as paper and crayons, trucks, dolls, and books, to use during the interview. Most children will be able to amuse themselves with these toys, although sometimes they need to be told that the toys are there for them to play with.

General Personality Characteristics: The clinician should note the child's mood, range of emotions, and ability to be comforted throughout the visit. Almost all preschool children are shy with a nurse or doctor, especially if they have had few regular or pleasant contacts with a health care practitioner. However, the ways that they seek comfort or express their anxiety are very significant indicators. Some children remain near their parents throughout the visit but do allow the clinician to complete the physical examination; some even gradually become more comfortable with the examiner. Occasionally a child will whine or cry and refuse to cooperate throughout the examination. It is important to find out if this behavior is restricted to the office setting or if it is a pattern that is manifested in other situations as well. Some children are even destructive or hostile during the visit, which should be addressed with the parents and looked into as a sign either of the presence of emotional problems in the child or of family problems.

The clinician should also observe the quantity and quality of the child's activity, attention span, and interest in people and toys. It is important in doing so not to miss noting a sad child, especially in the toddler period, when activity can be deceptive and may be erroneously interpreted as a sign of happiness.

Parent-Child Interaction: As with the infant, the examiner should observe both the child's and parents' behavior, and note how they all get along with each other in the waiting room and office. Does either parent behave in a way which is helpful for that particular child? Do the parents help to prepare the child during the visit, especially for threatening parts like lying on the examining table or painful parts like injections? Are they supportive to the shy child, or do they berate the child, push the frightened child forward, and shame the child because of his or her withdrawn behavior? When the child asks for help with toys, puzzles, or undressing, do the parents help in a kind way or do they act annoyed, threatening, punishing, or abusive? Do the parents hover over the child excessively, or do they allow the child appropriate independence? Do the parents seem to expect too much—for instance, do they ask the child to put on complicated clothing without assistance or become very stern about a small breach of self-control?

It is also very important to take note of how the child interacts with the examiner during the interview with the *parent*. Most children will interrupt the interview occasionally to show something, ask questions, or share some aspect of play. Sometimes a child is disturbingly withdrawn or preoccupied; others are excessively intrusive and interfere with the interview. Some children cannot control themselves even when parents or clinicians ask them to do so.

If a child becomes too noisy or excessively active, or in any other way requires discipline within the confines of the office, the clinician should resist the impulse to intervene and wait for the parent to set a limit on the child. This permits the examiner to see how, or if, the parent accomplishes this task. Some parents become overanxious about the child's misbehavior in the office and are extremely strict and severe in setting limits. Occasionally, a parent will even hit the child or threaten severe punishment. Other parents are unable to set limits effectively, and an occasional parent may even seem frightened of a four-year-old child. Sometimes parents wait for the clinician to set limits because they feel that the clinician is the one who should control what happens in the office. It may be necessary for the examiner to ask the parents how a similar situation would have been handled at home in order to assess the parents' apparent lack of, or overly strict, limit-setting in the office.

Large Muscle Skills: Most of a child's large muscle skills can be observed as the child sits, walks, bends over, and climbs up on the examining table. It is important also to note if the movements are well coordinated for the child's age, if there are any tremors or obvious spasticity, if there is weakness, or if there is an unusual preference for using one side of the body (as with hemiparesis) beyond normal handedness and foot preferences.

Small Muscle Skills (Especially Hand): The examiner can observe a child's manipulative skills as the child plays during the interview. One should note abilities to draw and to manipulate small toys such as trucks with movable parts, dolls and doll clothes, and puzzles (see Figure 7-1). The visit should be arranged so that the child can be observed undressing or dressing. Four-year-old children should be able to undress for the physical examination with a minimum of help with such items as slip-over shirts and shoelaces. They should be able to dress themselves, and the clinician may have the opportunity to observe muscle skills in their use

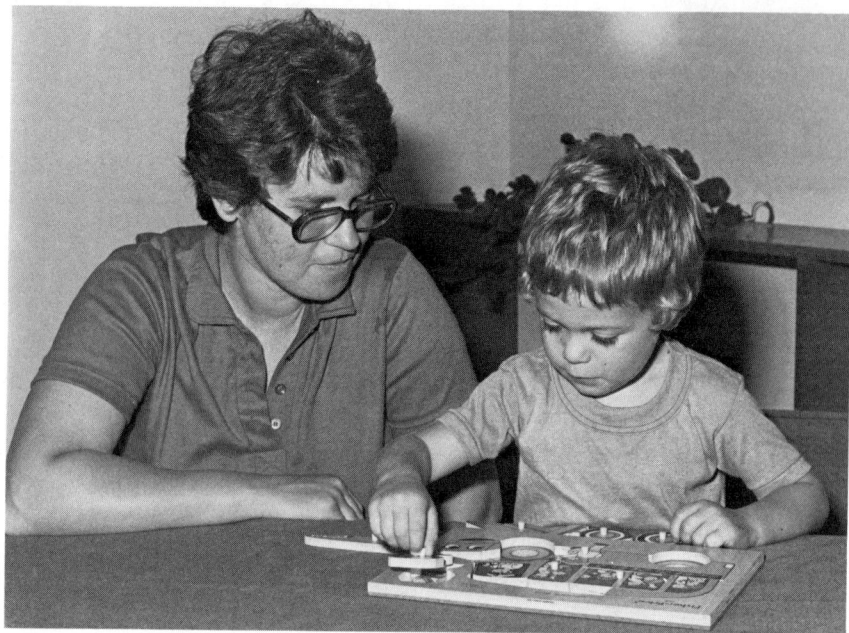

Figure 7-1. *Unstructured play.* A four-year-old boy works attentively to complete a puzzle. Puzzles and other toys should be available to the child while the clinician and parent talk. Observing a child at play can provide a wealth of information about cognitive skills, attention span, motivation to complete what is started, motor skills, and fantasy life.

of zippers and snaps and manipulation of large buttons. Most four-year-old children cannot tie shoelaces. Coordination, spasticity, and weaknesses will become obvious when these tasks are observed. Most children have a clear handedness at this age.

Problem-Solving (Adaptive) Behavior: In the preschool age group fine motor and problem-solving skills should be evaluated with a few structured tasks as well as unstructured observations. In fact, important aspects of a child's personality are often best revealed while the child is spontaneously using toys in the office or while she or he is working at structured adaptive tasks like those discussed in detail later in this chapter.

Language and Communication Skills (Both Receptive and Expressive Language): Many four-year-old children are comfortable enough with the clinician so that they feel free to talk to the practitioner about themselves; naturally, this is more likely when they have known the clinician for some time. This gives the examiner an opportunity to assess the child's ability to comprehend and communicate. The child's speech will demonstrate vocabulary, articulation, word usage, and concept formation. Sometimes the child will not be comfortable enough to talk with the clinician, but will talk to a parent in the clinician's presence. The practitioner can encourage this during the interview.

It frequently is useful to use a picture book, small objects, and toys as vehicles to assess a child's speech. One can ask the child to tell what certain pictures represent, to describe what action is occurring, and to identify some colors. This informal assessment may be perfectly adequate. Only if there is some problem that causes concern will the examiner want to supplement it with standardized structured tasks, which are discussed later in this chapter.

On rare occasions, the clinician will not get to hear a child talk at all. However, the child may follow directions and so demonstrate, grossly, adequate hearing and some elementary comprehension. If the child does not speak, it is crucial to ask the parent why, and one must try to determine if the child is mute in other situations.

A four-year-old child should be able to talk in full sentences, use pronouns correctly, and speak so that she or he can be understood fairly easily by people outside the family. Frequently, family members do not notice speech problems because they learn to understand a language-deficient child's speech, even if the sentence structure and enunciation are not so mature as they should be.

There is, of course, a tremendous range of variability in children's ability to speak; but practitioners should not be intimidated into thinking that they cannot evaluate it adequately. Mostly, it is a matter of pursuing the evaluation carefully and logically. For instance, if there are questions about a patient's language abilities, a crucial first step is to evaluate the child's hearing. Admittedly, a partial hearing loss may be difficult to diagnose based on casual observations of the child's speech and comprehension. But some gross testing may reveal it—testing through such simple devices as whispering words and having the patient repeat them, and asking the patient to listen for a watch tick at different distances and comparing the results to one's own presumably normal hearing. When a language problem is detected, the child must be tested by means of more sophisticated and reliable pure-tone audiometry, either in the primary health care site, or by referral to an audiologist. Other causes of expressive language problems must also be considered, and a complete developmental profile is essential.

Personal-Social Skills: At this age, social skills are evaluated mainly by data from the history; on occasion, however, they may be supplemented by observations during a home or school visit. Of concern here are the child's ability to take turns in play, to share, to play an assigned or chosen role, and to imitate parents in their domestic tasks.

The clinician should learn about the development of the child's self-help skills. This includes the child's ability to dress and undress alone, to use eating utensils, and to assist with simple domestic jobs.

School-age Child (nine years old): School-age children should be active participants in a health evaluation. Their language skills and ability to relate to the adults in the health care setting make them less dependent on their parents and more likely to be able to provide the clinician with a history. As a child gets older, the history provided by the child is of increasing importance in detecting problems. Older children usually are able to control their behavior in the office, even if they have psychological problems. Nevertheless, the clinician may observe unusual behaviors, or behaviors which are discrepant with the proffered history.

General Personality Characteristics: The practitioner should note especially the child's emotional state; that is, whether the child seems happy, angry, sullen, or depressed. Also, the attention span and level of motor activity are quite important as indicators of psychological well-being or lack of it.

Parent-Child Interactions: The kinds of observations made here are the same in this group as for younger children: whether the parents are supportive or critical of the child, whether they show enthusiasm and affection for the child, and whether the child seems able to ask the parents for support. The school-age child should be somewhat more independent of the parents and more able to care for his or her own needs. However, some parents infantilize their children and do not allow them enough privacy. On the other hand, some parents may have too high expectations. The clinician will have to rely heavily on assessing the quality of the interchanges between the parents and the child, much as one would judge interactions between adults.

Large Muscle Skills: To assess these skills one should note how the child holds and uses his or her body during the visit, especially during the physical examination. The developmental assessment will not be the place where deficiencies in large muscle skills are noted, as is the case with younger children. If large muscle skills have been delayed or are abnormal, this will have been noted in the history. Observations here and in the physical examination will aid in further assessment of these problems.

Small Muscle Skills (Especially Hand): At this age these skills are usually observed only casually in the examination setting. One can depend on the parents and the child to note any old or newly acquired difficulty with fine motor abilities. However, it is useful to ask specifically about handwriting and crafts. This is in contrast to what happens with the younger child, in which case the clincian is often the first to diagnose a delay or abnormality in both large and small muscle skills.

Problem-Solving (Adaptive) Skills: For the school-age child one can usually depend heavily on the history for data on the patient's achievements in reading, writing, and arithmetic. This should be supplemented by a narrative from the child describing activities and projects in which she or he is currently involved.

Language and Communication Skills (Both Receptive and Expressive Language): Frequently, we depend on the schools to diagnose speech and language problems. Nevertheless, the clinician should assess a school-age child's language comprehension and production in the course of their conversation together during the visit. One should note the complexity and level of abstraction of the matters discussed, the child's ability to form cohesive, complete, understandable sentences, and the presence of problems such as stuttering and enunuciation difficulties. If the patient has difficulties in comprehension, expressive language, or articulation, a thorough hearing evaluation and/or further speech assessment is indicated.

Personal-Social Skills: Most of the information in this area also comes from the part of the history that covers the child's relationships with family, peers, and school authorities. Self-help skills should be noted in the history; they include an assessment of the child's responsibilities for his or her own care, and degree of participation in family chores.

Adolescent: Adolescent patients usually assume the major responsibility for supplying clinical information, participating in the physical examination, understanding the reasons for laboratory tests and other studies, and learning about various clinical problems and their management. This participation in the health assessment provides much of the information in these observations.

General Personality Characteristics: The clinician should note an adolescent patient's emotional state, but should be prepared to find a wide range of variation. The patient may be relaxed and responsive during the interview and examination, or may be anxious, distractible, or reticent. Adolescents are quite labile: mood may change in the course of an interview and may vary from one visit to another. Some adolescents take an active, interested part in their health care from the beginning; others are more passive and distant in their relationship with the clinician. An adolescent's ability to tolerate frustrations and conflict and to plan for the near and distant future are both important aspects of his or her development.

Parent-Child Interactions: The clinician's impression of parent-adolescent interaction will largely be based on what one says about the other, and also the feelings which are conveyed with the information. If there are joint discussions with the adolescent and the parents, the qualities of the interaction should also be noted.

Large Muscle Skills: Observations about routine gross motor abilities are made during the entire visit, but especially during the physical examination. This is supplemented from the history with information about athletics, whether group or individual. Strength and endurance can generally be assessed from the history of the patient's capacity for sustained physical work.

Small Muscle Skills (Especially Hand): These may be assessed from reports of the adolescent's ability to work with creative media such as cloth or yarn, ceramics, metal, or wood, as well as pen-and-ink and various other graphics materials. Many other hobbies also require manipulative skills of hands and fingers. The adolescent who possesses good fine motor skills but whose handwriting is unintelligible or bizarre may have a specific language disability—or a psychological problem that merits investigation.

Problem-Solving (Adaptive) Skills: The clinician can base an assessment of the adolescent's problem-solving abilities on data about performance in mathematics and science in school, as well as on the patient's ability to assess and respond to a variety of demands and challenges provided by others. Often, the clinician also receives a good glimpse of the adolescent's ability to solve problems during a discussion of a clinical complaint and the patient's attempts to cope with the problem or the stresses it caused.

Language and Communication Skills (Both Receptive and Expressive Language): Instead of focusing on the adolescent's speech per se, experienced clinicians usually note the richness and expressiveness of the vocabulary commanded by the patient and also the ability to transmit information with clarity and animation. The adolescent's use of humor and his or her ability to verbalize abstract concepts should also be noted.

Personal-Social Skills: The information is drawn from the adolescent's relationships within the family, peer group, school, and job context. One should expect to see an adolescent take increasing responsibility for his or her own education, work, and long range plans. An absence of this development may signal emotional or other psychological problems.

HOME VISIT

A great deal can be learned about a child and his or her family from observing them in their home; this information may be difficult to learn from an interview and observations made in the office. For instance, one can learn about the neighborhood in which the child lives; the physical appearance of the home, including whether it is safe, well-organized, and clean and whether the family has made concessions to the presence of a child in the furnishings and toys they have about the house. The latter reflect both knowledge and the emotional ability to provide a child-oriented environment. Also, the mood of the household may be reflected in the cheerfulness or somberness of prevailing wall colors and lighting.

The child will probably be more comfortable in his or her own home than in the clinician's office. Therefore, a young child who would not speak with the practitioner or cooperate during the structured developmental assessment in the office might be willing and able to do both at home. Preschool-age and older children should be able to show the visiting clinician around the home and should be susceptible to active participation in conversation about his home life.

Sometimes, a parent who is extremely shy or uncomfortable in the office setting will be much more outgoing and comfortable at home. However, on rare occasions, a parent is more relaxed in the office than at home. This may occur if the spouse, in-laws, or other relatives are present. Occasionaly, the parent is ashamed of the home and is concerned that the visiting clinician will be critical of his or her efforts to provide a decent home for the family.

During a carefully planned home visit, the clinician may be able to meet other members of the family and see how they relate to each other and to the patient. This is particularly helpful when the clinician only sees the mother in the office; an introduction to the father, siblings, or a grandparent at home can be very informative, since signs of significant family discord may be readily apparent if the family members who are having difficulty are present.

The clinician may also want to visit the child when she or he is with a caregiver other than the parent, such as a sitter. This would be particularly important if there were a question about the adequacy of the caregiver or if the parent presented an unusual picture of the child which the clinician wanted to corroborate. The type of observation in this case would be similar to the unstructured observations made in the office and during a normal home visit: one should note the attitudes and feelings of the caregiver toward the child and the adequacy and safety of the environment.

It is very important to arrange a home visit in advance, either during an office visit or by a telephone call or letter. The purpose of the visit should be stated in terms of the problems as formulated (perhaps at a previous office visit) with one or both parents. Some examples follow: "I would like to visit so that I can talk and work with Robert where he is more comfortable than he was in the office. Often, children can work with me much better when they are at home and are relaxed." "I would like to visit so that I can meet Alice's father and sister. I think it would be helpful for all of us, in view of the difficulties your family has had in the past."

During an illness or in the first weeks after a child is born, a home visit may be very acceptable to a family. Although the clinician should initiate the idea of the visit, it is crucial to respect the parents' right to privacy. This means, among other things, being sensitive to cues that one is not welcome. These cues should be honored—but they also should be considered important data.

SCHOOL VISIT

"School" may mean nursery school, play group, day-care center, or any other institution where the child spends significant periods away from home and family. School visits give the clinician an opportunity to observe the child in a new and familiar context, and also to learn about the school itself. Usually, such a visit is undertaken if the parents or the clinician feel that the school may not be appropriate for the child. The clinician may offer school personnel information which is relevant to educational planning; it may also be useful to review the justification for the child's placement to be sure that the school accommodates the patient's special needs. Also, the teacher may have information to share with the clinician about the child's behavior in this setting and about the parents as well.

As with the home visit, the school visit should be arranged in advance. The teacher should always be a party to such an arrangement. It is important to plan for enough time to observe the child in a typical class (or even several classes), to talk with the teacher(s), and sometimes to interview other school personnel. For both ethical and practical reasons the child and parents should be informed about the visit before it occurs, and they should also know the proposed date. The clinician should be sensitive to the family's concerns about confidentiality. If necessary, he may explicitly tell them that he will not share any confidential information with school personnel. Upon arriving in the class the clinician should sit in an unobtrusive place and should follow the child's lead on whether or not to acknowledge his or her presence. Some children will greet the clinician openly and tell their friends who the clinician is; others are shy or embarrassed and will not acknowledge that they know the clinician.

Aside from information collected in interviews, a broad spectrum of data can be gleaned from a school visit. This includes the emotional and physical atmosphere of the class, including discipline, organization, noise, and distractions, and the equipment and learning materials available.

Clinicians do not visit schools frequently because it is quite time consuming. However, when children are having school problems, such visits are definitely called for and should be done more frequently than is usual practice. The student practitioner, in particular, can learn a great deal from school visits, even if there are no emotional or psychological problems. As a future child health clinician, she or he will be much better equipped to counsel families with children once familiarity with the locally available preschool programs and schools has been achieved, and one way to learn about some of the schools is to visit and discuss the progress of an individual child.

When either the patient or a parent is having a problem with school personnel, the clinician may be very helpful as a facilitator of communication. Sometimes it is necessary to go further and act as an advocate for the child vis-à-vis school officials. In any event, school visits have many uses—and all child health clinicians should be willing to consider undertaking them in given situations.

Structured tasks: general comments

As we have already indicated, it is possible to make the majority of one's pediatric observations in the unstructured manner we have been describing. However, the picture of the child is often not complete without data from a few tasks presented in a more structured way. These tasks give an accurate assessment of the child's success in areas which are difficult to evaluate from the history and unstructured observations alone, and they allow important clinical observations in a planned sequence of events. However, student clinicians should resist the tendency to be overly concerned with whether or not the child succeeds according to a precise testing protocol. In fact, it is often much more meaningful if the observer carefully notes not only the skills the child exhibits, but their manifestations such as emotional investment in the task, attention span and perseverance, sense of pleasure in accomplishments, responses to failures, and ability to learn a challenging task.

There are times when an examiner does not have an adequate opportunity to observe a patient at play in the office. This may happen if the interview is very complex and emotionally difficult, with the result that most of the clinician's attention must be devoted to the parent. It may also occur if the child is quite shy and stays with the parent instead of playing with the available toys. Therefore, it may be necessary to schedule more time for the formal, structured part of the developmental assessment.

This section will discuss the approach to the child and parent for a structured evaluation, a description of the setting of the structured assessment, and representative tasks for both a six-month-old and a four-year-old child.

AN APPROACH TO THE CHILD AND THE PARENTS

The examiner's manner is important in the developmental assessment, just as it is in the history and physical examination. A clinician who is calm, friendly, approving, and not rushed, will help put the child at ease and will be viewed as a friendly rather than a threatening figure. Indeed, the conditions under which a particular child performs best vary widely. Some children need firm containment, others need to feel in control of the situation. Some work best at a fairly rapid pace, and others need more time. A supportive, flexible examiner will help each child maximize his or her performance.

It is also valuable to consider the parent's feelings. Usually, if the parent views the clinician in a positive way, the child will also be more comfortable. Some children are especially sensitive to their parent's comfort or discomfort, and consequently the clinician's relationship to the parent may well influence such a child's performance. In order to allow for the building of a reasonably good working relationship with a parent, experienced examiners will present the formal developmental tasks to the child after the interview and before the physical examination.

THE SETTING

There are a number of reasons for placing the structured tasks between the interview and the physical examination. First, as we have just said, it allows the examiner time to establish rapport. Second, information from the interview will indicate which structured tasks should be presented and which areas are of special concern. Finally, the structured tasks are best done *before* the physical examination, because the examination procedures may be upsetting; consequently, a child is unlikely to do very well on the structured tasks while still in a state of upset or anxiety after the examination.

The child should be fully dressed when the tasks are presented. A parent normally should be present, just as for the history and the physical examination. A quiet, approving parent is a valuable asset in the evaluation. If the child is very upset by the parent's presence, the examiner can tactfully ask the parent to leave for a short time, just as for other parts of the health assessment. In fact, this is very rarely necessary.

Usually the child is comfortable if seated on a chair next to the parent's chair. However, not infrequently a toddler will only be comfortable when seated on the parent's lap. In some instances, a child is so frightened of the examiner that it is best to ask the parent to present the task to the child. This may mean that the parent will have to demonstrate building a tower or putting pegs into the peg board and will have to give the child directions. Then, as the patient becomes more comfortable, the clinician may be able to resume a more active role in the assessment. This procedure is not without pitfalls, however; some parents try to prompt the child, or even to do the task in the child's place. In such an event, one must ask the parent in a tactful manner not to invalidate the procedure: "It would be better if John did these things by himself, Mrs. Freeman. I will make sure to help him if he needs it." With coaching, most parents will be able to control the urge to help the child.

The patient and parent usually relax after the child has some successes. For this reason it is advisable to begin with a few simple tasks that the child will quite likely be able to perform easily. It is also very important for the clinician to explain the rationale and procedure for the developmental tasks to the parent. Parents generally need to know why the examiner is doing the structured assessment and to be reassured that it is part of the routine health evaluation—that it is not only for children who have problems. The parent should also be prepared for the fact that the child will not be able to do all of the items because the test will probe the patient's upper limits of ability.

As the child becomes old enough to understand (usually around two years of age) he or she should also be given a simple introduction to the testing. At the end of the interview and developmental history, the examiner might tell the child, "Now I would like you to work with some toys and puzzles I have." At the same time one should supplement those remarks by commenting to the parent, "I would like to see what John does with some of these toys." Then, going into some detail, one can continue, "It is helpful to combine this with the information you have already given me. I use these toys and puzzles with all the children in my practice. I will begin with simple items, and then proceed to more difficult ones, often above John's age level. Don't be concerned if he does not do all the items. At the end, we will be able to talk about it together." The parent may ask if it is a test. It is best not to use the word "test," but rather to describe the structured tasks as a part of "the ways in which one learns about a child's development." To this end one might say, "It is not a test with a score, but it is a group of problems to solve which helps me learn things about your child that I would not ordinarily learn from talking with you." If the parent or clinician is concerned that the child's development is delayed, the clinician might say, "These observations can help me to evaluate your (or our, or my) concern about John's language development."

It is very important for a parent to be present during the structured tasks so that she or he can observe the various things that the child can and cannot do. If there is reason to believe that the child's skills are not developing normally, the ensuing discussion about them is likely to be much more meaningful when the parent has observed the developmental assessment. Sometimes, it may help convince a parent that the child does have developmental delays or difficulties, even if the parent tends to deny the problem. In addition, some concerned parents are actually reassured by seeing the performance, whether it is normal or not.

REPRESENTATIVE TASKS*

The tasks described below are representative ones for each age. They are not intended to represent a precise, complete psychological test. The items have been chosen in many different areas of functioning. Also, particular items were selected because they are easy to administer and are designed so that it is easy to recognize whether or not the child is successful.

Six-month-old Infant: *Large Muscle Skills:* The clinician should note the infant's head and body control. This is easily done during the entire visit as the parent handles the child. However, if this was not achieved, the clinician can proceed to evaluate these skills specifically: In the prone position, a six-month-old infant should be able to lift his or her head completely off the table, lift the shoulders and chest, and look all around. In the supine position the infant should be able to raise his or her head off the table, although the infant usually cannot get to a sitting position without assistance. The infant can also raise his or her legs high and remove a diaper placed over the face when supine. When the examiner pulls the infant to a sitting position there should be no head lag,

---

* These tasks were selected from the Yale Revised Developmental Scales, which was developed by Sally Provence. The Yale Scales is a composite test protocol made up of items drawn from standardized scales: Gesell, Hertzer-Wolf Test from the Viennese Scale, Merrill-Palmer, and Binet.

and the child should anticipate the clinician's pull with tension in the arm and shoulder muscles. After the infant is in the sitting position the head should remain centered over the torso, and the child should maintain good muscle tone in his or her back. Many six-month-old infants will not be able to balance well enough to sit alone, although most infants at this age actually can sit briefly if their legs are spread out for them.

It is good practice to raise the child by placing one's hands under the infant's axillae and holding the child upright. The child should be able to support his or her weight and bounce actively on foot. The infant normally will not be able to balance alone, and should not be left unsupported. Again, the child's head should remain directly over the torso, and the back should be fairly straight and maintain good muscle tone. The infant should be neither too limp nor too rigid.

A six-month-old infant should have been rolling over—both prone to supine and the reverse—for many weeks. Occasionally, one direction of rolling is preferred over the other, but this need be no cause for concern if the child has equal strength and range of motion in both right and left limbs.

The clinician should determine, either by observation or by asking the parent, if the child can move from place to place using primitive motor skills. Frequently, the infant will move along the examining table on his or her abdomen to reach a toy. Sometimes she or he will roll over repeatedly to reach something. The infant should be able to use these primitive skills both to move toward interesting objects and to move away from things.

Fine Motor-Adaptive Skills: (These two categories are combined because most of the tasks demonstrate skills representing both areas at this age.) To begin with, an infant should be interested in objects within his or her visual field. The child should follow a moving object using the eyes, and look for a toy lost from sight.

If the child did not have the opportunity to play with cubes earlier, the examiner should present the infant with two blocks. At this age, the infant will just be learning to hold a small object in each hand simultaneously. As the child focuses attention on the second block, she or he may inadvertently release the first one. The ability to transfer a small object from one hand to the other is normally perfected between five and eight months of age. The child will use a raking motion to grasp a very small object such as a raisin, will use a radial palmar grasp for a larger object such as a cube, and may also bang an object on the table.

Four-year-old Child: *Large Muscle Skills:* One can expect a four-year-old child to be fairly competent in balancing and in coordinating his or her body. The examiner can ask the child to balance on one foot, hop on one foot, and catch a ball that has been bounced toward the child. The child normally should be able to follow the clinician's lead in walking forward with heel touching toe at each step, and even to walk

Developmental Assessment 169

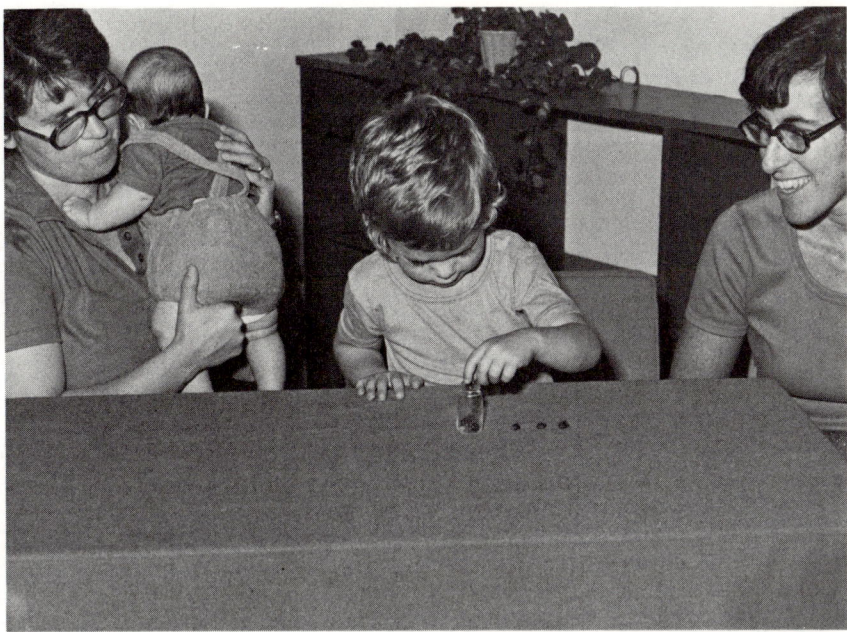

Figure 7-2. *Fine motor skills. The child is asked to use one hand to put the series of raisins in a bottle and then to repeat the task with the other hand. The clinician, at right, should note the child's use of the pincer grasp and ability to accomplish the task smoothly and quickly.*

backwards the same way. The child should also jump and may be able to skip, although somewhat awkwardly.

Small Muscle Skills: The examiner should ask the child to oppose thumb and forefinger on the same hand. A good way to evaluate finger dexterity is to ask the child to place raisins in a small bottle fairly rapidly (see Figure 7-2). It is also useful to note how much difference in performance there is between the right and the left hand. Usually, handedness is well established at this age, and some tasks, such as putting raisins into a bottle, are performed with more agility using the preferred hand.

The child's ability to use a crayon or chalk should be evaluated (see Figure 7-3). A child of this age should be able to copy a circle, and most children at this age can copy a cross. If the child cannot copy the cross, at the minimum end of the normal range she or he should be able to trace it. Squares are much more difficult, but many children can draw one after it has been demonstrated; and some can even copy one.

Problem-Solving (Adaptive) Skills: Many of these tasks require fairly well developed fine motor skills, but they also involve abstract thinking. The clinician should ask the patient to do simple puzzles. Children can also be asked to build a tower (see Figure 7-4) and to build bridges with small blocks (see Figure 7-5). This evaluates both small muscle coordination and problem solving. Knowledge of number concepts can be demonstrated by asking the child to point to objects while counting

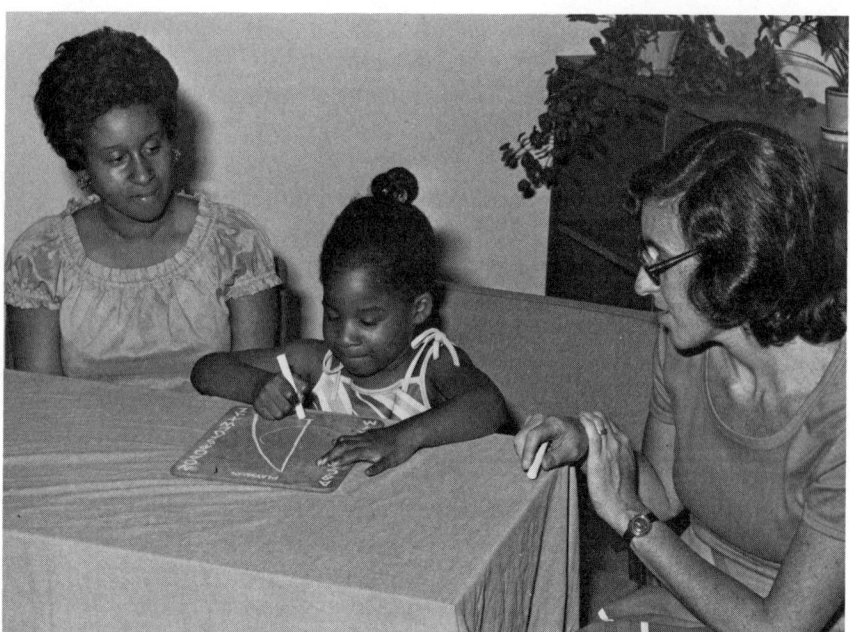

Figure 7-3. *Conceptualization and eye-hand coordination. The child is attempting to draw a square, which is quite a difficult task for a four-year-old. The clinician began with easier tasks, which the child would be likely to complete, in order to help the child experience success. This prepares the child to attempt the more difficult tasks with confidence.*

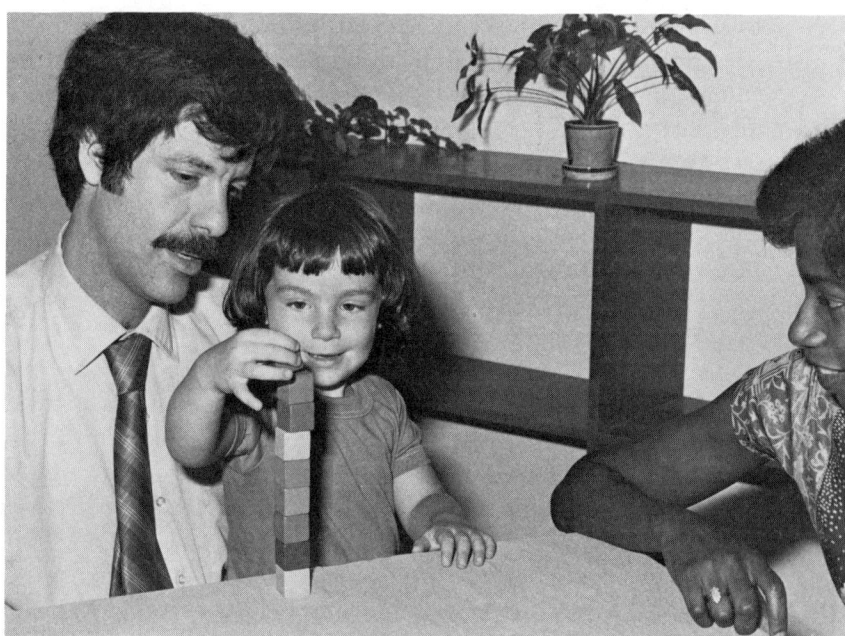

Figure 7-4. *Fine motor control and eye-hand coordination. A child building a tower. Things to note are her pincer grasp and her abilty to line the blocks up so that the tower is stable.*

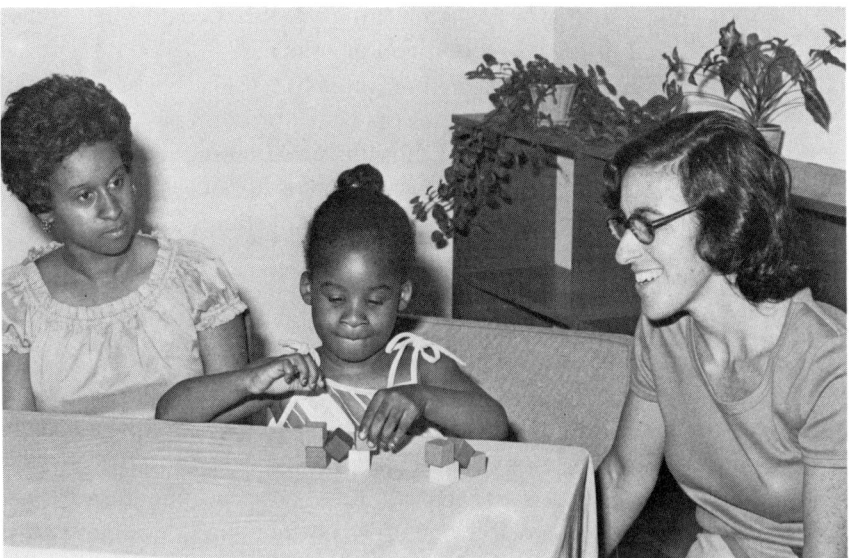

Figure 7-5. *Advanced fine motor control and conceptual skills. A four-year-old child is asked to build a "5-cube bridge" after seeing a model. Things to note are her finger and hand coordination as well as her ability to figure out how to build the bridge.*

them, at least to "three." Drawing humanlike figures also indicates perceptual and cognitive development. The child should be able to draw a person with two or three parts, and should be able to tell that a part is missing from a standardized predrawn rendering of an incomplete person. If the clinician has a board with shapes cut out of it (a form-board), she or he can ask the child to replace the shapes. The child should also have an idea of differences in size, as shown (for example) by an ability to pick the longer of two lines or the larger of two circles.

Language: If the child's conversation is age-appropriate, it is unnecessary to ask more than a few planned questions. If, however, there is some question about the child's vocabulary, grammatical competence, comprehension, or abstract thinking, more structured questions are appropriate.

A four-year-old child normally should be able to name at least three colors correctly. The less complex ability to discriminate colors (but not to name them) can be tested with a game made of variously colored boxes with same-colored discs; the child is asked to place the discs in the boxes that match their colors. A book with pictures can be used in place of formal test cards or papers to explore the child's knowledge of vocabulary and definitions. In order to evaluate a child's understanding of prepositions, the examiner can give the child something small and ask the child to put it *under* the table, *on* the table, *in front of* the chair, and *behind* the chair. Comprehension of simple questions can be determined by asking

"What do you do when you are hungry?" What do do when you are cold?" and "What do you do when you are sleepy?"

Between the ages of three and five years, a child normally is developing an understanding of opposites or contrasts. This can be evaluated by asking the child, "If mother is a woman, father is a ———?" "If a horse is big, a mouse is ———?" "If fire is hot, ice is ———?" "In daytime it is light, at night it is ———?" "The sun shines during the day, and the moon at ———?"

At the end of the structured tasks it is helpful for the examiner to make a brief statement to the parent and child to help them feel comfortable about the assessment. It is important to choose one's words carefully to ease their concern about any failures. If the child did well, the clinician might say, "John did a good job with the toys and puzzles. I see he particularly enjoys building with the blocks. Let's go on to the physical examination and then we can talk about everything some more."

If there is delay in some areas of the child's development, the clinician might reflect the parent's thoughts: "You may have noticed that Ann had trouble naming some of the pictures. We will talk about that after I do the physical examination. She did very well with the puzzles and she worked well for a long time." If the parent seems especially upset or needs to ask a question, it is essential for the clinician to engage in a little more discussion before moving on to the physical examination. For example, a parent might say, "Well, Tina is tired today, and she does name pictures at home." A facilitating response might be, "I know this is not a normal situation for her. Let's talk about it more afterwards."

In the clinical summary after the physical examination, the clinician should comment explicitly on the child's development, including strengths, delays, or problems. This is a process that requires judgment and tact. The way in which these formulations are presented can be just as important as their content. This is a sufficiently complex area that we have expanded on it at some length in Chapter 11, on the clinical summary.

CHAPTER 8

The History of One Day

Introduction
Illustration: A Typical Day

INTRODUCTION

The history of a full day is an interview which attempts to recreate the chronological progression of an "average" or "typical" day in a child's life, in order to provide the clinician with a picture of the child's current situation within the context of his or her family and social environment.*
In undertaking this interview the clinician inquires into the broadest range of information about how the patient passes through an average day including: which adults and peers are with the child, how developmental challenges are handled by the child, what areas are stressful, and how the adults guide, limit, and support the child.
This 24-hour history is a helpful supplement to the information gathered as part of the data base in the family social history and developmental history. It is more structured than much of the history presented earlier; however, within this highly organized sequence there is

---

* Sally Provence, Developmental assessment, in *Ambulatory Pediatrics II*. Morris Green and Robert J. Haggerty. Philadelphia, W. B. Saunders Company, 1977, p. 374.

ample room for open-ended questions, digressions, and opportunities to discuss feelings as well as physical and behavioral data.

The history of one day is particularly useful when a social problem is identified within the family or when the child seems to have a developmental or psychological problem. It is also helpful for the historian who feels uncomfortable with open-ended questions and prefers a preset structure for organizing information concerning specific events and facts. Furthermore, clinicians find this format useful in dealing with a historian who rambles excessively and does not answer questions directly.

In my own work as a consultant to child care programs, the 24-hour history has been especially helpful in the first appointment with parents whose child appears to have a psychological or developmental problem. In this situation I do not have the data base that a primary care clinician would have gathered, and the 24-hour history provides a valuable method for generating data quickly and in well-organized form. Also, the fact that it focuses attention on the child's daily life in the context of the family and other social interactions ensures that I will gather, in addition to data about the child, the kind of data that will indicate any other factors which may also be at work, factors that may indeed be causing the "presenting problem." Finally, the 24-hour history is a valuable supplement to the more routine pediatric history.

Although the scheme for the history presented below is quite structured, the clinician should feel free to digress from the chronological order—to explore any area, to listen carefully, and to elaborate upon concerns of the parents or child. It is easy to return to the sequence of the day at any time. Inexperienced or student clinicians frequently feel compelled to stick to the sequence, and so lose the flexibility afforded by a less structured interview. Another pitfall, although not limited to this history, is to feel that you *must* cover the entire day. Practitioners should use this history selectively, suiting it to their need to gather a useful data base. Whenever the interview becomes too cumbersome or burdensome, the clinician should feel free to alter or even terminate it.

As in any other interchange between practitioners and parents, the latter often request advice or reassurance during the interview process. Likewise, clinicians are often tempted to give advice or to quickly and facilely reassure parents about their child rearing practices. As discussed in the interview chapter, such temptations are best resisted at this time. Clinicians should not give advice, unless the matter is very clear-cut; rather, they should tell the parents that they will discuss the question further after a full picture of the child's day has been drawn. Subsequently, in the clinical summary, the clinician can have a well-organized discussion about the entire question, which can lead directly and logically into making a plan together with the parents. In the same way, clinicians should not criticize or attempt to correct parents' child rearing practices while gathering the history. Instead, these disagreements should be discussed in the clinical summary.

ILLUSTRATION: A TYPICAL DAY

The example presented here includes many areas, but not all that could conceivably be covered in the history of one day. Practitioners can alter the interview to suit the age of the patient and the characteristics of the family, and naturally will omit areas already familiar to them from other historical data. Through listening carefully and maintaining flexibility, clinicians will maximize the usefulness of this historical format.

The first 24-hour history can be introduced simply and directly: "As I get to know Daniel, it is helpful if I can learn about his average day. I'd like you to describe a usual day for him, and I may interrupt to ask you some questions. Think of an actual day in the past week." Then, one might begin the history with "What is an average day like for Daniel?" If the parent or older patient is not sure how to begin, it helps to suggest that she or he pick a specific but average day, perhaps yesterday. "Begin with the early morning, and go through the entire 24 hours until the next morning." As the person begins the narrative, the clinician can stimulate, supplement, and elaborate on it with the following questions:

At what time does Daniel usually wake up?
Does he wake himself?
How do you know he is awake?

This last question is quite helpful, especially for young children. Infants and toddlers may cry or call out; older children may come into their parents' room.

What does he do after he wakens?

The answer, depending on the child's age, will give the clinician a picture of the patient's abilities and perhaps his parents' expectations of him. Some school-age children make their own breakfast; others play quietly by themselves. Some watch television.

Where are the other members of the family at that hour?
What are mornings like for your family? Are they hectic?
What kind of mood is the rest of the family in at that time?

These questions provide information about the family as a whole—including how the parents share responsibility for the child, whether they meet the child's needs appropriately, and the quality of the emotional atmosphere. For example, there may be a problem if no adult gets up to be with a young child. Sometimes, the father has already left for work and the mother is depressed and does not get up. The parent who cares for the child during the day may work during the evening and, therefore, may try to sleep from 3:00 A.M. to 9:00 A.M. If the child wakes up before the parent, this may irritate the parent, causing a problem. If the child sleeps in a crib, she or he may be confined to the crib until the parent gets up. The clinician should try to determine if this is a reasonably short length of time and if the child seems happy in the crib. Many young children will in fact play contentedly with toys in the crib, "talk" to themselves, or be amused by an older child until the parents get up.

After investigating these issues, the clinician can continue:

> What is Daniel's mood when he wakes, both in the morning and after naps?

Some children awaken gradually and are happy. Others, especially young children, can be unusually cranky if they are not allowed to sleep until they waken on their own. Not infrequently, disturbed, irritable children have particular difficulty on first awakening. Also, some parents begin the day being irritable with their children, setting a tone that is hard to reverse.

> When does Daniel get dressed?
> Does he dress himself?

This question naturally is altered according to the age of the child. However, if he or she is a preschool or young school-age child, this question is particularly important. The answer will tell the examiner about the child's abilities, including fine motor coordination (with buttons, hooks, zippers, shoelaces) and self-care skills. If the child is old enough to dress himself, but the parents still do it, the clinician should be alert to learn more about the situation. It may represent a pattern of inappropriate infantilization of the child by his or her parents. It may be important to ask specific questions, such as "Does he need any help with dressing?" "Does he choose his own clothes?" "Can he manage buttons and zippers and tie his shoes?"

It is particularly important to ask the general question: "Are there any conflicts over dressing?" These conflicts may take the form of an argument about whether the child should get dressed without help, or whether the child should decide what she or he should wear. Children as young as two years of age will express vehement opinions about what they want to wear. The clinician should ask what the parent does if and when this occurs. In many cases, the parent will avoid a battle with an oppositional toddler by letting the child have his way, allowing a quick and simple resolution of conflict over an unimportant issue. If there are repeated, highly charged arguments which represent power struggles between parent and child, it is advisable to listen carefully for other data that may suggest a problem about the setting of limits and other conflicts between the parent and child.

> What is breakfast like?
> When does Daniel eat breakfast?
> Is breakfast a pleasant or a difficult time?
> With whom does Daniel eat?

Many families eat some meals together. Others never eat together, for a variety of reasons including conflicting work hours, disorganization, or a desire on the part of the adults to eat separately from the children. Since meals are inherently social occasions, both the pleasures and conflicts at meals can tell about the strengths and problems in a family.

Are there any problems associated with eating?

This is a convenient, open-ended question which may lead to information about concerns over the child's diet, battles with the parents about the quantity of food he eats, or conflicts over a young child's ability to feed himself. For the child under five years of age the clinician may ask specifically whether he feeds himself, uses a spoon or fork, and uses a cup, and how competently those utensils are handled. In this regard, it is useful to inquire whether an older child can cut his or her food.

How is Daniel's diet, in general?

This question can be asked in many places: here in the 24-hour day, at the end of the 24-hour day with an expanded discussion about diet and eating, or in the review of systems performed earlier in the course of taking the data base. Because children's eating habits can be erratic on a daily basis, it is often more accurate to inquire about the patient's dietary intake over a three- or four-day period.

What are Daniel's particular likes or dislikes in food?

Virtually everyone has particular likes or dislikes in food tastes. The clinician should note whether the child has an unusually narrow range of foods that she or he will eat. Some fussiness is within the range of normal variation; however, it may be excessive and associated with hypersensitivity to other stimuli, indicating an unusual psychological profile. Occasionally, a child's unusual likes and dislikes may raise concern about the nutritional adequacy of his or her diet.

What is Daniel's behavior like when he refuses to eat something?

How do you handle that kind of situation?

These two questions are intended to provide the clinician with information about parent-child interactions and possibly about limits and discipline. The information can best be analyzed when the entire developmental history and observations have been completed.

What does Daniel usually have for snacks?

When does he have snacks?

Are there any problems over snacks?

Many children have snacks during the day, both in the morning and the afternoon. Because most children like sweets, snack patterns can be a significant factor in the degree of dental caries. In addition, inappropriate snacks may interfere with the child's appetite and intake of nutritious foods. Snack patterns and how they are handled also tell a great deal about the parents' attitudes and ability to set appropriate limits. Some parents are very permissive, and allow the child to eat whatever and whenever he or she wishes. Other are not concerned about the timing of meals and snacks but are careful about the content, and do not have sweets or other nonnutritious foods available. Then again, there are parents who are very strict and severely limit both the timing of snacks and the foods their child may eat. Usually, family behavior related to eating is consistent with other behavior patterns; therefore, the practitioner can learn quite a bit about a family's values and style of child rearing through an inquiry into meals and eating patterns.

Continuing with the child's day, the examiner may ask: "What does Daniel usually do in the morning, after breakfast?"

If the examiner already knows that Daniel goes to school, this question obviously would be omitted; then questions about school would be appropriate. For a preschool-age child the answer may include a wide range of activities, including playing with neighbors or preschool-age siblings, going shopping with parents, being taken to visit friends, attending day-care, and watching television. Any answer should stimulate more detailed questions. If the child plays with neighbors, for example, one should explore the quality of the child's interaction with peers and other adults. It is also useful to inquire as well about the parents' role in these activities and how they feel about their participation.

How old are the neighbor's children?
Where do all the children play?
What do they do together?
How do they get along?
Are they able to take turns and share toys?
What kind of supervision do they need?
What do you do when you supervise them?
Is Daniel able to play independently, without adult or child companions?

If this history is *not* a supplement to the regular developmental history but rather stands alone as the initial history, it might be a good time to ask what the parent does with the child that is fun and how the parent feels about the time he or she spends with the child. Then one can return to the child's play:

Does Daniel have a chance to ride a bike or to play on a jungle gym?
Would you say he is confident about using those playthings?
Is he reckless in his play?
Does he have any fears about climbing?

If play is not mentioned spontaneously, the examiner should make sure to broach the subject at some time. Some additional questions concerning play include:

What are some of Daniel's favorite toys?
How does he play with them?

This last question helps the practitioner to find out whether the child's play is age-appropriate. It also provides information about the child's ability to engage in fantasy play and about whether the play is unusually narrow or possibly reflects a particular worry or concern the child may have. It is not which particular game is played that is of greatest interest. Rather, it is the meaning of the game to the child, and whether the style of play is indicative of problems, as when doctor-play is used excessively to express fear of bodily damage and to attempt to correct it.

Television viewing is a significant, often detrimental activity for children. The clinician should give it due attention and should discuss TV with the family. If the parents bring up television on their own, either at this point or later in the history, it is wise to gather more details. If the parent does not mention television, the clinician should bring it up.

What TV programs does Daniel watch?
Does he have any favorite shows?
How much time does Daniel spend watching television on an average day?
Does anyone in the family watch with him?
Does he watch adult shows?
Has he ever been frightened by any shows?
How did you handle that situation?
Does anybody at home monitor Daniel's TV viewing?

If the parent mentions shopping, the clinician might ask:
How does Daniel behave in the stores?
Does he like to choose things to buy?
What happens if he wants things he cannot have?
How do you handle it?

If morning activities include being at a day care center or a nursery school, that topic also deserves some inquiries.

Where is the day-care center?
What kind of center is it?

It may be a cooperative center at the local church, a family day-care program sponsored by the college where the parent studies, a commercial program, or a government supported center such as a Head Start Program.

What is Daniel's nursery group like?
What are the ages of the children?
What kinds of things do they do?
Are you and your wife satisfied with the center?
Is Daniel happy there?
What factors were involved in your decision to enroll Daniel in the center?
How did you pick this particular center?
How did Daniel adjust to the center in the first weeks?
Have there been any changes in his behavior (either positive or negative) since he has been in the program?
Do you or your wife participate in school activities?
What ones are you active in?

If the child regularly spends time with a sitter, one should ask whether the care is in the child's home or in the sitter's home and who else is with the child and the sitter (her own family or other children). The questions previously asked about a day-care center, with respect to the parents' reasons and satisfaction and the child's adjustment, are appropriate to ask here as well.

> Are you and your wife satisfied with Daniel's care at Mrs. Ludke's home?

If they are dissatisfied in any way, this should be discussed. The concern for continuity of care is a major one, especially for a young child, and naturally leads to more questions about the child's past experiences.

> What were the arrangements for Daniel's care when he was younger?

These can include family members, baby-sitters, day-care programs, and nursery schools.

A school-age child can answer direct questions:

> Tell me about your school.

This is a comfortable, open-ended question, which often serves as a convenient way to begin this part of the history. The clinician should learn the name of the school, the child's grade, and how long the child has gone there. It is important to interview the child before the parent. In this way, the clinician will have a more accurate view of the child's thoughts about the school than if the child first hears what the parents have to say about it. However, this approach unfortunately does not preclude the child's repeating what she or he has heard from the parents at other times.

> What is your teacher's name?

This and the next few questions are good ones to ask the young school-age child who is around five to seven years of age. It may also be necessary to be this direct with an older child who is uncomfortable or unable to answer more open-ended questions.

> Who are some of your friends in school?
> What is the most fun about them?
> What do you like to do the most in school?
> What do you like the least?

These questions provide an opportunity to engage the child in conversation and to assess his or her language abilities. The clinician can then turn to the parents and ask more questions about their view of the school.

> Can you tell me how you decided to send Daniel to the Prince Street School?

This question is a helpful one to start a discussion, especially if the school is special or unusual in some way. Most children will go to their local public school. If the child is in a special public school or in a private school, it is important to learn the reasons for that decision. The answer to this question may provide significant history about the child's special needs and any emotional or learning problems, or it may give the clinician insight into the family's aspirations and values with regard to education.

> What are your thoughts about Daniel's school and class?
> Are there things that you find particularly good or bad about it?
> Have you had an opportunity to visit the school in session, or to talk with Daniel's teacher?

This tells the examiner whether the parents have been able to visit the school and may indicate to what extent the teachers are available to the parents.

> Are you involved in any activities for parents or in school affairs?
> How is Daniel doing in school?
> Are you satisfied with his work?
> How does he get along with the other children and with his teachers?

All issues raised by the parent or child which indicate that there are school problems, either in academic performance or in adjustment, should be investigated thoroughly.

> Could you tell me about Daniel's problems in math?
> Tell me about his difficulties with the teacher.
> What have you done about it?
> How has that worked?
> Have you spoken to his teacher?
> What did the teacher say?
> How do you feel about it?
> Has there been any change since your conference at school?
> Has Daniel had problems in school before?
> What did you do about it then?
> How did it turn out?
> Have your other children had problems in school?
> Is there anything in particular you would like to ask me about the school problem, or anything you think I might do to help?

These questions help the clinician to learn the facts of the situation, the family's approach to problems, and their ability to resolve them. Incidentally, this way of gathering information can be used for any social problem that may arise. In some cases, the examiner may not ask if the family wants his or her help, but instead may say, "This is an area in which I can help you. We can discuss it further, later in the visit." Then the clinician can return to the chronological sequence of the history.

> When does Daniel usually have lunch?
> What kinds of things does he eat for lunch?
> Who eats with him at lunchtime?

The rationale and specific questions are similar to the ones used in asking about breakfast. If the clinician already has a good idea about the child's diet throughout the day, these questions can be abbreviated. If the child eats in school, in a day-care center, or at a sitter's home, the clinician may want to inquire into it specifically, especially if there is a problem about the nutritional content of the diet or if there are social problems concerning meals.

How does Daniel spend his afternoons?

Naturally, answers will vary widely according to the child's age. A preschool-age child may engage in activities similar to the ones that take place in the morning. The school-age child should have some opportunity to be with peers, and adult supervision should be appropriate to the child's age. Many children are in after-school day care, either with a sitter or in a program. As before, one should inquire about the arrangements—whether they are satisfactory—and the rationale for them if it is not obvious.

When does Daniel usually have supper?

With whom does he eat?

What kinds of things does he have for supper?

As was indicated under the breakfast discussion, the examiner should learn about the content and emotional environment at meals. If this has already been discussed, it can be omitted here.

What does Daniel do in the evening?

The stereotyped description includes a family dinner, family activities, and bedtime. However, one must be careful not to assume that this is the routine. In many families, because of work, school, or social activities of the parents—or because of social disorganization—this stereotype is not even approached. In a single-parent family, the parent may go to work at 7:00 P.M.; here it would be important for the practitioner to learn who takes care of the child, how long that arrangement has been in effect, and whether it is satisfactory. If the child watches television before going to bed, and if TV was not discussed earlier, the clinician may use this opportunity to ask questions about the content, amount, and supervision of the child's television viewing.

When does Daniel go to bed?

How many hours of sleep does he usually get at night?

This information, combined with the age of the child and amount of naptime during the day, will reveal whether the child has a reasonable amount of sleep. If the clinician or parents are concerned about this, the issue should be explored further with the parent.

Where does Daniel sleep?

Does he share his room with anyone? If so, with whom?

Does he share his bed with anyone? If so, with whom?

These questions provide information indicating whether the family makes appropriate decisions considering the resources available to them.

Are there any routines associated with going to bed?

Are there any problems at bedtime?

Going to sleep, whether for a daytime nap or at night, is a potentially difficult transition. Children of all ages periodically may have difficulty with sleep. Parents hear many kinds of advice about the amount of sleep children need, about appropriate bedtime behavior, about the length of time a young child should be allowed to cry in the crib or room without adult company, and about spoiling children. It is helpful to reassure them when this is appropriate and to give them simple guidelines. Generally, it is good for younger children to engage in a quiet activity, such as reading a story or quiet singing, before they go to bed. If there is no routine, and the child participates in noisy, exciting activity or stimulating and perhaps frightening television viewing before bed, she or he may have difficulty going to sleep. Ascertaining whether any conflicts about bedtime exist, and how the parents handle them, is an important part of the history.

Does Daniel sleep through the night?
How frequently does he wake up at night?
What does he do when he wakes up in the middle of the night?
How do you handle it?

This problem, like many others in child rearing, may be handled very simply, with no conflict, and a resolution may be found which is satisfactory for both the child and the parents. On the other hand, it may remain a source of conflict, and even become a battleground for the family.

This format has illustrated the combined use of open-ended and specific questions in a well-organized sequence. The history can be as rich and detailed as the clinician and parents wish. But it is difficult to exaggerate the importance of the detailed picture of the child and the family which is thus portrayed; indeed, it can be invaluable in health maintenance and managing problems, especially in cases where problems and family issues are complex.

CHAPTER 9

The Art of the Physical Examination

Introduction
Preliminary Considerations
    The Parent's Behavior
    Presence and Involvement of Siblings
    Alleviating the Child's Anxiety
        Infants and Toddlers
        Preschool-Age Children
        School-Age Children
        Adolescents
    What the Clinician Should Talk About
    The Clinician's Equipment
    More on Dealing with Anxieties
    The Need for Flexibility
Content and Order of the Physical Examination
    Introductory Comments Concerning the Five Age Groups
        Infants
        Toddlers
        Preschool-Age Children
        School-Age Children
        Adolescents
    Examination of the School-Age Child (six to ten years of age) and Adolescent
    Examination of the Infant (birth to six months)
    Examination of the Toddler (6 to 24 months)

Examination of the Preschool Child (24 months to 5 years)
Special Notes about Selected Elements of the Physical Examination
- Fontanelle
- Eyes
- Visual Acuity
- Ears and Throat
- Hearing
- Chest
- Abdomen
- Rectal
- Hips
- Nervous System
- Blood Pressure
- Height and Weight Measurements
- Head Circumference

INTRODUCTION

The main purpose of the physical examination is to detect illness. However, it also provides a valuable opportunity for the clinician and the child to build a good relationship with each other. How the examiner touches the child's body—an intimate and potentially intrusive gesture—is a very important factor in the child's experience of the relationship. Sensitivity on the part of the clinician to the ways in which a child is likely to subjectively experience any aspect of the physical examination is called for; and this kind of sensitivity is best developed by viewing the physical examination as a two-way communication process in which feelings, as well as factual data and instructions, are exchanged. The physical examination also provides the clinician with an opportunity to observe parent-child interaction and a chance to educate the older child about his body.

The physical examination of a well child does not take very much time; usually, about five to ten minutes is adequate. Naturally, if the child is uncooperative or if the parent has several questions it will take longer. In the case of a child with a normal history and developmental assessment, the physical examination rarely adds significant information other than that provided by a few parts such as the cardiac evaluation, the evaluation of the gait, spine, and feet, and the evaluation of growth. Screening tests are also important tools in the detection of illness in seemingly well children. If the examiner gathers a reliable history which indicates that the child is well, it pays to be selective about how thorough the physical examination will be: one should not feel bound to a ritual procedure.

Not all physical examinations will be cursory, however. When the patient or parent raises new concerns, if there are old problems (such as otitis media or eczema), or if the practitioner notices anything that might be abnormal, a thorough examination is required to evaluate the situation. Child health care practitioners must use their clinical judgment about how to set priorities in different situations. There is no set formula for clinical work, and flexibility is particularly important when examining children. Later in this chapter some examples of well-child evaluations are presented as suggestive guidelines for implementing the physical examination according to the particular circumstances of each case. It should be noted that each example is *more complete* than a usual examination, in order to show the variety of options that an examiner may elect to pursue for both the well child and one with a problem.

The physical examination can be a satisfying and positive experience for both children and parents. Children can learn to trust their health care practitioners and can feel proud that they have overcome their fears and completed an important task; parents can be pleased that their children are growing and developing well and proud of how the children are learning to cooperate and cope with a challenging experience. However, not all examinations are such unqualified successes. Many can be frustrating for the clinician, embarrassing for the parents, and frightening for the children. This is likely to happen when a child is overanxious or uncooperative, or needs to be restrained forcibly.

Children respond to the physical examination in many ways depending on their age, stage of development, verbal skills, state of health, and past experience with health care. Parents' attitudes about health care and evaluation and their emotional state at the time of an examination also are very important influences on children's behavior during a physical. (This is especially so with young children.) Other important factors are the clinician's manner and the physical environment. This chapter will discuss some of the factors which most pronouncedly influence the course of a physical examination. Additionally, it will present some techniques to enhance the quality of the whole experience for all concerned and to improve the efficiency of the examination itself. This chapter will not, however, enter into a discussion of the physical findings as such.

Even before the patient is examined, the tone of the experience for the parent and child is set by the physical environment and the behavior of the office or clinic staff (see Chapter 1). Clinicians should insist that children and parents be treated warmly and courteously by all staff and should ensure that the physical surroundings are neat, clean, and cheerful.

Experienced examiners will also take the trouble to learn about any previous unpleasant experiences related to health care practices the child or parent may have had. Although the clinician cannot alter the past, it certainly is possible to take advantage of present opportunities to assure the child or parent that the current examination will be different. When current anxiety is associated with negative past experiences, the clinician can clarify any misunderstandings and relieve unnecessary fears. It may be necessary to be especially careful to make certain parts of the examination as constructive and as pleasant as possible.

While taking individual variation into account, the clinician can predict from the child's stage of development which aspects of the examination may be most frightening and what internal resources the child quite likely has available to handle the stress. A toddler may be particularly frightened of strangers, or concerned about separation. Because of his or her minimal verbal skills anxiety will usually be expressed by being uncooperative and by crying. The older preschool child of around four years of age may not fear separation as much as the toddler, but probably will be afraid of bodily injury or pain from injections or from the examination. However, a four-year-old child has greater verbal skills and can benefit from explanations more than a toddler can. The child of school age is quite likely to be concerned about being undressed, especially in the presence of a parent. School-age children are generally quite sophisticated in their verbal skills, and thus are open to reasoned explanations of procedures and amenable to negotiated solutions for difficult aspects of the examination.

A child's state of health at the time of an examination affects his or her ability to handle stress. An ill child frequently regresses in the ability to communicate clearly, to wait for needs to be met, and to cooperate with a health care practitioner. The patient may become more infantile, including being more dependent on a parent, and also may be more sensitive to frustrations or anxiety of any kind. The examiner should consider these changes when evaluating an ill child, and therefore should be careful not to assume automatically that the child behaves that way under usual circumstances.

PRELIMINARY CONSIDERATIONS

The parent's behavior

The parent's emotional state during a child's physical examination can be the key to its success or failure. A calm parent can support even a very frightened child, whereas an anxious parent may cause a confident child to become tense. During the interview it is useful to learn about the parent's attitude toward the health evaluation, make an assessment of his or her emotional state (including how angry or nervous the parent is), and note how preoccupied the parent is with other problems.

If parents feel secure in their ability to perform adequately as parents, they usually will stay calm, support the practitioner in completing whatever parts of the physical examination are necessary, and comfort their children. This behavior can be furthered if the parent is given approval by the clinician. However, many parents feel some trepidation about this part of the visit; they may be upset, much as they would be for their own health evaluation. Thus they may find it very hard to tolerate a child's protest, and may be disturbed by whatever pain the child may experience. In addition, the clinician is an authority figure, and even a confident parent may feel embarrassed if a child regresses, becomes uncooperative, and whines during the examination.

Insecure parents must be attended to. If such a parent views the clinician as a critical person with whom he or she is not at ease, regression and uncooperativeness on the part of the child usually make the parent uncomfortable, often embarrassed, and at times angry. This may set in motion a chain of dysfunctional emotional responses: the parent may blame the child for his or her own embarrassment. Therefore, the child not only experiences failure in the physical examination itself, but also has to bear the parent's anger and rejection. This may cause the child to regress even more. If the parent then becomes more critical and less supportive of the regressing child, a destructive cycle will result which makes the health evaluation more difficult or even impossible. (It may also seriously impair future examinations.)

Frequently, a few supportive comments from the examiner to the parent in front of the child can help the parent to be more constructive and thus prevent the emergence of such regressive spirals. It is helpful to reassure the parent that he or she is not being blamed for the child's behavior and that the behavior is not abnormal. One should take care to show concern for the child and prepare both parent and child for each step and procedure. In the case of a four-year-old child, for instance, the clinician might casually tell the parent that "Checkups can be scary. Sometimes children don't act so grown up when they are having checkups. I don't mind if Robert wants to stay on your lap and suck his thumb." This does not *change* any of the underlying problems of the parent's relationship with the child, but it should help to facilitate the examination. It might also serve as a beginning for further discussions alone with the parent about the parent's expectations of the child and their relationship.

Occasionally, a parent will resort to threats of punishment or painful procedures as a way of coercing a child to cooperate. Such threats may even be an ongoing element of punishment for the child at home. Some threats verge on the bizarre: "If you don't shape up, I'll call the police!" or "I'll tell the doctor to give you a shot if you don't stay still!" This kind of behavior is often a sign of a disturbed parent-child relationship. It is very important for the clinician immediately to ask the parent not to make such threats and to tell the child that he or she will not be hurt punitively. One way to state this is, "John, while you are here there will be no police or punishments. I know you're feeling scared, but I will not do anything without explaining it to you first. Mrs. Denine, please don't threaten John. It only makes things worse. I'm not mad or upset at his behavior. He is frightened and it is hard for him to control himself." If, in fact, John will not be receiving any immunizations or having any painful laboratory procedures, it is very helpful to tell him explicitly that he "will not have any shots." Later, of course, during the clinical summary, the examiner will have to discuss this situation further with the parent.

On rare occasions, a parent will either threaten to or actually hit a child. The clinician should be firm and straightforward and take control of the situation. It is imperative to ask the parent to stop, to talk with the child, and later to talk at length with the parent alone. Nothing fancy is required. One can simply say, "Mr. Phillips, I don't allow hitting children in this office." If it seems appropriate, it may help to tell Mr. Phillips that one does not blame him for the child's behavior. For example, one might say, "Children sometimes become frightened during the checkup. It is not something they can easily control. Tina will do better if you do not hit her."

It is very important for the clinician also to reassure the child directly that there will be no hitting in the office. If Tina and Mr. Phillips cannot be reasonably calm together, it may be best for the parent to wait outside the examining room. It may be necessary to suggest this: "Sometimes it goes better if the parent waits outside, Mr. Phillips, and perhaps we should try it." Although this is in contrast to the usual principle of having the parent be present for the examination of a young child, separation may improve the situation if the parent is too upset to be helpful.

Parents frequently express concern about a particular part of the body while it is being examined. All parents have small concerns, but an examiner should be aware of the possibility that a question which seems casual and insignificant really may reflect the parent's serious concern about an abnormality or illness. If a parent expresses numerous concerns about an essentially well child, the clinician should recognize this as a clue to the presence of a significant underlying psychological problem on the part of the parent that may pose serious developmental problems for the child.

Sometimes the major task in a physical examination is to reassure a (possibly anxious) parent that no problems are present. This is especially true with parents of neonates. Parents want specifically to be told that the child does not have any abnormalities. It is frequently very helpful to point out to first-time parents some of the unique features of the neonate —such as the caput succedaneum, the umbilical stump, a vaginal discharge, and birth marks—which they might think signify abnormalities.

Certain procedures in the physical examination seem to arouse more than their share of parental interest and concern. When the clinician measures the child's blood pressure, for example, a parent may ask what the pressure is, what is considered normal for a child, at what age people begin to have high blood pressure, and whether the child should receive a low salt diet. In fact, a lot has been written in the lay press about hypertension, its familial patterns, and the theory that too much salt in the diet is a factor related to hypertension. If questions about such an issue are brought up, one should ask what thoughts the parent has had about it. If no particular reason for concern is given, the examiner is wise to ask specifically if the parent knows anyone with hypertension or if there is a family history of it (if it was not discussed earlier in the family medical history). In cases where no associated issues emerge, it still is a good idea to take the time to explain about the child's blood pressure at this point in the examination.

Another example of significant parent concern is the question frequently posed during the chest examination of an infant: "Is everything all right?" The examiner should answer seriously and honestly, and should also ask the parent whether there are any particular questions about the child's heart or chest examination that he or she wishes to bring up. There may be a significant family history of congenital heart abnormalities which prompted the parent to ask for explicit reassurance about the child's heart. If this or something similar is in fact the case, the parent should receive a thorough explanation about the child's heart and other related aspects of the child's health. A brief comment like "It's fine" is not adequate. This reassurance should then be reinforced during the clinical summary.

Occasionally, a parent is so anxious and so continuously intrusive, especially with an older child, that the clinician is best advised to ask the parent to remain in the waiting room until the examination is over. This may also be necessary with excessively overprotective parents who interfere with an examination. For instance, if a sick child refuses an essential part of the examination, the parent may undermine the clinician's efforts to be firm and to do what is necessary.

There are, of course, a myriad of other situations involving parents that will arise in pediatric examinations. Some parents will compete with the child for a clinician's attention, and the practitioner will need to find ways to limit involvement with the parent (see page 195 for use of examination tools). Some parents are utterly passive and will not offer comfort or other assistance to a child who needs it, necessitating firm directions from the clinician for the parent to help the child get dressed or to hold the child if he or she is upset. We can only alert the student to some typical situations here, but time and experience will be the real teachers of how to cope with such matters.

Presence and involvement of siblings

Not infrequently, siblings accompany the patient and parent to the health visit and are present in the examining room as well. Young children (under five years of age) do not usually express a desire for privacy from siblings, and older patients do not usually object if siblings under four or five years of age are present. However, the older patient may object if a sibling is present who is over five years of age, especially of the opposite sex. It usually is wise to ask a sibling to leave when the patient will undergo an uncomfortable procedure, such as a rectal examination, blood tests, or removal of cerumen from an ear canal. Children undergoing such procedures may get more upset when a sibling is present, and the procedure may make the sibling anxious as well. If the clinician detects discomfort on the part of a patient (even if the child says nothing overt), it is advisable to ask the sibling to step out of the room. Of course, if the health visit is a simple follow-up for an ear infection, perhaps, or for a rash on the arms, the issue of a sibling's presence may be unimportant.

Frequently, an older sibling who remains calm can be a model for a younger, more anxious child. The examiner can actually use such an older sibling as a demonstration model, to illustrate exactly what procedures will be performed on the patient. If the older sibling also has been scheduled for an examination, this can be done before the younger child is examined, with the younger child in attendance. The school-age child is often proud to be a role model for a younger sibling.

Younger siblings who accompany a patient are often interested in the examiner's tools: they may want to play with the hammer, light, and stethoscope during the visit. Even if this is not a scheduled visit for the accompanying child, it may be an excellent opportunity for the clinician to work on their relationship, to help the child perceive the clinician in a much less threatening way. It is very helpful to allow time for interacting with the younger sibling, so that at future visits the clinician and this child will not be strangers to each other.

Alleviating the child's anxiety

The practitioner's behavior is one of the most significant factors in helping the child and parent feel comfortable during a physical examination. Clinicians who are patient, interested, appropriately approving, honest, and sensitive to the child's concerns will have good rapport with most children and their parents, and so will be able to make them more comfortable during the physical examination. Abrupt, distracted, critical, dishonest, or inconsiderate clinicians will not develop the rapport and trust necessary for a successful evaluation and a constructive continuing relationship.

An examination should never be done in silence. Experienced clinicians talk to the child and parent during the examination, both to alleviate their anxiety and to give directions. In effect, the main purpose of such conversation is to facilitate the examination (not really to elicit information). Thus, it should begin as the physical examination is introduced, after the history and developmental assessment, and continue throughout the evaluation. Such conversing is an art and must be cultivated. It should not include irrelevant social conversation, nor extraneous medical history. Nor is it good for the examiner to talk just to relieve his or her own anxiety, since doing so will generally communicate these feelings to the family and make everybody uncomfortable. Some clinicians even joke or sing during the examination, which can be quite acceptable and often helps to relax everyone. However, it is very important that clinicians do not tease as part of their joking. Teasing, especially in a serious situation like a health visit, can be hostile and detrimental to a good relationship with the family.

Practitioners are also well advised not to talk down to their patients. School-age children will be insulted if they are spoken to as if they were four-year-olds. With experience, the student health care practitioner will learn to tell the degree of sophistication of a child and will develop several repertoires of explanations to suit the individual needs of each patient.

Infants and Toddlers: At the end of the history, the clinician should indicate to the parent of the infant or young toddler that the next portion of the visit will be the physical examination. It helps to ask the parent to partially undress the child so that the examiner can observe and listen to the child's chest. If the child is quiet and fairly relaxed, it is better to leave the child undisturbed in the parent's lap or on the examining table. (Of course, a child playing contentedly on the floor would have to be picked up at this point.) Toddlers should be examined either on the examining table with the parent next to it, or on the parent's lap. If the older toddler does not want to undress, the clinician should proceed as discussed below for the preschool-age child.

If the child is a toddler, the clinician will have to make a decision about how to treat the child: more like an infant or more like a preschool-age child. A child who is immature in terms of verbal abilities should be treated more like an infant, with most of the conversation directed toward the parent. A child who is more advanced in verbal skills can be spoken to directly, along with the parent. Frequently, clinicians underestimate the toddler's ability to understand conversation and so miss valuable opportunities to gain a patient's cooperation through verbal interaction.

Preschool-Age Children: If the child is of preschool age, the clinician might say, "Now we can do the checkup. I would like to look at your eyes, watch you walk, listen to your chest with my stethoscope (pointing to the stethoscope at the same time), and do a few other things. You can stay next to your father. As we go along, I'll tell you about each part of the checkup." It is unreasonable to *expect* the child to leave the parent's side, although many children will be comfortable enough to sit on the examining table. Many clinicians begin the examination by asking to look at the child's hands and feet and by examining the eyes with a flashlight. These maneuvers are relatively innocuous in that they do not require the examiner to touch the child immediately or the child to get undressed initially.

School-Age Children: It is always important for the clinician to use language appropriate for the child's verbal skills. School-age children understand directions quite well and will be insulted if the examiner speaks below their language level. One can say to the child, "OK, we're going to do the checkup now. I'd like you to take off all your clothes except your underpants, and put on this gown" (handing it to the child). It frequently helps for the clinician to leave the room while the patient undresses, especially if the child is of the opposite sex or is old enough to feel uncomfortable about disrobing. Sometimes older children who are the same sex as the examiner are also very self-conscious about disrobing, and this may be an indication of a problem. Clinicians should tell the child they will be back shortly to do the physical examination.

If a child expresses discomfort at having the parent present during the examination, the clinician should respect that feeling and ask the parent to wait in another room until the examination is completed. Sometimes it is necessary for a clinician to take the initiative in this if she or he perceives the child is uncomfortable about the parent's presence, but, for one reason or another, cannot articulate this. Many clinicians will ask the parent to leave in order to have some private time together with the patient, even if the child is not uncomfortable. This is especially helpful with older school-age children (about nine or ten years old).

Adolescents: Conversation with adolescent patients is essentially the same as it is with adults, perhaps with less use of technical terms. The examiner gives directions, acknowledges the patient's cooperation, and gives feedback when appropriate. The parent should not be present during the physical examination. After it is completed, the clinician can discuss his or her findings during the clinical summary.

What the clinician should talk about

Clinicians should choose their words carefully as they move from one part of the examination to the next. Sensitivity and forethought about what to say—or what not to say—are particularly called for with preschool and young school-age children, with whom misunderstandings can easily occur. For example, although taking blood pressure is a painless procedure, many practitioners forget how it might appear to a four-year-old child. If an examiner tells a four-year-old "I am going to take your blood pressure now," the child will probably think the clinician is going to draw a blood specimen with a needle. Therefore, it would be better to say, "I want to show you something called a pressure cuff. It has a piece of cloth, a rubber tube, a ball to squeeze that pumps air, and a special clock. Have you seen one like it before?" The clinician can adapt his or her description of the steps of the procedure to the level of knowledge indicated in the child's response. The extra effort put into an age-appropriate description will add greatly to the relationship between clinician and child and will help avoid unnecessary fear and uncooperative behavior.

Directions for each part of the examination should also be modified according to the patient's stage of development. In a cardiac examination, for instance, the clinician needs an opportunity to listen to the front and back of the child's chest while the child is quiet and not moving about. If the patient is an infant, the examiner will be able to give directions to the parent about how to hold or comfort and quiet the child. A toddler is generally treated much the same as an infant, except that the clinician may ask the parent to distract the child (with a toy, another stethoscope, or any other handy object); or it may be possible for the clinician to distract the child while doing the examination. A preschool-age child who is not particularly frightened should be able to stay still enough for the clinician to perform an adequate examination. The examiner may ask the child to hold his or her breath, breathe with the mouth closed, and turn around so that the back can be examined. Instructions may have to be supplemented by demonstration, with either the parent or the clinician holding his or her breath for the child to see. School-age children, on the other hand, should be able to cooperate with instructions that the clinician would use for an adult, but with words appropriate for the child's verbal skills. One might, for example, ask the child to "take a deep breath," instead of to "inhale deeply."

Toddlers and preschool-age children are particularly interested in explicit positive communication from the practitioner. It is very productive for a clinician to tell a child who has cooperated for an examination, for instance, "You did a good job with that. It helps a lot when we work together." A toddler may not understand complex sentences, but will appreciate the positive tone. As we mentioned earlier, the physical examination is a stressful event for almost all children, and they deserve recognition for their cooperation.

But, as always, the clinician should take care to act appropriately for a child's developmental stage. An older child might take an explicit comment as belittling or patronizing. However, even a teenager will appreciate some positive feedback at the end, especially if she or he was anxious about the examination. It certainly is appropriate to let the older child know that one recognizes how the child has been helpful by saying, "I appreciate your cooperation during the checkup."

Children as young as six or seven years of age are quite interested in how their bodies work. (Younger children are interested as well, but the task of overcoming their fears is usually more prominent.) They may be particularly interested in why their heart beats sound irregular, or what clinicians see when they examine the eyes with an ophthalmoscope. The clinician who allows time for such questions and answers them honestly, in a way that is appropriate for the child's intellectual abilities, will build a positive relationship with the patient as the child becomes more comfortable during the evaluation. Education about the body becomes an increasingly important function of the examination in the prepubertal and adolescent years, one that is quite separate from the efforts to allay anxiety about the physical examination as a procedure. The patient who has had satisfying discussions with a health care practitioner throughout childhood will be comfortable in asking about the body and its functions when he or she is older and is concerned about pubertal changes.

In certain cases, the examiner will feel that the parent, and sometimes the older child, should be given immediate feedback about a part of the examination. This is particularly true when the visit is for evaluation of a particular complaint or if it is a well-child examination for a very young child and the parent is concerned about a congenital abnormality. In cases where a family does need this feedback, and the part of the examination in question is normal, it is helpful for the clinician to give the family this information right away to alleviate anxiety and then to indicate that they can talk about it more when the entire examination is completed. If something is abnormal, the clinician will have to decide whether it would alleviate anxiety or be disruptive to mention it at that time during the examination. If, for example, the visit is to evaluate a fever, the family might well be relieved to learn that the child has an infected ear, which can be treated and cured easily. However, if the visit is a well-child health evaluation, discussion of a newly discovered heart murmur would best be left until the physical examination is completed and the clinician can enter into a thorough discussion with the parents.

The clinician's equipment

Many children like to handle the clinician's equipment during the interview and the physical examination. This should be encouraged, because it helps the child become more familiar with the tools and consequently less frightened of them. Frequently, parents feel uncomfortable when a child reaches for equipment, and they try to restrain the patient from doing so. It is helpful to tell such parents that "It is OK for John to play with the hammer and the stethoscope." One can then hand John the tools and observe what he does with them. Many children like to use the stethoscope on themselves. Some will initiate this, others will do it only after the clinician suggests it, and sometimes a shy child will refuse an invitation to listen to his or her own heart.

On rare occasions, a parent will ask to use some of the tools. In most cases, this parent is immature, identifies with the child, and even competes with the child for the clinician's attention. If a parent asks to use the tools, it is better to let this person use the instrument briefly, and then proceed with the examination of the child.

A clinician may want to invite a young child who is anxious to handle some equipment in order to assure the child that the tools are not painful. The blood pressure cuff is often not familiar to the preschool-age child, and so may be particularly frightening; therefore, the child may benefit from playing with it before the blood pressure measurement is taken.

Another way to alleviate the anxiety of the child from about 18 months to 7 years of age is to demonstrate the use of the equipment on the parent, on older siblings, or on oneself. For instance, the ear examination is often frightening. If a child sees the clinician examine the parent, and perhaps sees the parent look in the clinician's ears, and if the patient also can look through the otoscope into the examiner's ears, the child may be convinced that it is not so terrible. Although most children are usually still anxious, if they can control themselves enough to stay still, without particularly vigorous restraint by adults, the entire examination of the ears can be done painlessly within a few seconds. Once children have some positive clinical experiences, they will begin to trust the clinician and will be able to relax and cooperate during the remainder of an examination and in future examinations as well.

Sometimes children feel less anxious if they can help the clinician during an examination. Naturally, the opportunities for this are limited; they include having the child place a hand on top of or under the clinician's hand during the abdominal examination and during the perineal examination, and hold the "clock" of the blood pressure apparatus (if it is portable) while the practitioner squeezes the bulb. This type of participation is helpful for the older preschool and early school-age child.

Frequently the examining table is frightening to a child. It may represent alien territory where the patient gives up control to the examiner and child is separated from parent. Any frightened child should have the option of having as much of the examination as possible done while standing or seated next to the parent or seated on the parent's lap. A school-age child who is so frightened that she or he cannot be comfortable on the examining table should be allowed to remain near the parent. However, the clinician should evaluate the causes for this fear, and its broader implications for the child's emotional maturity. This should not be done during the physical examination, but during the clinical summary later in the visit.

More on dealing with anxieties

Children who are deaf or who cannot understand verbal instructions because they are mentally retarded frequently do understand simple demonstrations; certainly they benefit from being able to hold and touch the equipment before the clinician uses it. Even the opportunity to hold and feel a cotton swab will teach the child that it is not a needle and will not hurt. This can prevent much unnecessary fear and combative behavior.

On rare occasions, a child will be calm and comfortable during the entire interview, and even during the developmental assessment. Then, suddenly, the patient will become very frightened and obstinate when the physical examination begins. At this point the examiner should stop the proceedings and ask the patient (if the child is old enough) or the parent what is wrong or what the child is frightened of. The most common fear is of injections. Clinicians should be honest about whether or not there will be injections. It is important to ask the parent what the child's past experiences with previous health care practitioners have been like and whether the child usually finds health evaluations stressful. It may turn out, for instance, that the child has been frightened ever since being severely restrained in the course of having a laceration sutured in an emergency room, nine months prior to the current visit. If that is the case, one can talk directly to the child, explain how this checkup is different from the prior experience, and assure the child that there will not be any stitches or restraints. The child may be able to trust the examiner immediately, or may look to the parent for assurance. If the parent is reasonably calm and the examiner plans the order of the physical examination carefully, the child will probably be able to cooperate. This will be an important step in the child's growing up.

Occasionally, a patient, usually a toddler or young preschool age child, is so anxious and frightened that she or he cannot relax enough to cooperate with the clinician. Once again it is appropriate to balance the need for a complete health evaluation with the long-range goal of building a trusting, cooperative relationship with the child.

The need for flexibility

It is important not to be bound to a ritual physical examination; clinicians should separate what is necessary from what is useful but not vital. It is important to remain flexible in using one's judgment about deciding what data to gather from the history, developmental assessment, and laboratory tests; and there is no reason at all for an examiner to be inhibited about modifying the physical examination as well, to suit specific circumstances.

If—based on the history, developmental and physical observations—there is every reason to believe the child is well, there is no reason for a clinician to feel obliged to complete the physical examination at that visit. If the patient is especially anxious, it may well be to the patient's advantage to have time to "acclimate"—to play in the clinician's office, listen to the conversation with the parent, and have a limited examination, even without undressing. The health care practitioner and parent together may decide to schedule another appointment in several weeks and to complete the examination at that time. Nonurgent booster injections and laboratory tests should also be postponed in this situation. Some children may need several office visits before they are comfortable.

If the history or observations reveal any information which suggests possible problems, it is imperative that the clinician be conscientious about gathering all the necessary data to assess the child's health adequately. This must take precedence over concerns about the child's anxiety. The patient-clinician relationship is preserved by being honest at all times, even when the clinician decides that the child must be held and forcibly examined. Although the child will probably not feel or act very friendly to the clinician, it is usually a great relief to have the dreaded examination finished and important for the child to know that the clinician was honest about the discomfort. It is when practitioners feel guilty about restraining a frightened child that they may become very angry, apologetic, or inconsistent.

CONTENT AND ORDER OF THE PHYSICAL EXAMINATION

A clinician's goal is to gather whatever data are necessary to provide the patient with adequate care while causing the least amount of distress. Consequently, in planning each examination the clinician must consider both the order of the components and how thorough the examination should be. In every case it is necessary to individualize the physical examination to fit the needs of the particular patient. The plan or strategy must take into account both the medical importance of the data elicited in each part of the examination and the degree of anxiety that each procedure is likely to cause the patient.

If a child or parent has a specific complaint, the clinician must gather enough information to make an adequate decision about diagnosis and management. A three-year-old child who has a cold does not need to be examined for hernias, strabismus, or abnormal gait. However, a thorough evaluation of this patient's nose, throat, ears, and chest is called for —even in the face of possible resistance by the child. A full physical examination should also be peformed if this is the child's first visit, if she or he has not yet had regular health care, or if the history or initial parts of the examination suggest physical problems more serious than a mere cold.

If a child is severely ill, only the measures necessary for diagnosis and immediate treatment should be done initially. For example, a child with asthma might be in severe respiratory distress. The examiner should evaluate the airway, lungs, heart, and vital signs first. The patient should then be given whatever medication or cardio-respiratory assistance is indicated. The clinician should complete the examination only after the respiratory distress is treated.

If there is no presenting complaint and the examination is part of a general health evaluation, the physical examination will evaluate the patient's entire body in an order which is appropriate to the child's stage of development (see the following section). The components of the physical examination should be arranged in a sequence that takes advantage of the child's resources and minimizes the stress on the patient. Hence, components which are the least upsetting and which require the most cooperation from the child should be near the beginning of the examination. Components which seem intrusive, upsetting, or uncomfortable to a patient are best left until later in the visit or until the end when the child is more accustomed to both the experience and the examiner, and everything else has been accomplished in a satisfactory manner.

Introductory comments concerning the five age groups

As we have just indicated, the order in which the components of a physical examination are best undertaken will vary according to each child's age and stage of development. The details of the examination will be presented separately for five different age groups: infant, toddler, preschool, school-age, and adolescent. The five groups are used here as rough guidelines; flexibility in application is crucial because there are areas of overlap between age groups and individual variations within each group.

Infants: Infants from birth to six months of age are generally quite easy to examine—they have minimal stranger anxiety, little memory, and are distractible and easily comforted. Although the six- to twelve-month-old child is not yet quite considered a toddler, the physical examination needs to be modified from about six months on because the child becomes more wary of strangers and frequently reacts more negatively when touched by a clinician. These changes occur even before the child begins to "toddle" or ambulate.

Toddlers: Children from 6 to 24 months of age, or "toddlers," are probably the most difficult age group to examine. They are acutely aware of strangers, have a memory for recent events (including frightening or painful clinical procedures), and limited verbal skills. It is difficult to distract a toddler who is anxious or frightened. In addition, clinicians frequently underestimate the ability of older toddlers to comprehend language, and thus lose valuable opportunities to help their toddler patients understand what is happening. Simple statements like "I want to touch your tummy" or "Look at my light" can aid immeasurably in smoothing out an examination. The older toddler can benefit from demonstrations of parts of the physical examination, such as the use of the otoscope on a parent, older sibling, or even the clinician. Toddlers enjoy imitation, and may want to manipulate instruments and equipment along with the examiner.

Preschool-Age Children: This group—from two to five years of age—are still vulnerable to stranger anxiety, fear of bodily injury, and the desire to control the world around them. However, they have more resources than do toddlers, including verbal skills which help them to understand what is happening and to express their feelings and concerns. They also have good memories for past events, including past visits to health care practitioners. Preschool-age children can understand directions and cooperate with the examination much better than can toddlers. Demonstrating parts of the examination and giving the child permission to handle the examiner's tools can be extremely helpful in alleviating the patient's fears. A child of this age usually wants to act "grown-up," will try to cooperate, and will experience pleasure from a successful visit with the clinician.

There are some important developmental changes during the preschool-age period which affect the course of an examination. The average child who has not had unusually frightening experiences or memories of past health evaluations will be cooperative and easy to examine at two and one half to three years of age. However, as some children approach four or five years of age, they become much more afraid of bodily mutilation. They view the examination as an attack and are more frightened and uncooperative than when they were younger. Parents are surprised when their child, who was "so good last year," is now difficult to examine. They usually feel ashamed and/or guilty about what they assume is their failure in child rearing, and they may become angry at the child. It is very important for the clinician to explain this change to the parents and to reassure them that this difficulty is usually transient. One way to put it is "Sometimes children are frightened at this age, even if they were not frightened when they were younger. It's not something Ruthie does on purpose, and there's nothing you could have done to avoid this. We'll do the checkup as well as possible." At the same time, it helps if the clinician takes a little time to talk to the child, to try to alleviate her anxiety and tell her what they will do together.

School-Age Children: Children between six and ten years of age still have many fears and concerns but also have much more sophisticated resources with which to handle their anxieties. As they grow older they develop advanced verbal skills; they usually have had more positive experiences (it is hoped!) with health care and can call upon memories of these past experiences to reassure themselves; and they understand the difference between routine health evaluations and medical and nursing care during illness.

Throughout this age group fear of bodily injury persists, but it usually is less frightening than for the younger child of four to six years of age. Additional issues for school-age children are the desire for privacy and increasing independence from parents. The child may not want a parent to be present during the examination and usually does not want to undress in front of a parent, especially of the opposite sex. As the child nears puberty, he or she may become more uncomfortable about being with a parent and also with a clinician of the opposite sex. Occasionally, a sensitive patient feels so strongly about it that only a clinician of the same sex should care for the child.

Most children from six to ten years of age are better able to sort out current circumstances from fearful memories and are thus more capable of cooperating and participating actively than the younger preschool-age child. However, the concerns and sensitivities of school-age children are just as important and often more complex than those of the younger child. The practitioner who remembers these sensitivities, and takes the time to make the child comfortable early in the visit, will usually find it easy to perform a very complete physical examination.

Adolescents: Adolescents should be treated individually, according to their maturity, degree of comfort, and reason for the examination. The major difference in the examination of the adolescent patient is evaluation of pubertal changes. Not infrequently a patient is uncomfortable and/or confused about these changes. In all cases, this part of the physical examination provides an excellent opportunity to educate the adolescent about bodily changes during this period. The examination may also provide a shy adolescent with an "excuse" to ask questions not mentioned previously.

The examination generally follows the procedure presented for the school-age child. However, the breast examination and evaluation of the external genitalia are performed to carefully evaluate the stage of pubertal development and the presence of pathological conditions of adolescence. Pelvic examinations are much more frequently performed in this age group, usually when the adolescent is sexually active.

We now proceed to a somewhat detailed discussion of each of these stages in relation to the physical examination. The examination of the school-age child and adolescent is presented first, since it is most like that of an adult and the reader can use it as a baseline for comparison with the examinations for the other age groups of children described subsequently.

Examination of school-age child (six to ten years of age) and adolescent

The examination discussed here is for a thorough health evaluation of a healthy prepubertal school-age child (for the sake of convenience we shall use a girl) who is comfortable with the examiner. She has the usual concerns about privacy and independence but is a competent child without handicaps. This examination is essentially the same as one for an adult, except that certain components which are important for the adult would not be done here: prostate, rectal, internal gynecological, and extensive breast examinations.

♦ The patient should be sitting on the examining table at the beginning of the examination. She would be wearing underpants and, since she is a girl, a gown as well.

1. Observation of general appearance. Although the examiner has had the opportunity to observe the child throughout the interview, she should be observed more thoroughly now that she is undressed, with a special focus on physical features.
2. Measurement of blood pressure, pulse, and respiratory rate.
3. Observation and palpation of the head, scalp, and hair.
4. Observation and palpation of the face, eyes, ear pinnae, and mouth, without any equipment. Tests for six cardinal directions of gaze, accommodation of pupils and strabismus. Optional: visual fields by confrontation, usually only done in evaluation of possible intracranial tumor.
5. Examination of the eyes with light: conjunctivae, and reaction of pupils to light.
6. Examination of the nose, mouth, and throat with light. Use of tongue depressor only if necessary; avoid posterior one third of tongue, where gag reflex is triggered.
7. Examination of ears with otoscope.
8. Examination of eyes with ophthalmoscope.
9. Examination of head and neck for cranial nerve function. This may be reserved for the end of the physical examination and then incorporated into the neurological examination.
10. Observation and palpation of the neck.
11. Palpation of the axillae.

♦ At this point, the child's gown should be moved for each part of the chest examination, so that the chest is exposed and the examiner can observe and listen to the chest directly; the chest examination cannot be done adequately through clothing.

12. Observation, palpation, and auscultation of the anterior chest.
13. Observation and palpation of the breasts (especially in the pubescent child).
14. Observation, palpation, percussion, and auscultation of posterior chest.
15. Palpation of the neck for enlargement of the thyroid gland. Examiner is behind the patient and the examiner's fingers are on the patient's anterior neck.

♦ Now the child should be asked to lie down, so the examination can proceed in the supine position on the examining table.

16. Percussion and auscultation of anterior chest.

♦ The patient should roll slightly to her left side.

17. Auscultation of the left anterior chest.

♦ The child should roll back again to the supine position. Her underpants should be lowered, although not removed, so that her abdomen is uncovered.

18. Observation, auscultation, percussion, and palpation of the abdomen.

19. Palpation of the femoral pulses.

20. Palpation of the posterior flank, bilaterally.

♦ Next, the patient should roll to her right side.

21. Palpation of the spleen.

♦ The child should return to the supine position.

22. Observation and palpation of the lower extremities.

♦ Since the patient is a girl, she should remain supine with the hips and knees flexed or be in the frog-leg position. Her underpants should be lowered below the pelvis, or removed.

23. Observation and palpation of the external genitalia and anus, and evaluation for hernias.*

♦ Boys should stand on the floor facing the practitioner; the underpants should be below the pelvis, or removed. For visualization of the anus, a boy should bend at the hips, leaning on the examining table or supporting his arms on his thighs. Examination of the anus for both girls and boys can also be accomplished in the left lateral position with the hips and knees flexed, for the right-handed practitioners, or the right lateral position for a left-handed practitioner.

Continuing with the physical, the examiner asks both boys and girls to sit on the examining table with their feet over the side; they may keep their underpants on; female patients may keep on their gowns.

24. Observation, palpation of the upper extremities.

25. Neurological examination; include head and neck for cranial nerves, deep tendon reflexes in upper and lower extremities, tests of coordination and sensation. NOTE: the extent of the neurological examination will vary, depending on clinical circumstances (see p. 221 of this chapter).

♦ The patient should now stand with her back to the clinician.

26. Examination of the back for scoliosis, both standing straight and bending at the hips.

27. Evaluation of balance, stance, and gait.

♦ The legs, feet, and gait should always be evaluated without any shoes, socks, or leg coverings, since these may obscure the view of the parts being examined.

♦ The child should be invited to get dressed and should join her parent and the examiner during the clinical summary.

Examination of the infant (birth to six months)

The examination discussed here is for a thorough health evaluation of an infant (this time a male) who is presumably well. Children this young do not usually have stranger anxiety, nor do they sustain, for long periods of

---

* The pelvic examination will not be elaborated upon here. It is not a routine part of the evaluation of the school-age child and is usually only included for the sexually active adolescent or one with symptoms in the pelvic area. See suggested readings for relevant references.

time, vigorous objections to specific parts of an examination. The infant should remain where he was during the interview, if he is comfortable and if the health care practitioner can observe him adequately. Usually, this position is on the parent's lap or on the examining table. The clothes should *not* be removed initially.

1. Observation of the infant. Especially note general appearance, nutritional status, skin color, respiratory pattern, pulsation of the fontanelle, facial features, and spontaneous movements. If the child is asleep, it is important to observe the quality of sleep, including the startle response. If he is alert and content, one should note orienting behavior, including the directing of eyes, at the beginning of the examination.

2. Observation and auscultation of the anterior chest. This should be followed by palpation of the anterior chest and percussion (with child supine), if indicated by a history of medical problems.

• The parent should support him in the sitting position on his or her lap, or on the examining table, or the infant may be held over the parent's shoulder.

3. Auscultation of the posterior chest. Palpation and percussion as indicated by medical problems.

4. Palpation of fontanelle, if the child is not crying (see p. 212 of this chapter).

• At this point there are two options: for the young infant, it is easiest to take off all the clothes, to weigh and measure him, and to place him on the examining table in the supine position. The parent should be next to the table so that the child cannot roll off and the parent can observe the examination. Alternatively, if the child is particularly restless or irritable, the examiner may prefer to leave the infant supine on the parent's lap and to postpone the height and weight measurements until later.

5. Observation, auscultation, percussion, and palpation of the abdomen.

6. Palpation of femoral pulses.

7. Examination of the hips (see p. 221).

• If the child had earlier been examined on the parent's lap, this maneuver would be performed after the eye examination, when he is on the examining table.

8. Examination of the eyes for directions of gaze and ability to follow a moving object with the eyes; use a brightly colored object or a light.

9. Examination of the eyes with a light for the appearance of the conjunctivae and for the reactions of pupils to light.

10. Examination of the eyes with the ophthalmoscope.

• The child should next be placed in the supine position on the examining table.

11. Observation and palpation of the head, fontanelle (if not done earlier), scalp, hair, face, and ear pinnae.

12. Observation and palpation of the neck.

13. The child's muscle tone and strength in his upper and lower extremities should be evaluated next. Then evaluate the strength of his grasp. Deep tendon reflexes may be tested if the child is relaxed. Patellar reflexes are the easiest ones to elicit, but the heel (Achilles), brachial, and triceps reflexes may be observed. The feet should be dorsiflexed to test for the presence of clonus. NOTE: transient clonus in the neonate is considered normal.

♦ At this point the child should be placed in the prone position on the examining table.

14. Auscultation of the posterior chest, if not done earlier.
15. Observation of the child's gross motor skills, including his ability to raise his head and shoulders from the table, to crawl or creep, to roll over, and to move toward an object out of reach.
16. Examination of the lower extremities, in particular their symmetry and the symmetry of the gluteal folds.

♦ To proceed, the clinician should hold the child up in the standing position with his hands under the child's axillae.

17. Evaluation of body tone, head control, and the ability to bear weight on his legs.
18. Several infant reflexes can be evaluated in different positions in the child under five months of age: tonic neck, sucking, stepping, parachute, and back incurvation. The test for the Moro reflex can be upsetting and so should be done later (see #22, below).

♦ A child over four months of age should now be propped in the sitting position, with support from the examiner. (This may also be done after #4, before the infant is placed in the supine position for the abdominal examination.)

19. Evaluation of the child's ability to sit alone, or the beginning components of this skill, such as back support and head control.

♦ The child should be placed in the supine position on the examining table.

20. Observation of the mouth, with light and tongue depressor.
21. Examination of the ears with the otoscope. NOTE: detailed discussion of restraint positions for the examination of the ears and mouth are on page 214 of this chapter.
22. In the child under six months of age, the test for the presence of the Moro reflex should be performed. It is usually not present after four months of age.

♦ To finish the examination, one can seat the child on the examining table, or on the parent's lap, with whatever support is needed.

23. Measurement of the head circumference. NOTE: see page 224 of this chapter for comments.
24. Measurement of the height and weight, if not done earlier in the examination.

♦ The child can then be allowed to relax on the parent's lap or examining table, so that the clinician can talk with the parent. (It is better not to feed the infant at this time if he will be getting injections later. Not infrequently, the child will vomit when he cries as a result of an injection.)

Examination of the toddler (6 to 24 months)

The toddler (once again a male) has increasing verbal abilities and a new interest in people and things in his environment. He also is more wary of strangers and is concerned about separation. More than in any other age group, the physical examination of the toddler is best done on the parent's lap and with the parent's help. The order of the examination is different for the toddler because it is wise for him to get to know the clinician through the most playful parts at the beginning of the examination. Thus it is best to undertake those elements which require the most cooperation in the middle of the examination and to leave the most threatening or upsetting parts until the end. In general, it is best not to undress the child completely before the examination begins, but to undress only the part of the body being examined. This is especially true if the child actively objects to being undressed. Here the clinician should specifically ask the parent to undress the child only when necessary, as the examination proceeds. However, if the child has been very comfortable during the interview and developmental assessment, he can sometimes be completely undressed, except for the diaper or underpants, at the beginning of the examination.

Discussed here is the complete examination of a moderately shy toddler who is healthy. He is comfortable near his parent, and he will allow the clinician to perform the examination. The child is seated on his parent's lap, or is playing nearby in the examining room.

1. Observation of the child. The clinician has been observing the child throughout the interview and developmental assessment. However, she or he now has the opportunity to focus these observations on physical features including the child's general appearance, growth, body proportions, nutritional status, skin color (including cyanosis and pallor) and respiratory movements, and on whether he appears healthy or acutely or chronically ill.

▸ At this point the child should be seated on the parent's lap or on the examining table, with the parent nearby.

2. Observation and palpation of the hands and feet. This provides a nonthreatening, playful way for the child and clinician to make their initial contact during the physical examination.

3. Examination of the eyes for cardinal directions of gaze, strabismus, and pupillary reactions to light. The flashlight serves both as an attractive, noninvasive object of interest for the child and as a useful tool for the clinician.

4. Observation of the mouth. If the child is particularly comfortable, he may respond well to requests for a "smile" to show his teeth, and then to open his mouth wide and say "ahhh" so that the clinician can observe the oral cavity and pharynx. The tongue depressor should not be used at this time (it is too intrusive and upsetting); if necessary, it can be used near the end of the examination.

5. Examination of the eyes with the ophthalmoscope. The toddler cannot follow complex instructions, and so the routine eye examination usually is limited to a rapid examination of the eye for opacities, red reflex, vessels, and sometimes the optic disc.

6. Observation and palpation of the head, scalp, face, ear pinnae, and neck. This procedure brings the examiner closer to the child, but still will generally not frighten him.

• If the child was not completely undressed at the beginning of the examination, his chest should be exposed at this time. If he is completely nude from the waist up, the examination will be more efficient. If, however, the child is particularly shy or frightened, the clinician may have to examine the chest by holding up the shirt but not removing it completely. It is never acceptable to examine the chest through the clothes. The child should be kept seated for the chest examination.

7. Observation, palpation, auscultation of the anterior and posterior chest. Percussion is not routinely performed on an otherwise well toddler with a normal chest examination; however, if it is called for, this would be the appropriate time to do it, on the posterior chest.

• Next, the child should have the clothes below his waist removed, except for the diapers or underpants. He should be in the supine position, either on the examining table or on his parent's lap.

8. Auscultation of the anterior chest (palpation as indicated).

9. Observation, auscultation, and palpation of the abdomen and femoral pulses.

• The examiner should now proceed to take off the child's diapers or underpants while he is in the supine position.

10. Observation and palpation of the external genitalia and anus.

11. Evaluation of symmetry and anatomy of lower extremities.

• The child's underpants or diapers should be replaced, and the child returned to the sitting position. He should be either on the examining table or on the parent's lap.

12. Neurological examination. In the "average" case, assessment of the child's muscle strength and tone and evaluation of the deep tendon reflexes would be appropriate at this point in the examination. Of course, other observations from the developmental assessment in the preceeding physical examination contribute to the neurological examination. (See page 212 for a detailed discussion of how to determine what is an appropriate neurological examination.)

13. Observation and palpation of upper and lower extremities. (The

evaluation of the lower extremities supplements that in #11 but does not replace it.) This can be done at any time during the examination, but it is placed here because it does not require very much cooperation from the child; it could also be somewhat upsetting if it were placed earlier and the child was not yet ready for the clinician to handle his body.

◆ To proceed, the examiner should have the young toddler stand up on the examining table with whatever support he needs; he should stand on the floor if he is learning or able to walk.

14. Observation of the back, symmetry of the lower extremities, anatomy of the lower legs, feet, and gait. Frequently, the parent will have to walk beside the child, either to help him balance, or for psychological support.

◆ Now the child should be seated on the parent's lap.

15. Examination of the ears with the otoscope.

16. Examination of the mouth with light and tongue depressor. Omit mouth examination if it was successfully performed earlier. If the patient is at all fearful, for both the ear and mouth examinations, the clinician will probably want to use some demonstrations with the parent before looking in the child's ears. See page 215 for a detailed description of techniques of holding the child and ways to help him feel more at ease.

◆ If the ear and mouth examinations were performed on the examining table in the supine position, the child should now sit, either on the table or on the parent's lap.

17. Measurement of the head circumference. A demonstration of the tape measure on the clinician's head may reassure the child that the head measurement is not uncomfortable. If the child is frightened or irritable, the parent may have to hold the child's head still. Head circumference should be measured at each well child visit until the child is 24 months of age, and subsequently every two years.

18. Measurement of height and weight.

◆ After this, the child should be dressed. While the clinician and parent talk, the child may play while seated on the parent's lap, on the examining table, or on the floor. As with the infant, it is best not to feed the child if he will be having injections before the end of the visit; this is to prevent vomiting in the event of vigorous crying.

Examination of the preschool child (24 months to 5 years)

The child at this age has more verbal skills and more patience, and increasingly relates directly to the health care practitioner instead of making contact through the parent. As with younger children, any part of the examination that might be frightening is best left until the end. Parts which require more cooperation are done after the child is familiar with the clinician and before any upsetting sections of the examination are performed.

The child's comfort with the examiner will determine whether the examination is done on the parent's lap, next to the parent, or on the examining table.

It is most efficient if the child is undressed, except for underpants or diapers, at the beginning of the examination. If, however, the child has been particularly uncomfortable during the earlier parts of the visit, or if he or she objects to being undressed, the examiner can allow the child to disrobe gradually as the examination proceeds.

The examination presented below is for the complete evaluation of a moderately shy preschool-age child (girl) who is healthy. She is comfortable with her parent nearby and is willing to let the clinician examine her.

1. Measurement of height and weight. (If the child is particularly unwilling to leave the parent's lap and to get undressed, these measurements can be done at the end of the examination.)

▸ The child should be seated on the examining table, on a chair next to the parent, or on the parent's lap.

2. Observation of the child. The clinician has been observing the child throughout the interview and developmental assessment; however, she or he now has the opportunity to focus observations on physical features, including the child's general appearance, growth, body proportions, nutritional status, skin color (including pallor and cyanosis), respiratory movements, and whether she appears healthy or acutely or chronically ill.

3. Observation of head and face. It is best *not* to palpate the head at this time, because the child may not feel ready to have the clinician handle her body.

4. Examination of the eyes for the cardinal directions of gaze, tests for strabismus, pupillary reaction to light and accommodation, and appearance of the conjunctivae. Children usually find these maneuvers interesting and nonthreatening.

5. Examination of the eyes with the ophthalmoscope. Most preschool-age children can follow directions well enough to focus on an object so that the clinician can see the anterior and posterior chambers of the eye and the fundus. The examiner usually can obtain a brief glimpse of the disc, and may even see the macula. (If the child has too much anxiety to cooperate, the clinician can try this later, perhaps after listening to the chest or during the neurological examination. Occasionally, the examiner will have to be satisfied with a rapid glimpse of a clear lens and the red reflex.)

6. Observation of the mouth with the light. The clinician should ask the child to show her teeth and then to open her mouth and say

"ahhh." A tongue blade should not be used at this time because it is generally quite upsetting to a child.

7. Observation and palpation of the head, scalp, ear pinnae, face, and neck. This portion of the examination is best postponed until this point because the child may not want the clinician to handle her body at the beginning of the examination.

♦ If the child was not undressed at the beginning of the examination, her chest should be uncovered.

8. Observation, palpation, and auscultation of the anterior chest.

9. Observation, palpation, percussion, and auscultation of the posterior chest.

♦ If the child was not completely undressed previously, at this time she should remove all clothing below the waist except for underpants (or diapers). The child should now lie in the supine position on the examining table. If she refuses, as the younger preschool-age child may, she can be examined in the supine position on her parent's lap, as described on pp. 219–220. This is not ideal but is acceptable.

10. Observation, percussion, and auscultation of the anterior chest.

♦ Now the child should turn to lie on her left side.

11. Auscultation of the heart, especially the mitral area.

♦ The child should return to the supine position.

12. Observation, auscultation, percussion, and palpation of the abdomen.

13. Palpation of the femoral pulses.

14. Palpation of the posterior flank, bilaterally.

♦ Next the patient should roll to her right side.

15. Palpation of the spleen.

♦ The child should return to the supine position.

16. Observation and palpation of the lower extremities.

♦ The clinician or parent should remove the diaper or help the older child to pull her underpants down to her knees. The child may flex the hips and knees or be in the frog-leg position.

17. Observation and palpation of the external genitalia and anus, and evaluation for hernias.

♦ A boy should stand on the floor facing the clinician so that he can be examined for the presence of hernias. The younger preschool-age child can stand on the examining table.

Following the preceding examination, the child should have her pants (or diapers) replaced and then should sit on the examining table.

18. Neurological examination. Deep tendon reflexes and coordination may be evaluated at this time.

♦ The patient should stand on the floor, with her back toward the examiner.

19. Observation and palpation of the back.

‣ The child should stand upright, then bend at the waist, then resume the upright position once again.

20. Observation of gait.

‣ The patient should be instructed to walk away from and then return to the examiner. The parent may need to accompany a shy child.

21. Observation of gross motor skills such as jumping, hopping, skipping.

‣ Next, the child should return to the sitting position either on the examining table or on the parent's lap.

22. Measurement of blood pressure. This is usually not done routinely before three years of age. If the child is very cooperative, it may be done earlier—before she is asked to lie down for the abdominal examination or after the neurological evaluation. The blood pressure measurement may be unfamiliar and therefore frightening, although in fact it is only mildly uncomfortable. See p. 222 of this chapter for a description of how to introduce the blood pressure measurement to a child.

23. Examination of the ears with otoscope. The child may be able to handle this calmly much earlier in the examination, as with the blood pressure measurement. If the child is comfortable early in the physical examination, the clinician may ask the parent, "How does Robin manage with the ear examination?" If the ear examination is not usually difficult or upsetting for the child, it can be done earlier, just after the head, face, and neck are examined. If the parent reports that the child does not like the ear examination, or if the child is not very comfortable, it should be left until the end. In rare cases, especially if there is a question about ear problems, the child may have to be restrained on the examining table, possibly with the help of an aide in addition to the parent.

If an adequate examination of the oral cavity was not performed earlier, it can be repeated now, with a tongue depressor and restraint from the parent if necessary. The ear and mouth examinations are less frightening if done on the parent's lap or with the child standing next to the seated parent.

‣ The child should now be dressed, and she may play in the office while the clinician and parent talk.

SPECIAL NOTES ABOUT SELECTED ELEMENTS OF THE PHYSICAL EXAMINATION

A number of terms have been used to refer to specific elements of the physical examination. Most of them are self-explanatory, but a few need further explanation, especially with regard to pediatric practice. These and some other items are discussed in this section.

Fontanelle

The term "fontanelle" usually refers to the anterior fontanelle; however, the posterior fontanelle is also examined during the neonatal period since it may remain patent, normally, until two months of age. The anterior fontanelle can only be adequately evaluated when the child is upright or seated and is not crying. If the child is recumbent or crying, the fontanelle is not as flat as it normally is, and this leads to the false impression that there is increased intracranial pressure. The anterior fontanelle usually closes between 8 and 18 months of age, although the normal range is even wider.

Eyes

The ophthalmological examination for a child who is well varies with the child's age, how comfortable the child is with the examiner, and his or her ability to follow instructions. An infant's eyes are best examined when the child is asleep. However, an infant who is awake and comfortable may spontaneously keep the eyelids open enough to allow a brief but adequate view of the fundus. The clinician should avoid touching the infant's forehead or eyelids, since these maneuvers are likely to cause the child to grimace and try to move away. It is sufficient to know that there are no cataracts or tumors and that the red reflex is present. A view of the vessels, the optic disc, and the macula may be obtained but are not required parts of the examination in this situation.

Toddlers and young preschool-age children cannot follow directions well. As a result, the examination may be somewhat unpredictable. Again, it is best to look in the eyes quickly with the ophthalmoscope when the child is awake and not crying. It is adequate to obtain a good red reflex without abnormalities in the anterior or posterior chamber, plus a glimpse of the vessels. Sometimes it is possible to see the disc or macula as well.

Older preschool and school-age children can almost always cooperate with an examiner's instructions. They can usually focus their eyes on a picture or special mark on the opposite wall, or even on the parent's hand. In this manner they are able to hold their eyes still long enough for the examiner to see the fundus, including many vessels and the disc. At this point, it is frequently helpful to tell the child *not* to look at the ophthalmoscope light since following the light hinders the clinician's attempt to see the optic disc and vessels. At the end of the eye examination, it is important to look to the lateral part of the fundus and to ask the child to look at the ophthalmoscope light; this enables the examiner to see the macula.

It is helpful to dim the lights in the room during the eye examination. However, in rare instances, a child will be upset by this.

If there is a complaint which suggests the possibility of an eye abnormality or an intracranial lesion, a complete eye examination is mandatory. Medication will probably be needed to dilate the pupils.

Visual acuity

For the child under three years of age, examiners must depend on several kinds of observation to estimate the child's ability to see. These include the child's ability to follow an attractive object with his or her eyes; to recognize the faces of familiar people without hearing their voices; to manipulate small objects; and to see the environment clearly enough to move around without bumping into things. For the child from three to five years of age, clinicians can use the Snellen illiterate "E" test or equivalent screening tests using pictures of familiar objects. After five or six years of age, the standard Snellen chart should be used. The screening of visual acuity is routinely performed at the end of a visit, after the physical examination. However, to ensure maximum cooperation from the child, it is best to do this before any injections or laboratory procedures are performed, since these are likely to upset the patient.

Ears and throat

A child's early experiences with throat and ear examinations, as well as procedures like removal of cerumen from the ear canals, are generally important determinants of the child's future reactions to these aspects of the physical examination. A clinician can make the throat and ear examinations less frightening by performing them while the patient is seated on the parent's lap. Other helpful devices for an older toddler include letting the child hold the tongue depressor, play with the otoscope, and watch the light go on and off. This can be followed by having the parent and/or child look into the examiner's ears, and then having the examiner look in the child's ears. Of course, one's clinical experience is the best guide. There are some children who need a minimum amount of demonstration, while others never really feel comfortable, even after they have been given may opportunities to get accustomed to a procedure. In general it is good to give some demonstration, elaborate if needed, and proceed with the examination. On subsequent visits the child will usually remember if the previous experience has been positive (or negative!), and likely will be more comfortable and cooperative.

If cerumen blocks the view of the tympanic membrane, the clinician must decide whether or not it is important to clean out the canal at this time. If the child is very fearful, and if there are no symptoms or signs of respiratory, ear, or hearing problems, the examiner may decide not to clean out the ears at this time. See page 233 for a description of this procedure.

It is almost always preferable to have the parent rather than an aide restrain the child, except in the rare situation when the parent is so anxious that he or she cannot hold the child adequately. Usually, any stranger will add to the child's feeling of being attacked or violated, and the presence of an aide will probably provoke more vigorous resistance from the child.

For the infant and young child, the position of choice usually is the supine position on the examining table. Parents can hold the infant's arms straight over the child's head using their hands, and simultaneously hold the child's head with their thumbs (see Figure 9-1). This frees the examiner to lean over the child and to see into the ears. The same position is used for the throat examination, except that the head is held in the midline. Right-handed clinicians can hold the light in their right hand and the tongue depressor in their left hand (reverse for a left-handed clinician).

When the child can sit well, usually around seven or eight months of age, it is practical to attempt to examine the child on the parent's lap. This position is preferable to the supine position because the child is much less likely to feel so vulnerable to attack.

The parent should hold the child firmly, with the child's back against his or her chest. For the examination of the left ear, the parent should hold the child's forehead with the right hand, turning the child's head to the right. Simultaneously, the parent's left arm should be used to

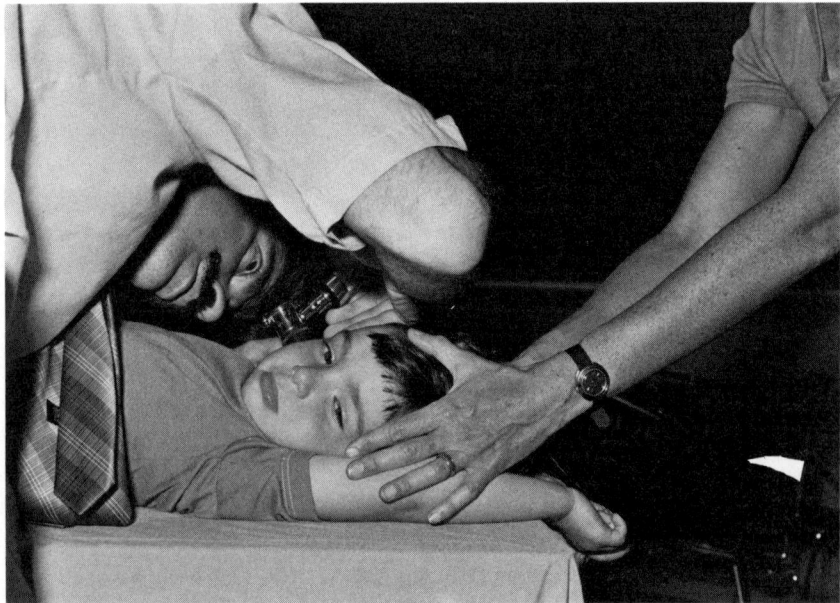

Figure 9-1. *Ear examination for a two-year-old—supine. A young child is restrained with arms and head immobilized. The examiner may have to restrain the child's torso by leaning over her, or may need an aide to hold the child's legs to prevent the child from moving.*

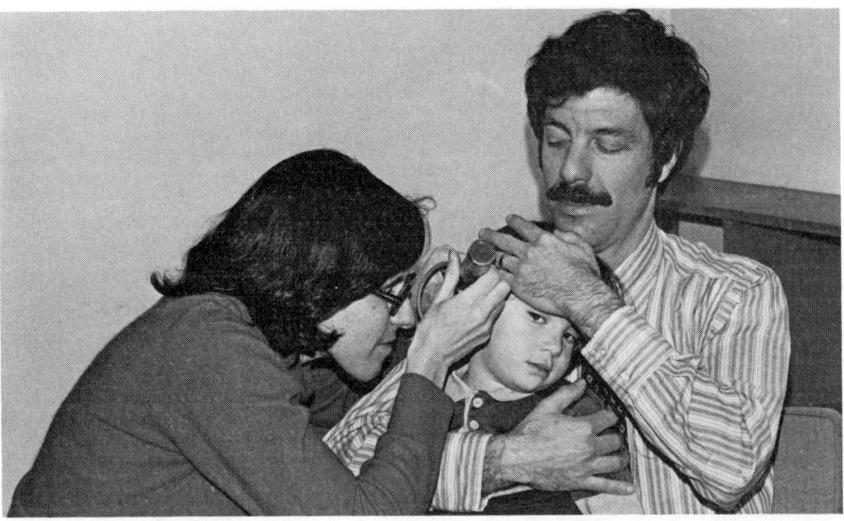

Figure 9-2. *Ear examination for a three-year-old child, on parent's lap. A parent holds his child on his lap, using his hands and arms to immobilize both the head and the arms. In order to examine the child's left ear, the examiner will move around to the other side and the girl's father will reverse his hand grip.*

hold the child's arms along the trunk, so that the child cannot grab the otoscope. It is best if the clinician is seated at the same level as and facing the parent, with their left sides adjacent and parallel (see Figure 9-2). The directions are reversed for the examination of the left ear. It is very important that the parent hold the child firmly; if this is not done, the child will probably move and likely will exacerbate an already stressful situation.

This same position can also be used to perform a throat examination, except that the head is held in the midline. The examiner can be on either side. A very frightened child may kick vigorously in an effort to get free. In the seated position, parents can immobilize the child's legs between their own. In the supine position, the examiner is best positioned over the child in such a way as to hold the child's legs with his or her own chest. In rare cases, a child will need additional restraint by an aide either at the head or the foot.

The older, cooperative child can be examined without restraint in the sitting position (see Figure 9-3).

Hearing

In the healthy child under three or four years of age, hearing is grossly evaluated by observing the child's response to a number of stimuli including normal sounds in the environment, the noise of crackling paper, a bell (see Figure 9-4), and certain voice sounds like s-s-s, k-k-k, and t-t-t. As the child becomes older, good indicators of the child's ability to hear include responses to verbal instructions and to his or her name, especially

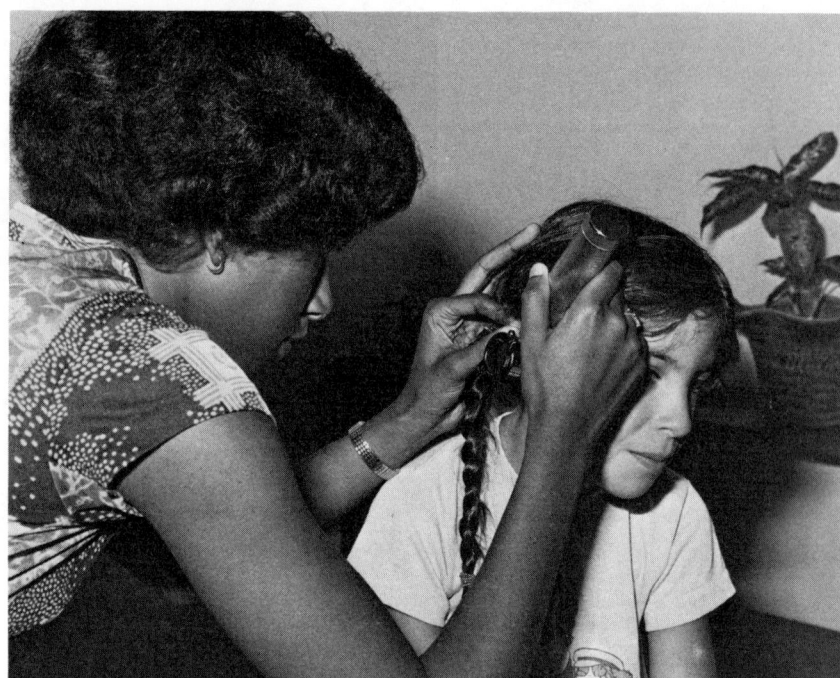

Figure 9-3. *Ear examination for a composed eight-year-old. The patient, sitting on the examination table, requires no restraints. Note how the clinician holds the fingers of her right hand to control how deeply the otoscope will penetrate the ear canal in the event that the patient suddenly jerks her head.*

when the speaker's mouth is out of view, and the child's ability to speak. All children who can cooperate, usually around three or four years of age, should have their hearing screened with a pure tone audiometer.

Hearing deficits, even severe ones, are much more likely to go unnoticed than are visual impairments. Hearing-deficient children are amazingly competent at learning to lip-read and to speak, even some with major hearing losses. Therefore, the clinician should be particularly conscientious about evaluating children who show any delay in preverbal vocalizations and speech, inadequate response to verbal communication, and in whom illness (such as meningitis) or use of ototoxic drugs occurred.*

Chest

The chest examination includes evaluation of the skin, musculoskeletal structures, and intrathoracic respiratory and cardiovascular structures. In infants and young children it is often difficult to examine the respira-

---

* Infants with severe hearing loss vocalize fairly normally until about six months of age. Subsequently they suffer a delay in progression of their preverbal vocalizations.

tory and cardiovascular systems because the child very often cries when the clinician listens to the chest. A thorough examination requires a child who is quiet much of the time and who is not resisting the clinician. With experience, examiners use information from the history, the physical examination thus far, and observations to decide which parts of the chest examination are essential. Usually observation and auscultation are the most important procedures in an otherwise well child. Percussion and palpation can be helpful, but usually do not add significant information to the data if no pathology is suspected on other grounds.

For young children, observation of the child at rest, especially with

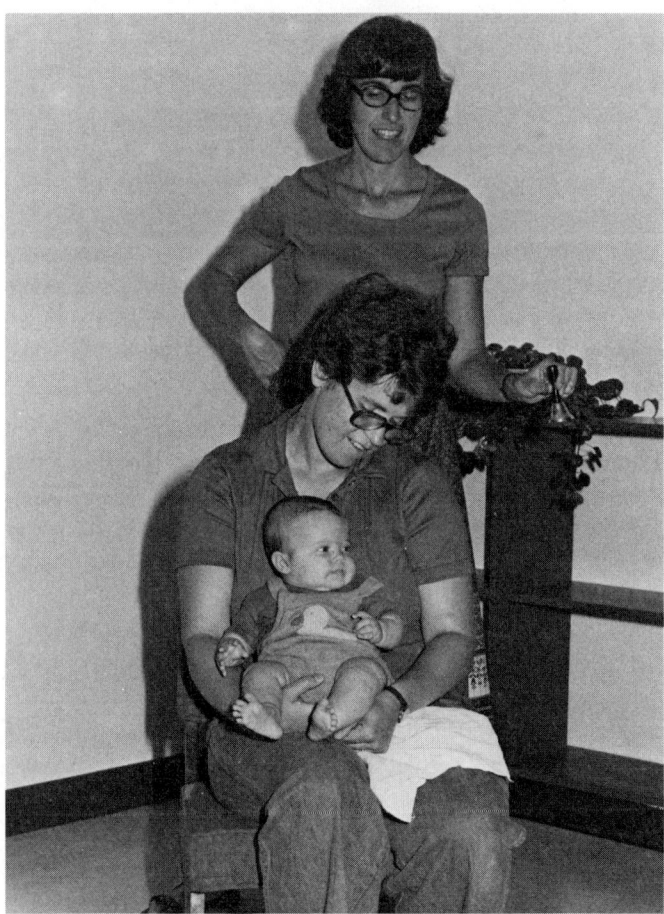

Figure 9-4. *Gross hearing test for an infant. A gross test of an infant's hearing is to ring a bell which is held outside his line of vision—behind and to each side of his head. It is important for students to recognize the frequently subtle signs by which an infant will indicate that she or he has heard the bell. The infant's response may be nothing more than a brief cessation of activity, an opening of the eyes, or a hand gesture. Sometimes an infant will turn both the eyes and the head toward the sound.*

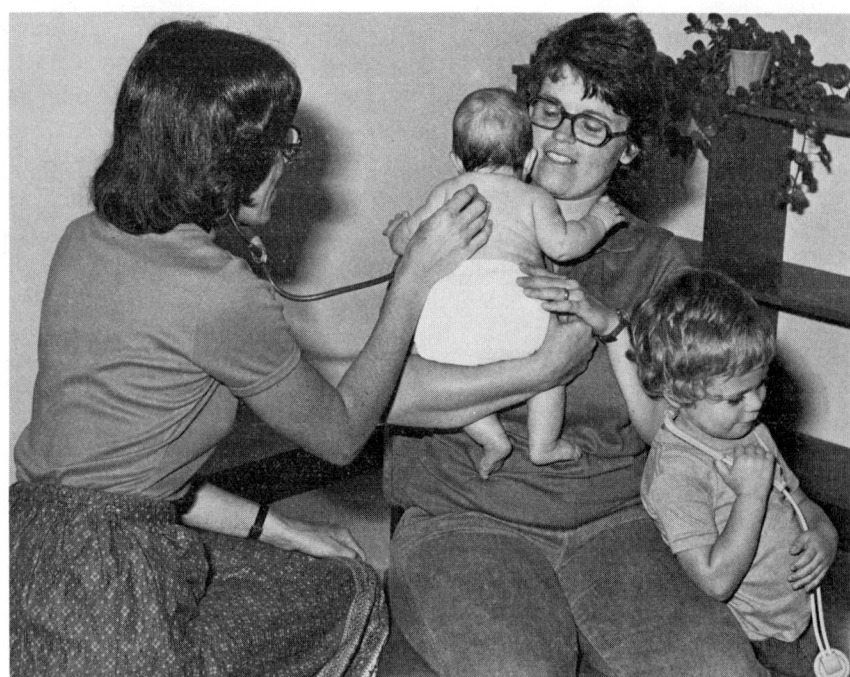

Figure 9-5. *Using the stethoscope on an infant. The examiner listens for heart and lung sounds in all areas of the infant's posterior chest. Note the sibling's interest in play equipment and in remaining near his mother and sister.*

the chest uncovered, is an extremely important part of the examination. It should include the gross appearance of the child, the presence of cyanosis, nasal flare, any unusual noises, and the use of accessory muscles.

There are a few ways in which it is possible to improve one's opportunities to listen to the chest adequately. The child usually is most comfortable reclining on a parent's lap, and may be more relaxed with a pacifier or a bottle. It will probably be easiest to listen to the posterior chest if the child is held against the parent's upper chest with the child's head resting on the parent's shoulder (see Figure 9-5). The clinician should prewarm the stethoscope and try to hold it in one position for 15 to 30 seconds in order to give the child a chance to relax and become quiet. After listening in that area, the practitioner can move it to another part of the precordium and hold it in place again until the child becomes quiet.

As always, it is the clinician's responsibility to be thoughtful in selecting what information is vital and what is optional in any particular clinical circumstance. For the young child who is presumably well, it is adequate to know that there are no signs or symptoms of cardiac or respiratory disease; that the breath sounds on inspiration are normal (as with the crying child); that the cardiac sounds are normal; and that there are no heart murmurs. Naturally, if signs or symptoms of possible problems are detected, a thorough evaluation is mandatory.

Abdomen

The abdominal examination should be done with the child in the supine position, preferably on the examining table (see Figure 9-6). Some children feel particularly uncomfortable in the supine position, presumably because they feel vulnerable and unable to move away from the examiner. If the patient (usually a toddler or young preschool-age child) refuses to lie down on the examining table, the clinician should offer the alternative of lying down on the parent's lap. For a child beyond the infant period, the examiner can sit facing the parent with the child's torso resting on the parent's lap and the child's legs on the examiner's lap (see Figure 9-7). Some children who will not relax on the examining table can manage to relax in this position—at least enough to permit an adequate abdominal examination.

Sometimes the child feels better if the examiner places the child's own hand over (or under) the examiner's hand. Even if the child's hand is under the clinician's palm, the clinician's fingertips are still free to perform the examination. A child who is moderately anxious and has difficulty in relaxing the abdominal muscles can be helped to relax if the examiner engages the child in a conversation about his or her family, friends, school, or favorite activities. This is an exception to the rule against social conversation during the physical examination.

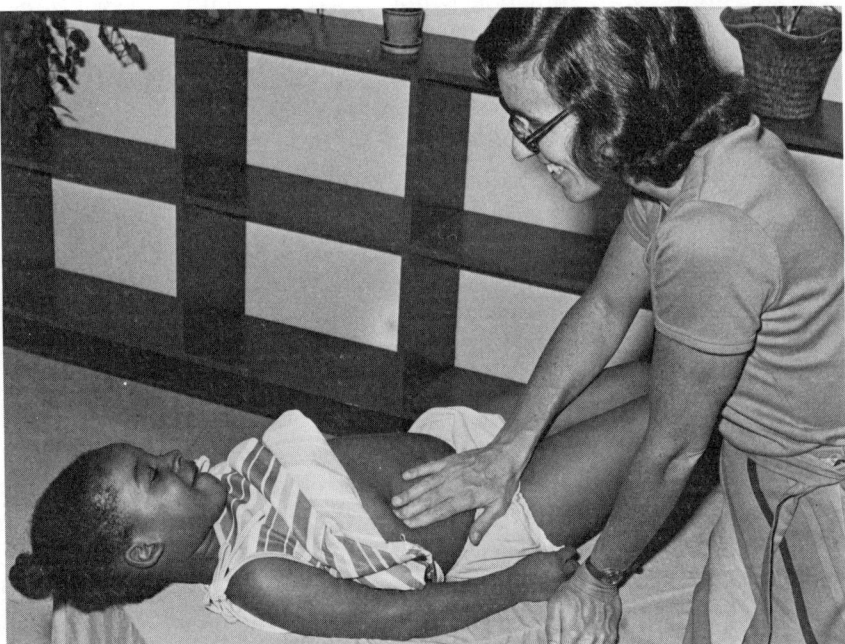

Figure 9-6. *Palpating the abdomen of a four-year-old girl. This child is relaxed, with her knees flexed and arms at her sides. The examiner is able to palpate this child's abdomen, just as it would be done on an adult.*

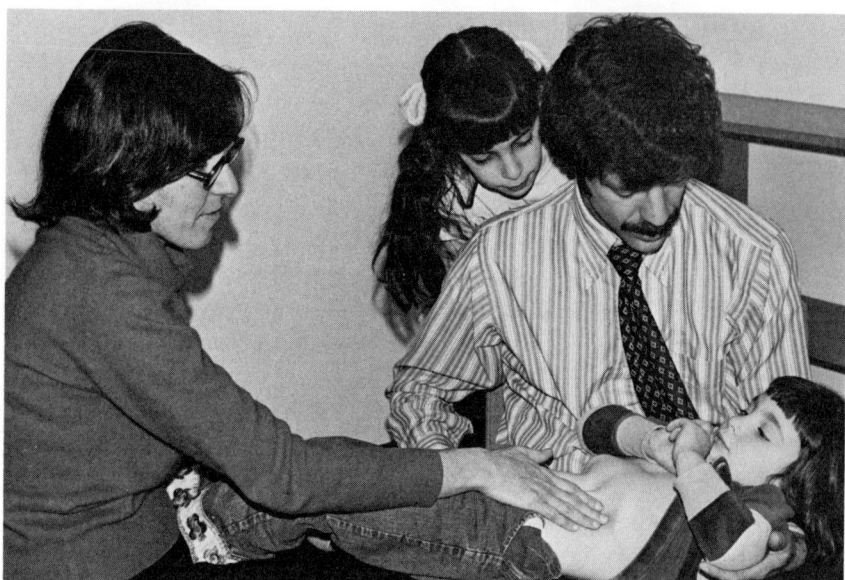

Figure 9-7. *Palpating the abdomen of a three-year-old girl. The examiner palpates the child's abdomen while the child is resting on the parent's lap. Note the apprehensive look on the girl's face and the intense interest of the older sibling.*

Rectal

The rectal examination is not part of the routine pediatric evaluation. However, if the history or physical findings (such as abdominal pain or a mass) indicate a possible abnormality, the rectal examination is called for.

There are two positions used for the rectal examination in children: the supine position with the hips and knees flexed or (for the right-handed clinician) the left lateral position with the knees and hips flexed (reverse for left-handed). Either position is acceptable. However, the lateral position may remind the child of unpleasant previous experiences, including injections. If the child can understand, she or he should be told there will be no injections given during the rectal examination.

As soon as the patient's verbal skills allow any comprehension, the clinician should provide the child with an explanation of the rectal examination. An analogy to the experience of the rectal thermometer may be helpful. The child should see and feel the examiner's finger and rubber glove or fingercot. A child even as young as two and one-half years of age should be told that she or he may feel like making a bowel movement, but will not, in fact. Often, children at that age or older are afraid that they will lose sphincter control when they feel the pressure from the intruding finger. The clinician's explanation before the examination can save the child from experiencing panic and anxiety over an anticipated embarrassment because of this loss of control.

Hips

A newborn infant should be evaluated regularly for the presence of a dislocated hip (Ortolani's test) or an unstable hip (Barlow's sign). After the newborn period, asymmetry of abduction and of leg length are more reliable findings than the above maneuvers. These tests should be done on a flat surface rather than on the parent's lap. The hips should be evaluated at every visit until the child walks; not infrequently, a hip abnormality is missed in early examinations.

NOTE: *Ortolani's test* involves abducting the legs (with the hips and knees flexed) and feeling for a "click" as the femoral head slips into the acetabulum, in a dislocated hip (see Figure 9-8, p. 222).

With *Barlow's sign* the femoral head slips back into the acetabulum after the examiner has forced the unstable, dislocatable hip out of the socket by exerting outward and backward pressure on the flexed hip (see Figure 9-9, p. 223).

Nervous system

The neurological examination, perhaps more than any other part of the physical examination, must be altered significantly with each age group. For this examination, the clinician observes the child during the interview, the developmental assessment, and the physical examination itself in order to gather data about the patient's neurological status. For example, the examiner will be able to evaluate a child's ability to speak while conversing with the child. Gross motor strength and coordination can be evaluated as the child climbs up and down from the examining table.

The neurological examination of the older preschool-age child and the school-age child is similar to that of the adult, with the addition of some age-appropriate tasks to test cognitive skills. Since the toddler and younger preschool-age child cannot follow complex directions, observations during other parts of the examination are even more important.

With infants, the examiner must evaluate several reflexes in addition to making the usual observations of cranial nerves, motor, and sensory functions. An infant examination usually includes the testing of a few of the many infant reflexes which have been described, such as: Moro, tonic-neck, back incurvation, stepping and placing, and vertical suspension reflexes. (Students should consult a pediatric physical diagnosis test for details about these reflexes.) The clinician should note if the reflex is present, if it is normal in its form, and if it disappears at the normal age. Absent, abnormal, or persisting reflexes indicate central nervous system pathology and require further evaluation.

Testing for the deep tendon reflexes is of limited value in the young child because it is difficult to elicit them in a reliable, reproducible way and because they are virtually never an isolated sign of pathology. The

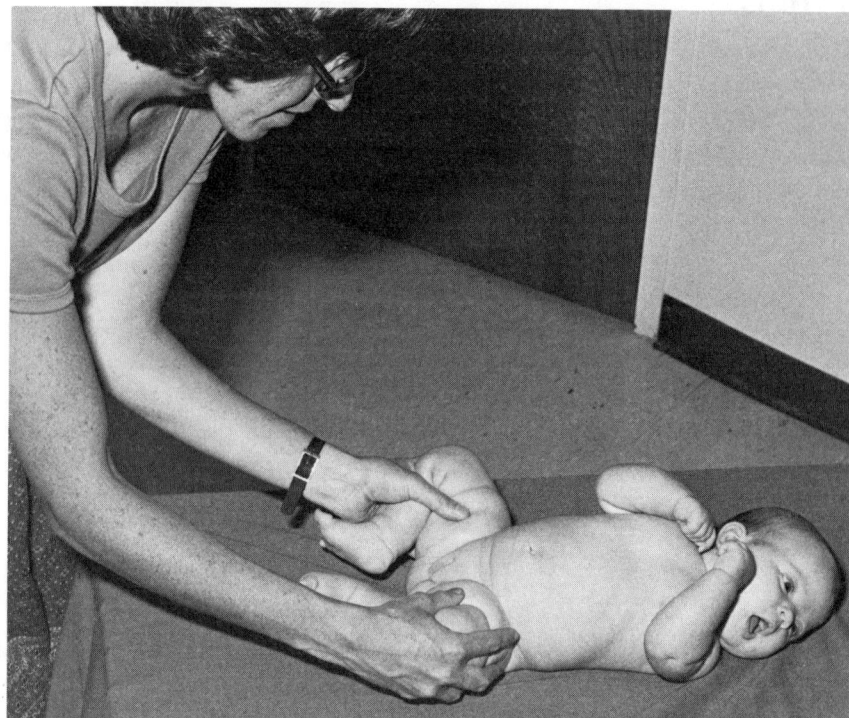

Figure 9-8. *Ortolani's test. The examiner feels for the "click" with her index and middle fingers, which are over the head of the femur as the hip is abducted and adducted.*

patellar reflex is usually present at birth, and the Achilles and brachial reflexes develop in the first months of life. The triceps reflex appears around six months of age. In the school-age child, reflexes are comparable to those in adults, and they are more reliable physical signs than in younger children. Whenever there are signs or symptoms of abnormalities, a thorough neurological examination is mandatory.

Blood pressure

The child's blood pressure should be measured routinely beginning at three years of age. This requires quite a bit of patient cooperation, and there are many three-year-old children for whom the entire health evaluation is so upsetting that an attempt to measure the blood pressure is unlikely to be successful. Nevertheless, it is important to introduce the cuff to the child around three years of age, even if no measurement is made initially. As mentioned earlier in this chapter, the clinician should avoid words that might frighten the child unnecessarily, and it is helpful if the practitioner knows whether the child has had experience with the blood pressure cuff prior to the current visit.

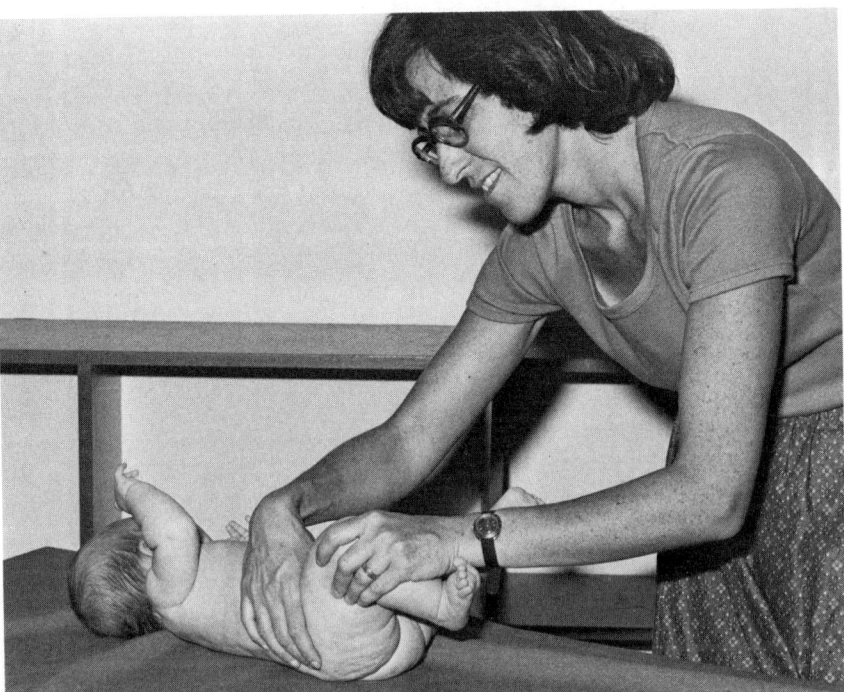

Figure 9-9. *Examination for Barlow's sign. The examiner evaluates whether the hip can be dislocated by stabilizing the pelvis and exerting pressure posteriorly on the flexed hip.*

The clinician can look to the parent, who may indicate that the child has never seen such a device before or had the blood pressure taken; conversely, it may turn out that the child has seen it many times before and is not afraid of it. The examiner can quickly demonstrate the cuff on a parent's arm, describing the process to the patient. If the child is not particularly anxious, the examiner can proceed with comments like "I will put this around your arm. It will squeeze a little, like this (gently placing a hand on the child's upper arm and squeezing). You can help by holding the clock and watching the pointer (NOT needle!) with me. I will listen to your arm, just as I did for your father, while we do this." Usually the examiner will have to repeat the blood pressure measurement several times because of artifacts produced by movement of the tubing or the child's arm.

After the blood pressure measurement has been taken, the clinician should tell the parent the results. If they are normal, this should be stated. Parents often want to know the numbers of the measurement and what they mean. The clinician should explain that the normal blood pressure for children is much lower than for adults. If this is neglected, the parent may worry that the child has abnormally low blood pressure.

Height and weight measurements

These measurements are two of the most important parts of the pediatric health evaluation. They should be performed carefully so that they are accurate, and they also should be done in such a way as not to upset the child. In many offices and clinics the child is undressed, weighed and measured, and seated in the examining room to wait for the clinician. As we indicated in Chapter 1, this is not conducive to good clinician-parent-patient rapport, and is not fair to the child. It is very simple to weigh and measure a child after the history and developmental assessment and before the physical examination begins.

If the child is very anxious, the measurements may be postponed until later in the visit as we described in the preceding sections for the examination of children of different ages. Some toddlers and young preschoolers are afraid to stand on the scale; they may be reassured if the parent or clinician stands on it for a demonstration. In rare cases, the examiner will have to weigh the parent alone, then weigh the parent holding the child, and subtract the former weight from the latter.

Young infants should be completely undressed when they are weighed. Older infants and toddlers can wear a clean dry diaper or underpants. Preschool and school-age children can be weighed wearing underwear or very light clothing, without shoes. If there is a possibility of inadequate weight gain, the child should be weighed on the same scale at each visit, consistently wearing only underpants and/or an examining gown, and the scale used should be noted in the record.

Height measurements are less complicated by clothing, but are difficult to measure accurately. Infants are measured in the supine position. Frequently the examiner will need the parent's help to hold the child still or to extend the legs to obtain an accurate measurement. Older children should be in stockinged feet and should stand as straight as possible.

Height and weight are information which parents and school-age children like to know. The clinician should tell the parent and older patient the measurements in pounds and inches (most people are not familiar with the metric system) and should plan to discuss these measurements once again during the clinical summary, using a growth chart.

Head circumference

This measurement can be obtained most accurately by placing a pliable, nonelastic tape measure (a paper tape is excellent) at the largest frontal-occipital circumference. The child should be held still by the parent, and the clinician should take a few extra seconds to be sure the tape is at the largest circumference. False large measurements may be obtained if braids, ribbons, or barrettes are included under the tape.

If there is any indication that the head circumference is abnormally small, or especially if it is large or growing too rapidly, transillumination of the head is indicated as a supplement to the usual physical examination.

We end this chapter by reminding the reader that we have been principally concerned here with how to go about a physical examination of a child in such a way as to maximize the possibilities of patient and parent cooperation and also to make this a positive experience for the child. This is the **art** of the examination. Other books and manuals should be consulted for details on techniques for performing the physical examination.

CHAPTER 10

The Art of Performing Painful Procedures

Introduction
Talking to the Family
Role of the Parent
Restraint
Concluding the Procedure
Examples of Painful Procedures
    Injections for a Child under 18 Months of Age
    Injections for a Child between 18 Months and 5 Years of Age
    Injections for the Older Child, Approximately 5 Years and Older
    Venipuncture
    Finger-Stick or Skin Test on Lower Arm
    Removing Cerumen from Ear Canals
    Suturing a Laceration
    Foreign Body in the Eye
    Throat Culture

INTRODUCTION

It is very important to keep in mind that an uncomfortable procedure is a real and consequential experience for a child. The child's experience of such a procedure depends on its painfulness and duration, the child's development, the ability of the parent to be supportive, and how the clinician prepares both the child and the parent. The child's age, verbal skills, past experience, and trust in the examiner all contribute to his or her ability to cooperate during the procedure. A child is likely to be less anxious and more cooperative if the parents are calm, supportive, and tolerant of anxiety than if they are nervous, critical, and impatient because they do not want their child to be frightened. Naturally, the same comments apply to the clinician as well.

A sensitive clinician will remember that many factors go into making a procedure uncomfortable. Of course, all painful procedures are uncomfortable by definition, but each patient will have his or her own threshold of pain. Additionally, procedures on certain parts of the body may be frightening because the child cannot observe them (e.g., suturing a face laceration) or because of past experiences (e.g., having cerumen removed from the ear canals). The better examiner and patient get to know each other, the more the clinician will know about how any given procedure is likely to affect the child.

Painful procedures should be done at the end of the visit, just before the patient leaves the office. If the clinician delegates the procedure to another member of the health care team, there should be a carefully thought out plan about preparation of the parent and child and about performing the procedure.

This chapter will present some specific procedures commonly performed in primary pediatric practice and discuss how to manage them. The principles of management are very similar to those which guide the clinician in carrying out painful or frightening parts of the physical examination, such as the ear and rectal examinations discussed earlier.

TALKING TO THE FAMILY

It is very helpful for the examiner to tell the child and parent about the procedure before it is performed, and also to give them an opportunity to ask questions. This description should be directed toward both the parent and the child, which involves repeating portions at a level that the child can comprehend. A two-year-old child can understand more than many clinicians think possible, and a three-year-old child can comprehend a great deal. It is wise to be completely honest with the child and make it clear that the procedure will hurt. This may make the child less cooperative, but she or he will have no reason to be angry or feel deceived or to mistrust the clinician in the future. It helps for the examiner to make such a statement early in the discussion, before the parents are tempted to say, "Don't worry, it won't hurt."

Many children will cry or become tearful before or during a painful procedure. Although this is a healthy expression of anxiety and physical pain, both children and parent may feel uncomfortable with the crying expressed. (Indeed, clinicians are not immune to feeling such discomfort themselves.) This issue should be addressed directly. Ms. Jordan, for example, might tell Judy that it is okay to cry, and that she will not be angry if she does so. Should Judy's parents threaten to punish her, either in anticipation of crying or poor cooperation or after she has begun to cry, Ms. Jordan should tell them not to threaten her and that it is quite acceptable for Judy to cry. Observations about a child's behavior in relation to his or her age and stage of development and the parent's reaction to this behavior are valuable in understanding how the child and the family respond to stress. If the response is exaggerated or unusual, these observations should be noted in the medical record, making due allowances in the interpretation for diverse cultural styles in the expression of stress or excitement.

It is often important to ask the child to hold still or to assume a certain position. This can be done firmly, without threatening the child, by telling the child that the parent or an aide will help her or him remain still "because sometimes it is hard to do it alone." The child should never be picked up suddenly and restrained without preparation; and if restraint is needed, the child should be introduced to whoever will assume the role of restrainer if the person is a stranger.

ROLE OF THE PARENT

In most situations, it is best if the parent is present during a painful procedure. Occasionally a parent may be very anxious and ask to be excused. In other cases, the clinician finds it advisable to ask the parent to leave: perhaps the parent is being punitive or shaming, or is so anxious that by being present makes the procedure more difficult for the child. In any event, if the parent does leave the room, the child should be told that the parent is leaving but will wait nearby and will return as soon as the procedure is completed. A parent should never sneak out of the room without informing the child that he or she is leaving.

There are certain instances in which a parent should not be asked to restrain a child. These include cases where the procedure is lengthy (e.g., suturing a laceration), where successful restraint requires experience (e.g., venipuncture), or where the child or parent is very upset. However, the parent may assist in other ways; for example, during a venipuncture, the parent can talk to the child, restrain the arm not being used for the test, and even restrain the legs if necessary. Most parents can restrain the young child for an injection without excessive stress, and this is the routine in most settings. Nevertheless, the arrangements should be individualized according to the needs of the child and the parent.

Sometimes practitioners may want the parent to leave the room because they feel the parent will be critical of their technique in performing a painful procedure. However, it is crucial for clinicians to learn to feel comfortable while being observed by parents, peers, and supervisors—even when they perform painful procedures, such as giving injections or drawing blood. Supervisors and teachers may be expected to help student clinicians become comfortable proceeding in the presence of a parent and so prevent needless separation of patients from their parents.

The older school-age child and the adolescent are generally comfortable if their parent is not in the room. In fact, they may feel unnecessarily infantilized if the parent is present. If the clinician is unsure about whether the patient wants a parent to be present, it is a simple matter to ask the child directly and let the patient decide.

RESTRAINT

Restraint should be adequate to prevent unnecessary movement, trauma, and failure of a procedure, but it should not be excessive. It is desirable for the child's face to remain uncovered if at all possible, because covering it increases the child's fear and the panicky feeling of loss of all control. If there is any latitude in the position in which the child may be restrained for a given procedure, experienced practitioners choose the sitting position because the child feels more vulnerable to attack when supine than when upright. If a patient is likely to be combative, it is wise to remove the child's shoes so that the person restraining the child will not get hurt. When one arm is needed for a procedure such as a venipuncture, the other arm should be restrained so that the patient cannot grab the needle or otherwise interfere with or endanger the procedure.

CONCLUDING THE PROCEDURE

At the end of a painful procedure, the patient should promptly be released from the restraint, allowed to sit up, and reunited as quickly as possible with his or her parent. It is never useful to chastise a child for poor behavior or crying. Instead, the patient should be told clearly that it is all over. Then the clinician can make some supportive comments such as complimenting a child who "did a good job" or sympathizing with the child who had a hard time. It is a nice gesture and strongly recommended to offer a Band-Aid to any child who has had an injection or a procedure to draw blood. Children as young as 18 months of age use Band-Aids to make themselves feel better and to reassure themselves that their body will recover. Preschool and young school-age children also use Band-Aids as a symbol of their ordeal and a badge of their courage.

In the situation where the child lost control and was difficult to restrain, the practitioner should talk with the parent, in the child's presence, after the child has calmed down. A brief discussion of why the child at this particular age and with his or her past experience could not control the anxiety will usually alleviate the parent's concern and feelings of self-criticism.

Anyone who performs a painful procedure on a child should realize that often the child will not feel friendly for a while after the procedure and should allow the child time to smooth out ruffled feelings. It is not useful to ask the child to show affection or to ask to be forgiven. Not infrequently, the parent wants the child to demonstrate "good manners" and strongly encourages the patient to say thank you and good-bye to the health care practitioner who gave the injection. It is helpful to the child and parent when the clinician shows understanding and acceptance of the child's bad mood. Sometimes it may help if the clinician verbalizes the child's feelings; for example, one might say to the child, "It sure is hard to say thank you to someone who just gave you a shot. I don't blame you." Then, one can tell the parent, "I don't mind if Susan does not want to talk to me now."

EXAMPLES OF PAINFUL PROCEDURES

Common procedures in the primary health care setting that are typically painful for a child include: injections for immunizations, intramuscular medications for illness, venipunctures in the antecubital fossa or the dorsum of the hand, and finger-sticks for blood tests such as the hemoglobin and hematocrit measurements. Other painful procedures which occasionally occur are: having cerumen removed from the ear canals, suturing of lacerations, and removal of a foreign body from the eye. Here are some suggestions for restraint of a child undergoing a number of typically painful procedures. Naturally, there are other acceptable methods.

Injections for a child under 18 months of age

These are usually given in the anterolateral thigh. The position of choice is for the child to be on the examining table, with the parent helping to restrain the child (see Figure 10-1). The child up to about two years of age

The Art of Performing Painful Procedures 231

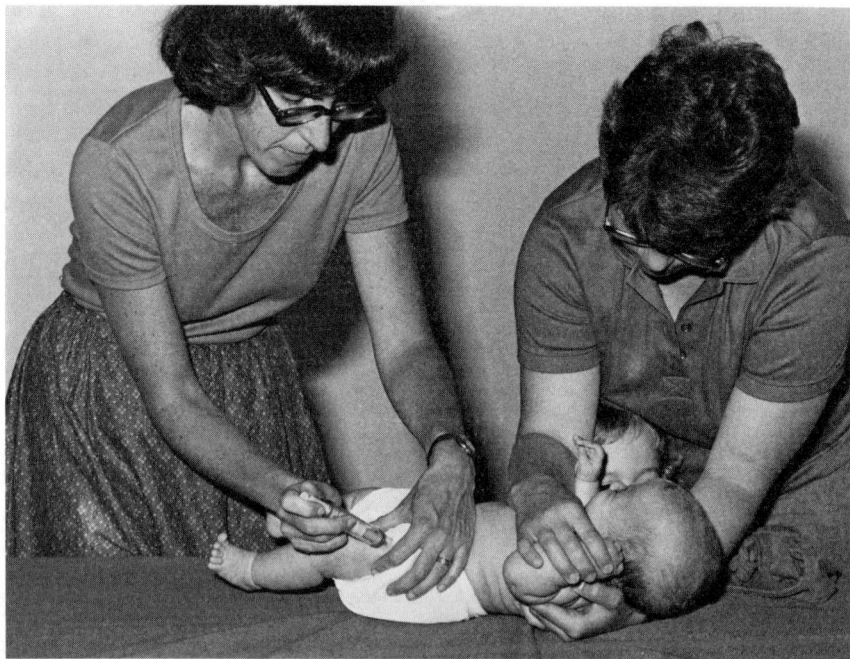

Figure 10-1. *Giving injection to infant. The clinician gives the injection in the thigh while the parent helps to restrain the child. Note the close proximity of the sibling to mother and infant.*

has little ability to understand the procedure, and so it should be explained to the parent and performed as efficiently as possible.

Injections for a child between 18 months and 5 years of age

If these injections are given in the thigh, the child should be restrained (much as the younger child) on the examining table. If the child (over three years of age) receives an injection in the arm near the deltoid or subcutaneously in the upper arm, the patient may be adequately restrained and less frightened while seated on a parent's lap. If necessary, the child's legs may be restrained between the legs of the parent. *It is important to secure the arm that is not receiving the injection so that the child cannot grab the needle.*

Injections for the older child of approximately five years and older

It is often helpful if the parent can sit next to the patient, either on a chair or on the examining table. This may help the patient psychologically and also make the parent available if restraint is needed.

232   Clinical Assessment: Sources for the Data Base

Venipuncture

More time is needed for this procedure than for an injection, and adequate immobilization is crucial in order to keep the needle in the vein, obtain the specimen, and avoid a second venipuncture. Some people prefer to wrap the patient in a sheet, leaving exposed only the child's head and the arm on which the venipuncture will be done. This is generally more frightening than the restraint shown in Figure 10-2 and it may not be necessary. Since it takes a great deal of self-control to hold still for this procedure, up until about eight or nine years of age the child should be restrained in the supine position, as shown in the illustration. A mature eight- or nine-year-old can, however, be given this test independently in the sitting position, like an adult, without much risk of the child moving the arm or flexing the elbow (see Figure 10-3). In any event, venipuncture is generally less difficult when children are able to see their parent and, whenever possible, have the parent nearby rather than across the room.

Finger-stick or skin test on lower arm

For these procedures a child under eight years of age should be allowed to remain seated, preferably on the parent's lap. The parent should hold the arm just below the elbow with one hand, and the (right-handed) clinician

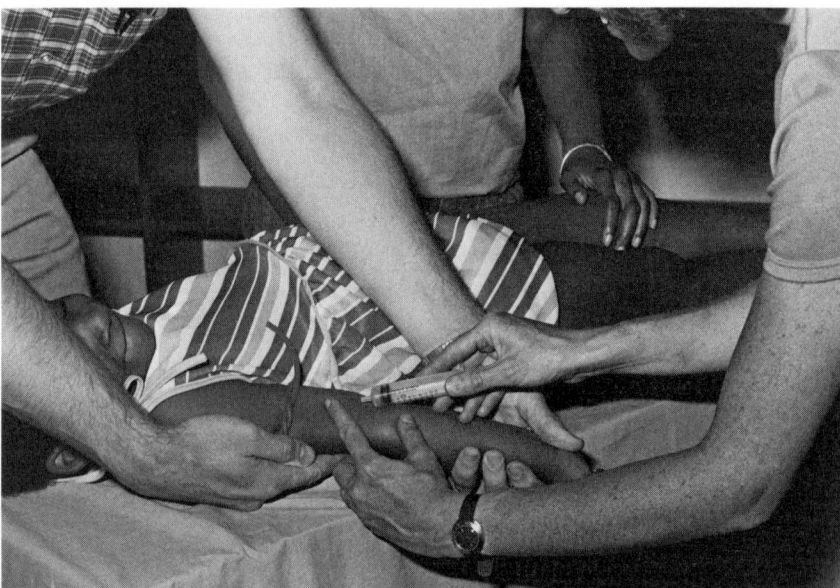

Figure 10-2. *Venipuncture for a child under eight years of age. An assistant restrains the child's arm so that the clinician has clear access to the antecubital vein. The child's parent is within view of the child and can talk to her during the procedure. If necessary, the parent can restrain the child's legs as well.*

The Art of Performing Painful Procedures 233

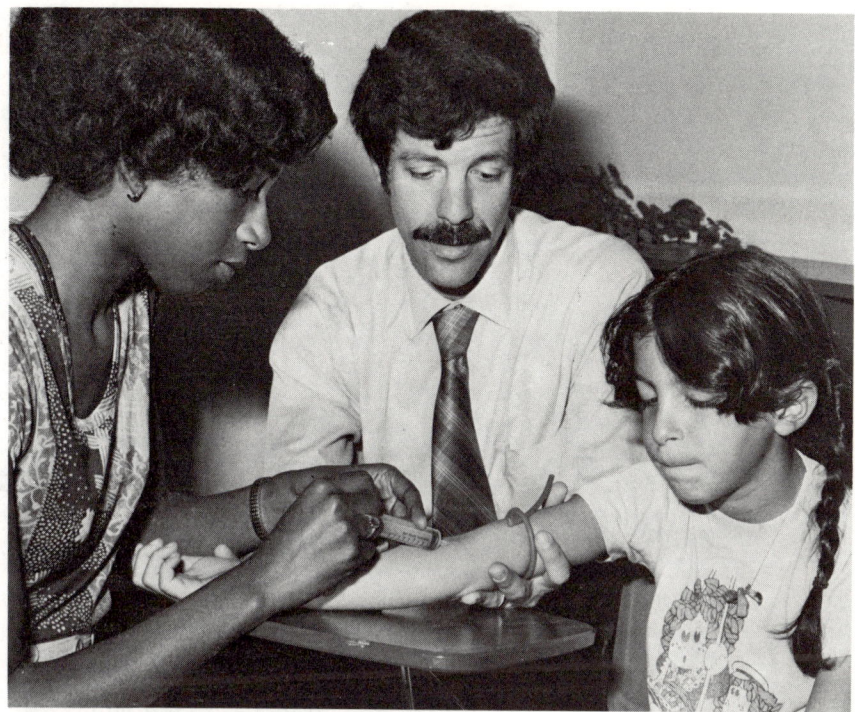

Figure 10-3. *Venipuncture for a child over seven years of age. The parent can help restrain the older child's arm if it seems necessary. Usually, the child who is old enough to sit up for a venipuncture needs no restraint. In fact, many preadolescent and older children may prefer to have their parents wait in another room during the procedure.*

should hold the lower part with his or her left hand. It is helpful if the parent can also hold the child's free hand and/or shoulder. If necessary, the child's legs can be restrained between the parent's knees (see Figure 10-4).

Removing cerumen from ear canals

A child who needs to have cerumen cleaned out of the ear canals should usually be restrained in the supine position. If a curette is used, the advisable position is similar to the supine position for ear examination (see page 214). Experienced clinicians find that it usually helps to have the parent nearby, talking to the child. Since it may take several minutes to complete the procedure and it is frequently quite upsetting for the child, the parent should usually not be asked to restrain the child because he or she is not likely to hold the child still enough to prevent the child from being hurt with the curette. If it is absolutely essential to enlist the parent's aid in restraining a child, it is wise to have the parent hold the child's legs; the clinician or a clinical assistant should secure the head. If

234   Clinical Assessment: Sources for the Data Base

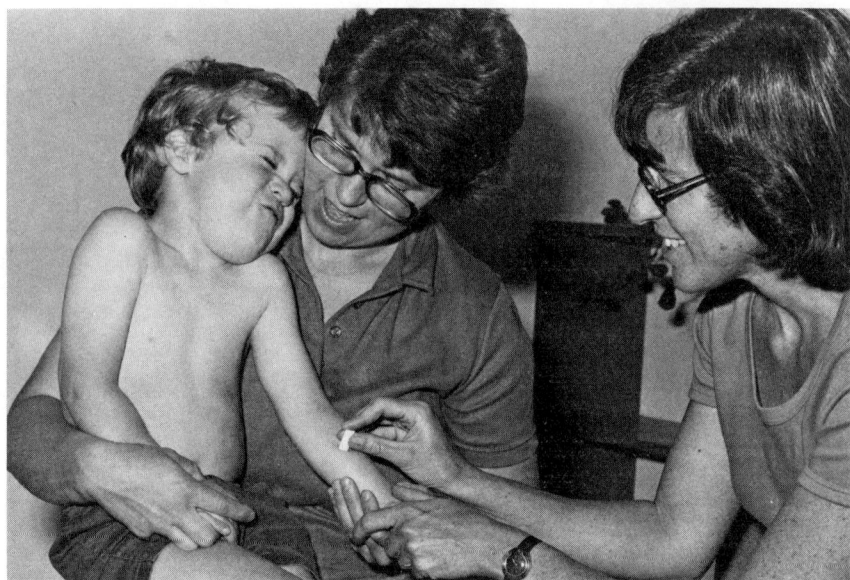

Figure 10-4. *Skin test for four-year-old. The mother restrains both of the child's arms and his legs (between her own) while the clinician places a Tine test.*

the water-pick machine is used, the positions are the same as for the ear examination with an otoscope: preferably sitting, and supine for a young or combative child.

Suturing a laceration

In suturing, the optimal position naturally will depend on the location of the laceration. Usually, a child will need more restraint for administering the local anesthetic than for the actual suturing. If a child has not been too badly frightened, she or he may need no restraint at all after the anesthetic has been injected. The procedure of suturing a face laceration is particularly frightening because much of the face may need to be covered by the sterile drapes. Someone who is familiar to the patient can be very helpful in explaining the procedure and talking with the child as the suturing progresses. Children, like adults, may be comforted by being told that things are going well and how soon the procedure is likely to be completed.

Foreign body in the eye

The restraint would be the same as that used for the supine ear examination, but with the face turned up rather than to the side. It is less frightening if the parent can be present to talk to the child. Once again, because it is so important to immobilize the child's head completely, it is preferable if the parent is not asked to restrain the child, and especially the head.

Throat culture

It is best if a child who is beyond infancy is sitting instead of supine. The preferred position is the same as for the throat examination (see page 215). Young children are best restrained on their parent's lap. Experienced examiners give the child an extra cotton swab to hold; this frequently reassures the patient that there is no needle hidden inside it. It also helps to tell the child that he or she might choke or gag but that it all will be over quickly.

Suggested Readings Unit III: Clinical Assessment

Chapter 5: The Interview

Francis, V., Korsch, B.M., and Morris, M.J. Gaps in doctor–patient communication. Patient's response to medical advice. *New Eng. J. Med.* 280:535–540, 1969.

Gozzi, E., Morris, M., and Korsch, B. Gaps in doctor–patient communication: implications for nursing practice. *Am. J. Nurs.* 69:529–533, 1969.

Korsch, B.M., Gozzi, E.K., and Francis, V. Gaps in doctor–patient communication. 1. Doctor-patient interaction and patient satisfaction. *Pediatrics* 42:855–871, 1968.

Chapter 7: Developmental Assessment

Anyan, W. Changes in personal and interpersonal spheres during adolescence. Pp. 27–31 in *Adolescent Medicine in Primary Care*. New York, John Wiley and Sons, 1978.

Levy, D.M. Observations of attitudes and behavior in the child health center. *Am. J. Public Health* 41:182–190, 1951.

Lewis, M. *Clinical Aspects of Child Development*. Philadelphia, Lea and Febiger, 1971.

Provence, S. Developmental assessment. Pp. 374–383 in Green, M. and Haggerty, R.L. *Ambulatory Pediatrics II*. Philadelphia, W.B. Saunders, 1977.

Provence, S. Developmental assessment: Principles and process. In Brennemann's *Practice of Pediatrics*, Vol. I. Hagerstown, Md., Harper & Row, 1972.

Provence, S., Lipton, R.C. *Infants in Institutions*. New York, International Universities Press, 1962.
Senn, M.J.E., Solnit, A.J. *Problems in Child Behavior and Development*. Philadelphia, Lea and Febiger, 1968.

Chapter 9: The Art of the Physical Examination

Alexander, M.M. and Brown, M. *Pediatric Physical Diagnosis for Nurses*. New York, McGraw-Hill, 1974.
Anyan, W. Physical examination. Pp. 7–10 in *Adolescent Medicine in Primary Care*. New York, John Wiley and Sons, 1978.
Barness, L.A. *Manual of Pediatric Physical Diagnosis*, 4th ed. Chicago, Year Book Medical Publishers, 1972.
Bates, B. *A Guide to Physical Examination*, 2nd ed. Philadelphia, J.B. Lippincott, 1979.
Cohen, S. Patient assessment: Examination of the female pelvis, Part II. *Amer. J. Nurs.* 1–28, Nov. 1978.
McGee, J. The pelvic examination: A view from the other end of the table. *Annals of Internal Med.* 83:563–564, 1975.
Omni Education System. Ortho Pharmaceutical Corp. Module: Breast Examination, 1974.
Prechtl, H.F.R. *The Neurological Examination of the Full Term Newborn Infant*, 2nd ed. Philadelphia, J.B. Lippincott, 1977.

UNIT FOUR

The Clinical Summary

CHAPTER 11

General Principles and the Typical Clinical Summary with No Problems

General Principles
    Purpose of the Clinical Summary
    Setting
    Participants
    Conduct of the Summary
    Time Constraints and Priorities
The Typical Clinical Summary with No Problems
    Statement about the Child's Current Health Status
    Anticipatory Guidance
    Screening and Immunizations
    Plans for Future Care

GENERAL PRINCIPLES

Purpose of the clinical summary

A good clinical summary is a conversation and not a monologue. It is a time for discussion about the visit among the clinician, parents, and patient. If successful, the summary will address all salient issues raised during the course of the visit, and should be conducted in a way which will help the patient and parents feel attended to and hence inclined to be active participants in future visits and/or treatment plans.

It is best if the clinician introduces the summary in an explicit manner by presenting, first, the findings, then opinions about the child's health and development, and finally a formulated plan or proposal for treatment. The summary should also include more complete responses to any previously mentioned concerns whose discussion was deferred to expedite the examination. When the child is well, the primary purpose of the summary really is education and guidance for heath promotion.

It is important to recognize any concern of the parents, child, or clinician as a problem and label it as such. This will aid in gathering further data, making a plan, and remembering to follow the problem's course. For an essentially well child, minor problems can be discussed at some length. Of course, if there is a major problem, it should be the primary focus of the summary discussion, while preventive care and health maintenance are deferred for future discussions. If the parent is very worried, but there does not seem to be any medical problem with the child, the concern should still be treated as a problem—in the parent.

Setting

The proper setting for conducting the clinical summary is essentially the same as that for taking the history. It should be undertaken in a comfortable, quiet place where privacy is ensured. In some pediatric examination settings, the same room is used for both discussion and examination. If the examining room is separate from the consultation room, the participants may return to the consultation room after the physical examination has been completed. The older child should be dressed, and the younger child should be clothed enough so that she or he is warm and comfortable during the discussion, even if this means pausing after the physical examination to dress the child. There should be appropriate furniture for both the adults and the children, and some toys as well. It is not good enough to conduct the summary standing beside the examining table.

Participants

The clinician must decide in each individual case who should be present during the clinical summary, just as in all other parts of the health evaluation. Usually the parents and child are kept together for the final discussion, especially when they have been together throughout the visit. If the parents were not present for the physical examination, it may be a good idea to take a few moments for a brief discussion of one's findings with the child and ask if there are any questions. Then the practitioner can invite the parents in for a full discussion of the health evaluation and whatever plans need to be made.

In some cases, the parents and patient have been together

throughout the history and physical examination, but the clinician wishes to speak with either the parents or child separately. This may occur, for example, when one needs to talk to the parent about family problems such as marital difficulties or when it seems appropriate to talk to the child about his or her feelings about the parents' impending divorce. It is best to approach such situations directly by stating one's intentions: "I would like a few minutes to talk with your mother alone, Ronnie. Would you please stay in the waiting room?" If a child asks why, one should explain briefly, in terms appropriate for the child's age.

If the child is under six years of age, the clinician should be sure a staff member is given responsibility for supervising the child in the waiting area. For the child who is comfortable without his or her parents, an aide can perform nonpainful screening procedures such as vision and hearing tests while the parents and clinician are in conference. If the patient is uncomfortable about the separation, it may be reassuring to let the child see the room where the conference with the parents will be.

When it seems appropriate to talk to the child alone, the examiner should ask the parent to wait in the waiting room. If this is the first time the clinician has chosen to do this with a particular family, it might be helpful to say, "I find it productive to talk alone with children when they get to be Herman's age. This helps children learn to take responsibility for their own health care, and I am able to get to know them better." This kind of separation may be called for even if there are no problems, simply to build rapport with the patient. (See page 102, Chapter 5, about separation of the parent and child during the interview.)

At the end of the clinical summary, the examiner should be sure to say an appropriate good-bye to all the participants, just as a proper greeting is given at the beginning of each visit. This may be done either in the conference room or in the waiting area, depending on the circumstances.

If an interpreter has been involved in the previous parts of the health visit, it is very important for this person to be present during the clinical summary. If the interpreter does have to leave after the initial interview, she or he should be asked to return so that the conclusions and plans will be communicated clearly and the parent and child can ask the practitioner questions effectively.

Sometimes the adult accompanying a child to the examination is not the child's primary caregiver. If the escort is a mature and competent member of the patient's family, it is appropriate to relate to this individual as one would to a parent. However, if the data base in inadequate, or the escort cannot be relied upon to relay the information from the clinical summary to the parent or primary caregiver, the clinician will have to make special arrangements to communicate with the responsible party. This may occur when the escort is not a close relative, when an older sibling brings the patient for health care, or when a very young or immature teenager is the parent, but the grandparent is the responsible caregiver.

If the clinician cannot talk to the responsible person by telephone, he or she can write a note and ask that individual to call or perhaps arrange for a home visit. It might also be useful to request, if at all possible, that one of the responsible caregivers accompany the child at the next visit. If the child is with a foster or adoptive family, the clinician naturally should discuss health care directly with the substitute parents. However, when a serious physical or psychological problem is detected, and the child has not been legally adopted, the agency which placed the child should be informed.

Perhaps the least clear case is that of an adolescent who comes alone for health care. Here the clinician must not rush to judgment; only after evaluating the whole interview and examination should the clinician decide what his or her relationship will be with the parent in each individual case.

Conduct of the summary

As the concluding interaction of the health evaluation, the summary affects the family's feeling of satisfaction; thus it influences their understanding and willingness to carry out plans for the child's health maintenance and care. Therefore, the summary must be individualized, and the clinician should be very sensitive to each family's particular needs. In general, the clinician's manner during the summary should be consistent with the principles discussed for the interview.

The summary, as we have already indicated, should not be a solely didactic presentation of information, but rather an exchange with the family. If additional data remain to be collected during the summary, modified open-ended questions are called for. The practitioner should present his or her opinions, conclusions, and advice in a straightforward fashion. A good presentation is precise and specific, and does not make use of generalizations or oversimplifications. Accurate, although not necessarily scientific, terminology should be used, and it should always be explained further, if necessary, in language the family can understand. If it seems appropriate, either because the parent and patient may hear the medical terminology in the future or because they seem to be interested in that terminology, the practitioner may use those terms also. For instance, one might say, "Joseph has fluid behind his ear drums. It is not very serious, and can be treated with some medicine. You may hear it called serous otitis media, which is the medical term for that ear fluid." Information about the etiology, treatment, and course of serous otitis media should follow.

The child should be included in the conversation as much as his or her verbal skills allow. At times, the clinician may want to speak first to the parent, and then rephrase the information so that the child can understand it. Needless to say, there should always be a sufficient opportunity for both the parent and child to ask questions.

It is crucial that the clinician be aware of the impact of the summary on the family. Nonverbal cues which indicate that the family members are upset, do not understand the presentation, or disagree with it should be noted. Sometimes the parents or child are too shy to say that they do not understand something, but are relieved when the practitioner "reads" this in their reaction and offers further explanation. Patients and parents are often reluctant to disagree with the clinician openly but can accept an opportunity to talk about disagreements when the clinician initiates the discussion.

Occasionally, the clinician must tell the parents and child something that is very upsetting. A serious physical or psychological problem may be identified, hospitalization or a painful diagnostic or therapeutic procedure may be necessary. Upsetting information should be presented in a clear manner that is neither evasive nor blunt and, if possible, positive information should be offered along with the negative. In general, the clinician should be honest but appropriately hopeful and encouraging. It is important to remember that it may take a family a long time to assimilate complex or upsetting information fully, and adequate arrangements for follow-up discussions should be made.

The clinical summary for a family without major problems should be conducted with the same care as for a family that must adjust to upsetting information. Too often, when there are no major problems, the health care practitioner is tempted to say, "Everything is fine; see you in six months." When the clinician thus neglects to make a clear statement about the child's growth and development or to discuss unresolved issues which were mentioned earlier, lack of concern may be communicated and the parents and child are left unsure about the outcome of the health evaluation. Such an abrupt ending also omits counseling about a child's physical and psychological development, crucial aspects of health promotion. Every parent and child, including the most healthy, should have an opportunity to present questions and to clarify health care plans.

Time constraints and priorities

Ideally, there should be enough time available for the clinical summary to permit an adequate discussion of health promotion and problems. When the child is physically well, and when there are no psychological or social problems, a complete clinical summary can be fairly brief. More often, however, there will be concerns or problems which the practitioner needs to discuss with the parent and child. This will take longer, but naturally practical considerations will keep the summary confined to a reasonable length of time.

Not infrequently, the entire health assessment takes more time than expected, and so the clinical summary must be shortened. This may occur if the historians give a history slowly, if an interpreter is involved, or if the child is uncooperative during the developmental assessment and physical examination. Occasionally, a parent will bring up a problem at the end of the evaluation, often in a "by-the-way" question. This may be a very important concern, and the practitioner should take the time to evaluate its urgency. If for some reason, the clinician needs to shorten the summary, a quick decision should be made as to how to use the time available. Any urgent physical or psychosocial problem should be handled immediately, however, regardless of time pressures.

Problems or concerns which are important but not urgent may be handled later, either by telephone or in a subsequent office visit. In general, psychological and social problems frequently require several visits for adequate evaluation. It is far better to evaluate these problems at an appointed time that is explicitly set aside for them than to do a hurried and incomplete evaluation at the end of a visit. A rapid evaluation may omit important information, and so jeopardize management. The clinician should not recommend consultation or therapy until the pediatric evaluation and assessment of the parent's and older patient's ability and motivation to follow a plan has been completed.

THE TYPICAL CLINICAL SUMMARY WITH NO PROBLEMS

The clinical summary includes (1) a statement about the child's current health status encompassing physical health, growth, development, psychosocial strengths and weaknesses, and stresses; (2) anticipatory guidance about development and health promotion, including accident prevention; (3) plans for screening and immunizations; and (4) plans for future health care. As with previous sections of the health evaluation, the clinician needs to be flexible and to alter the format to suit particular circumstances. Minor problems, when present, are usually discussed after the statement of the current health status. However, when there are major problems requiring further evaluation or complex management, the clinical summary is the most appropriate time for a discussion of the problem. In such instances, anticipatory guidance and discussion of other important issues in well-child care may be postponed.

Statement about the child's current health status

The clinician should make a clear statement about the child's health, growth, developmental achievements, and psychological adjustment. An example of such a brief statement for a four-year-old well child might be, "Louise-May is a fine, healthy girl. She is growing well and is learning the things she should be for her age. She seems to be a comfortable, happy child, although somewhat shy in new situations. But she adjusts appropriately. I enjoy seeing her growing and developing like this."

It might be helpful at this point to show the parent and older child a growth chart and briefly discuss the child's growth in relation to the percentile curves on the chart. Parents are frequently concerned that their child is "too fat," "not tall enough," or "does not eat enough." Growth charts can be a helpful adjunct in this discussion because they serve as a concrete, scientific indicator of the child's growth and body proportion. However, use of the chart is not always appropriate or helpful; some parents have difficulty in comprehending charts and are confused by them, even with a full explanation. For such parents, a presentation with a growth chart may therefore be embarrassing and hence counterproductive.

After presenting the evaluative statement about the child's health, growth, development, and psychosocial adjustment, the clinician should give the child and parents an opportunity to comment or to ask questions. If they do not respond spontaneously or mention their concerns, one can encourage an exchange by saying, "I would be interested to know if there are other things you would like to discuss," or "Are there any questions, either about what we have discussed or about other things that you would like to talk about?"

Anticipatory guidance

This part of the clinical summary is a presentation of the health care practitioner's ideas concerning how to foster the patient's health and development. Some of this information may have been discussed earlier, during the interview (see Chapter 5), however, the majority of it is usually presented at this time. Anticipatory guidance requires careful thought about priorities and which areas should have priority at a particular visit. With repeated visits, as the child grows and develops, most areas will be covered.

Anticipatory guidance includes providing information about likely changes in daily habits, such as the sleep–wake cycle of an infant or appetite changes in a toddler. A brief discussion about developmental changes which the child and family are likely to experience in the near future can be most helpful; it should include such items as the oppositional attitude of a toddler or the assertiveness of an adolescent. In addition to stage-specific challenges and stresses, the examiner should discuss situations relevant to the particular family at this time; appropriate items include possible reactions to the birth of a sibling, the patient's entrance into a day-care program, the death of a close relative, or a change in the occupation of a parent.

Recommendations about diet, dental care, television viewing, and accident prevention are important components usually brought up in this section of the clinical summary.

Guidance also includes advice about child rearing, such as toilet training for a toddler and fostering independence and self-care for a school-age child. However, as we have emphasized before, a clinician's advice about child rearing should communicate that there may be several satisfactory alternatives for handling a particular stage and that the parents should trust their own judgment about what is best for their family. In addition, the health care practitioner can offer to be a continuing resource for the parents when problems do emerge and suggest that they get in touch even if it is not time for a routine visit. When there is disagreement, the discussion of child care is much more complex. (See Questions about Child Rearing and Disagreements in Chapter 5, pp. 93 and 96.)

To illustrate the approach to anticipatory guidance that we advocate, we have selected some examples chosen from various stages in a child's development. In the *prenatal visit*, for instance, the clinician will discuss the parents' plans for feeding the infant. Here parents frequently ask for information and advice on whether to breast or bottle feed. These should be given, as should information about accident prevention, such as car restraints for infants and crib safety. It is also helpful to give advice on how to tell other children in the family about the expected baby and on optimum arrangements for the children when the mother delivers the infant. Finally, it is appropriate to mention plans for immediate postpartum health care and routine visits to the office or clinic beginning at two weeks of age.

During the health evaluation of an *18-month-old* child, it will be important to talk about the child's vulnerability to poisoning with household chemicals and medications (if this was not already discussed at the 12-month visit), the need for Ipecac as an emergency measure in poisonings, and the beginning oppositional stage becoming more pronounced at around two years of age. The clinical summary for a *four-and-one-half-year-old* child should include discussion of the most common hazards, such as fire, drowning, and bicycle accidents. And it may be appropriate to recommend ways to handle the transition to kindergarten.

The *older school-age* child can benefit from information about the effect of sugar on teeth and bodily changes to anticipate during growth. The child and parents may need advice on how to monitor the amount and quality of television viewing and how the child can become increasingly responsible for self-care and household chores. The *adolescent* may benefit from information about current and ongoing body changes during puberty, the issue of sexuality and birth control, skin care and control of mild acne.

The child should be included in the discussion of anticipatory guidance. As the child matures, increasing responsibility will be taken for his or her own physical health and social relationships. Even four-year-olds take responsibility for their own safety much of the time, and by school age, most children essentially control their own diets, protect themselves from accidents, and choose their playmates. In addition, adolescents are responsible for their own sexual activity, use of drugs, and social relationships.

Written materials can be a helpful adjunct to this guidance; however, they should never replace discussions between the health care practitioner and the family. These materials are especially useful when they contain specific details and instructions such as information about children's car seats, suggestions for low-sugar snacks, and recommendations for accident prevention and emergency treatment. They should be available in English, and in any other language prevalent in the patient population. The clinician may recommend books for children or for the parents, including books about preparation for the birth of a sibling, moving to a new house, sex education, hospitalization, effective parenting, and child development.

Screening and immunizations

Many well-child health evaluations include immunizations and screening tests (see Chapter 4 regarding the data base and recommendations for screening tests). Most parents know about these procedures, but frequently they have inaccurate information about their purpose, indications, or side effects. In addition, the current medical recommendations change frequently; this means that younger children may well have different immunizations and tests from their older siblings. As in other discussions with a parent and older child, the clinician should present the facts and provide an opportunity for questions.

For example: "Robert is due for his combined measles-mumps-German measles immunization today. He will not have the sore leg and fever that you mentioned he had with the last DPT injection, but he may have a low grade fever or rash 6 to 14 days from now. These side effects occur occasionally, and I want you to know about them so you will not be surprised if they do occur. There is no special treatment for the side effects, and they usually disappear on their own within a few days. But, if for some reason you feel Robert's reaction is unusual, or if you have any questions, please call me about it. Do you have any questions now about all this?" A parent who has an older child in addition to the 15-month-old toddler receiving the immunization, may comment that her 6-year-old daughter had the immunizations for those illnesses separately, and therefore she is wondering about the change. The clinician might explain that studies done in the last few years show that children get as good protection with the combined immunizations as with the individual ones. In this way they need only have one injection instead of three.

Screening tests, such as the hemoglobin and hematocrit measurements, urine culture on toilet-trained girls, and vision and hearing tests all occur repeatedly throughout childhood. The clinician should provide the parent and older patient with a brief explanation about such tests, their purpose, and how they are done.

Parents should have a written record of the child's immunizations and screening tests. In many health care facilities the parents are given a record with this information, beginning with the first immunizations in infancy. This card is used for repeated entries as immunizations and screening tests are performed, and it is particularly helpful for the examiner to remind the parent to bring it along at each visit. This record is very helpful if the child needs health care when away from home, or if the child transfers to a different health care facility.

Many health care practitioners find that written information about the common side effects of immunizations and their management is helpful for parents. But here again, the pamphlet should never replace the clinician's brief teaching about side effects and the opportunity for all parties concerned to ask questions.

Plans for future care

Plans for future health maintenance visits should be discussed briefly at the end of the clinical summary. The parents should know when to return and the expected content of each subsequent visit, particularly when there will be any immunizations or tests. A lot of unnecessary anxiety can be avoided when the parent can tell the child that "shots" are not due. When painful procedures are planned, however, it is better for children to be prepared before the visit than to be surprised at the time they are performed.

Parents should be reminded that they do not have to wait until the next scheduled appointment to talk with their clinician. If they are concerned about anything with regard to the patient, they should call. Most parents will call when their child becomes ill; however, relatively few will call to discuss psychological or developmental issues. This is unfortunate, since a good deal of anxiety and emotional discomfort for the family may be avoided if they do call the clinician before the next scheduled visit, which may not be for many weeks or even months. If a minor problem has been discussed in the clinical summary, the practitioner may help the family a lot by specifically telling the parents to keep in touch about the situation. In some cases, the clinician may decide that it is best to call the family on his or her own initiative to give special support. In other cases it will become necessary to call because the parents fail to keep the clinician informed about a recognized area of concern.

CHAPTER 12

The Clinical Summary With Minor Problems

Minor Physical Problems
    Introduction
    Examples
        1. Inadequate Primary Care
        2. Poor Dental Care
        3. Small Deviation from Normal Growth
        4. Infant with Thrush
        5. Recurrent Eczema
        6. Asthmatic and Allergic Problems
    Follow-up
Minor Psychological Problems
    Introduction
    Examples
        1. Sibling Rivalry at Different Ages
        2. Toilet Training
        3. New Situation—Kindergarten and Bus
        4. Budding School Avoidance

MINOR PHYSICAL PROBLEMS

Introduction

Minor physical problems are those which the clinician decides do not require complex diagnostic or therapeutic procedures and which are not likely to have serious consequences. A discussion of minor physical problems is best included in the clinical summary, after the statement about the child's current health status. It should include a brief statement about the diagnosis, treatment, and course of the problem, followed by a discussion of management, follow-up and questions.

It is important to keep in mind, however, that an illness which a clinician defines as minor because of its benign course and simple treatment may be experienced as a major illness by the parent or child. Consequently, when either the parents or patient give clues that they are concerned about a problem, the clinician should try to find the source of that concern. The illness may have consequences for the social or economic welfare of the family, cause the family inconvenience, or be one of a series of burdens on the physical and psychological resources of the family. The parents may also worry about a serious underlying illness. For example, a parent may worry that recurrent nosebleeds are a symptom of a bleeding disorder or that "swollen glands" associated with mononucleosis are a sign of leukemia. An adolescent may consider his or her acne to be very disfiguring, although it is mild in comparison to other cases which the clinician has seen. A toddler may have "only" an ear infection. However, the parent worries that when he has to stay home because the child is not able to attend day care as a result of the infection, he may lose his job.

Even when a problem is medically minor, the health care practitioner should be sure that the management plan is clear and that an adequate rationale for the plan is given. Minor problems may become complicated if they are not handled appropriately. For example, a minor case of diarrhea may quickly worsen if a parent, not hearing or remembering the clinician's precaution against it, gives the child milk because it is "nature's perfect food."

Follow-up is crucial because major problems in children and their families may masquerade as minor ones. For example, a fever may be a short-lived symptom of a minor viral infection; but a prolonged fever may be a symptom of a urinary tract infection, which requires treatment and evaluation. Arrangements for continuing contact with the clinician are simple, but they should never be omitted just because the clinician thinks the problems are minor or because the parents seem to be competent and will know when to call. It is advisable to describe the expected course of any problems and arrange for a visit or telephone contact.

The following situations illustrate a variety of minor problems and how the clinician can include discussion of them in the clinical summary.

Examples

1. **Inadequate Primary Care:** Sometimes inadequate primary care is a problem in itself, with its accompanying incomplete immunizations and sporadic well-child care. The evaluation would be handled by learn-

ing the reasons for the problem, educating the family about the purpose of primary care, and suggesting appropriate resources. Inadequate well-child care should be labeled explicitly as a problem, with specific management and follow-up arrangements.

2. Poor Dental Care: In some situations, a specific physical abnormality or disease will result from inadequate health maintenance. Here is a suggestive case:

Hubert is a six-year-old who is a new patient in the practice of pediatrician Dr. Louise Harris and Ms. Ellen Green, a pediatric nurse practitioner. At his routine health visit, Ms. Green learns that Hubert does not brush his teeth regularly, has never been to a dentist or dental hygienist for dental care, eats a large quantity of sweet foods, and has many large cavities which are grossly visible. Ms. Green tells Hubert's father about the cavities. She learns why the child has never been to a dentist and if and where other family members receive dental care. There are many possible reasons for this problem, including cost, fear of the dentist by the child or parent, and lack of information about a dentist who works well with children. If the family needs advice about dental care for Hubert, Ms. Green should give them information about suitable resources for pediatric dental care.

Ms. Green talks with Hubert and his parents about the importance of limiting the amount of sugar in his diet, and she may suggest ways to decrease sugar, especially in snacks. She should also ask about the source of drinking water; if it is not fluoridated city water, the family should be advised to consider fluoride supplements. This may be necessary for some municipal water supplies, for well water, and for a child with little water intake although the water supply has adequate fluoride. Dental hygiene should include regular brushing twice a day and regular visits to the dentist or dental hygienist to have the teeth cleaned and caries repaired.

This lack of dental health maintenance and the associated caries should be noted in the record as a problem, and explicit follow-up should be planned.

3. Small Deviation from Normal Growth: A common problem is a small deviation from normal growth patterns. In the case of Ann, a one-year-old girl, the clinician's initial statement to her parents in the clinical summary could be: "Ann is a healthy girl who is learning new things very well. I am a little concerned about her fast weight gain in the last few months. What are your ideas about her growth?" The parents' answer will lead into a discussion about Ann's growth, her dietary habits and those of the family, any history of obesity in the family, possible long-term implications for rapid weight gain in infancy, and a plan for her diet and follow-up.

4. Infant with Thrush: A newly diagnosed problem in an infant may require a fairly detailed discussion, but it can still be included in the clinical summary. John, an eight-week-old infant, comes for a routine health evaluation and the clinician makes the diagnosis of oral moniliasis (thrush). When the clinician notes it during the physical examination, she or he may ask the parents if they had noticed the white plaques in the child's mouth. Frequently, the parents will answer "yes," and may wonder if the plaques are milk. At that point in the physical examination the clinician can say, "The patches are called 'thrush.' It can be treated easily and is not serious. We'll talk more about it later in the check-up." Later, in the clinical summary, after a general statement about the child's growth and development the examiner might say, "I would like to talk a bit more about the white patches in John's mouth. As I mentioned, it is called thrush. It frequently occurs in young babies and is caused by a germ called monilia. Have you ever heard of this before?"

The mother may recall that she had vaginal moniliasis during her pregnancy and that the obstetrician had prescribed a topical medication for her. The clinician should ask if her condition is still present, because it may be a source for the infant's thrush. If it is present, the clinician should mention that this is a frequent pattern and that if both she and the baby are treated, the problem will clear up completely. Then, one would continue with specific instructions for management of the problem, such as medication for the child, advice to boil all nursing bottles and pacifiers (to prevent reinfection of the child from these sources), and plans for the mother's treatment. At the end it would be good practice to inquire, "Are there any questions you have about John's thrush? (pause) It should disappear after a few days of treatment. Please use the medicine for the full week to ensure that all the germs are gone. If it doesn't seem to be clearing, or if you have any other questions, please call."

5. Recurrent Eczema: A manageable problem, such as recurrent mild eczema, can be included in the statement about a patient's health without focusing the clinical summary too much on this one issue: "Robert is a healthy boy who is growing well. I am glad to hear that the rivalry with his brother has lessened. His only problem today is the eczema, which has been bothering him a bit more lately. I think it is important to treat it vigorously now, before it gets worse. From our past experience with Robert's skin, I'm confident that we can get it under control and he will be more comfortable soon. The rest of the check-up was fine." The management of the eczema should be attended to, and the summary can then proceed to anticipatory guidance or screening tests.

6. Asthmatic and Allergic Problems: An asthmatic episode is a fairly common problem which may be either minor or major, at any particular time; depending upon the severity of the symptoms, the physical findings, and the child's previous response to treatment.

Diane, a nine-year-old girl complaining of a "cold," is seen by Dr. Harris. The physical examination reveals watery rhinorrhea, a slightly wet cough, and mild expiratory wheezes in all lung fields—but also good air exchange. A review of the child's medical history reveals a past history of seasonal hay fever.

At the end of the evaluation, Dr. Harris should talk with both the parents and the child. The conversation might proceed as follows: "Diane, the tight feeling you said you feel in your chest is wheezing. This is a symptom of asthma, which we can treat with pills or liquid medicine. It is difficult to know exactly what makes the wheezing begin for each person, but in you it is probably related to the cold you have. Your current wheezing is related to the hay fever that we talked about earlier. Many children who have hay fever later develop asthmatic wheezing without colds." Diane might ask some questions, which should be answered. Then Dr. Harris might turn to the parents to ask them what they know about asthma, and inquire, "Do you know anyone with this problem?" If they say, "Yes, an uncle of Diane's on her mother's side," Dr. Harris should find out about that person's illness, especially its course over time, and whether he was ever hospitalized for it. She can say, "What was the asthma like for your brother? Do you know what treatment he had? Did it keep him from doing any of the things he wanted to do?" The reason for asking these questions is to find out if the family had an experience that might give them a particularly atypical and severe picture of what it means to have asthma, and to learn whether they have any misinformation about the illness. It would be helpful to continue, "It is very difficult to predict the course of a person's asthma. However, most people have relatively mild cases, which are usually well controlled with medicine. Also, most children outgrow their asthma."

Sometimes parents ask whether asthma is inherited. It is best to answer truthfully, but in a way that does not increase any guilt the parent feels. The answer might be, "Asthma, like allergies, does tend to run in families. It is common for a person with asthma to have relatives who also have asthma or other allergic problems. However, this is not always true. In addition, there is no way to predict who in the family will develop asthma, nor can we prevent it from happening. There isn't anything you could have done to have kept Diane from developing asthma. All we can do is to treat it now and whenever it recurs. (pause) Are there other questions I can answer for you?"

Then, along with a prescription for the appropriate medication, the clinician should provide instructions for its use in the next few days. Here it is important to discuss how the parent will decide to give the medication for future episodes of wheezing, how to decide when to get medical consultation, and the side effects of the medication. A visit to the office should be scheduled for some ten days hence and the parents can be urged to telephone if the child is not feeling better by the following day. The follow-up appointment allows further opportunity to discuss the family's reaction to the presence of this new problem in their lives.*

---

* The need for consultation about this patient would depend on the medical expertise of the primary clinician and the protocol followed in the particular clinical setting (see Chapter 14 on Consulation).

Follow-up

Follow-up is extremely important to ensure the early detection of treatment failures, complications, and erroneous diagnoses. Minor physical problems are ubiquitous in children, but fulminating serious conditions appear capriciously. In young children, especially, changes occur rapidly, and serious problems may become life-threatening if they are not treated early in their course. On follow-up the clinician may realize that the problem was not resolved with the treatment prescribed and that the concerns were symptoms of severe pathology which need more vigorous intervention. Serious errors occur in pediatric health care because of inadequate follow-up of what initially appeared to be common and minor disorders.

In order to avoid these errors, clinicians should be explicit when discussing the expected course of a problem with a family and should instruct the parents to call (or return to the office or clinic if they have no telephone access) if the problem does not progress as anticipated. An example is the typical case of a six-month-old infant with mild gastroenteritis. The health care practitioner gives routine advice about early diet restriction, followed by a gradual return to the child's regular diet during the next several days. This advice should, however, be followed by the clear recommendation that the parents should contact the clinician if the child's symptoms fail to improve within 24 hours or if at any time the vomiting, diarrhea, and systemic signs such as fever, lethargy, or irritability worsen. For some parents, the clinician may even need to initiate follow-up contact.

MINOR PSYCHOLOGICAL PROBLEMS

Introduction

Minor psychological problems are ones which the clinician thinks are likely to improve fairly quickly with pediatric counseling—without the necessity for intensive mental health intervention such as psychiatric therapy or medication. As in the case of minor physical problems, these psychological problems are best included in the clinical summary after the statement about the child's current health status.

This section will discuss those psychological problems which can be handled in the clinical summary. (Those that require further visits for pediatric evaluation and management are discussed in Chapter 13 with major psychological problems.) Minor problems include the challenges which most families normally encounter as their children grow and develop. However, a family may need help in solving a particular problem, although in general they manage such issues adequately. Sometimes it is difficult for the clinician to decide when to label a concern or stress as a "problem" because there is such a wide range of perfectly adequate child rearing patterns, life events, and possible responses. However, the purpose of labeling and recording a minor problem is to ensure adequate follow-up whenever the clinician is concerned that it may lead to further difficulty. Certainly when one has known a given family over a long time such an assessment is more likely to be accurate and useful for that family without the necessity of an extensive evaluation. Naturally when a patient is new to the practitioner, more time is needed for the health evaluation; this may necessitate scheduling another visit.

Minor psychological problems show themselves to the family and the clinician in different ways. Sometimes the parents and children are concerned about a situation and ask for help. In other situations, one parent is concerned, but the other one feels the behavior at issue is "just a stage." Occasionally, it is a teacher or another unrelated adult who first brings the child's behavior to the parents' attention, indicating that it seems to be problematic. Sometimes, an older child or adolescent may tell the clinician about a problem directly, occasionally in confidence. Not infrequently, however, the clinician decides that there is a minor problem based on the developmental history and observations, even though neither the patient nor a parent has mentioned any concerns. The clinician may also recognize that certain stresses—such as a difficult pregnancy, marital separation, or a death in the family—put both the child and the family at risk for psychological problems. Hence, although there is no active problem, it is wise to note such circumstances and plan future well-child psychological assessment and care appropriately. What all this amounts to is that whenever there is a minor psychological problem, or the patient is at risk for such problems, good health care practice requires that the problem be approached systematically, in the same way one would evaluate a physical problem.

Although the clinician considers a problem minor, the child or parents may experience it as major. Their anxiety should never be dismissed. It may only reflect their insecurity about psychological problems, in which case counseling might be very helpful. However, the reaction may well reflect more complex problems, requiring further inquiry and possible intervention. In either case, the clinician should approach the discussion with care and sensitivity for the family's concerns.

Management of minor psychological problems may be accomplished in large part simply by talking over the situation with the child and parents. One can draw attention to the specific difficulty and help the family to appreciate its importance. Usually, the family already has some ideas about how to manage the situation. The clinician can help the older patient and parents sort out their options and decide what is the best solution for the family by discussing the situation with them and suggesting alternative ways for the parents to respond to the child's behavior. Frequently clinicians help parents to communicate more clearly with other family members and to work more effectively with people outside the family. However, the most important task for the clinician is to clarify the problem and support the family in their own efforts to solve it.

Follow-up is very important because the clinician can never be sure, at the beginning, which concerns will resolve themselves and which are symptoms of more severe disturbances. Complicated psychological problems sometimes seem deceptively simple initially. With adequate follow-up, serious problems which first presented as minor problems will be detected early, before severe or irreversible damage has occurred. Clinicians' failure to record minor psychological problems is often a factor in poor follow-up.

Examples

The following examples illustrate the management of minor psychological problems.

1. Sibling Rivalry at Different Ages: Rivalry between siblings is universal, and it occurs at many ages. However, sometimes it is excessive, or the parents are particularly upset by it, and consequently needs some form of intervention. Excessive rivalry may be a minor problem, or it may be a symptom of more severe psychological problems in the family. The following helps to demonstrate the potential range of the problem.

Mrs. Hutchins comes for a health evaluation for her 12-month-old daughter, Sally, and she brings along her two-and-one-half year-old son, John. Roger Kingman, the nurse practitioner, notices that John repeatedly provokes Sally by taking her toys, pushing her down, and shoving her away from their mother's lap. Mrs. Hutchins seems uncomfortable, but never mentions the obvious conflict; she does not limit John's behavior and tells Mr. Kingman that the children get along well together. In this situation, Mr. Kingman should gather more data about the sibling relationship before sharing his own impression. He may ask the mother to describe the children's behavior together at home in more detail. He may ask her opinion of John's behavior in the office, and then give his own impression. He also needs to know how both parents handle the jealous behavior and how they feel about it. He should ask the mother if she has any ideas about why the family is having this difficulty and what she thinks could be done to help.

Mr. Kingman should discuss his assessment and make suggestions about how to manage the situation. For example, he could recommend that the parents protect the younger child from being harmed by John, that they improve the amount and quality of the time John has with his parents, and that they talk with him about his feelings of jealousy and help him verbalize these feelings, instead of expressing them with aggressive physical behavior.

Excessive quarreling between school-age children is frequently related to the quality of their earlier relationship. If this problem exists in a family, their health care practitioner should be sure to talk with both the children and the parents. It is not uncommon for the children's conflicts to reflect those of the parents, especially if one child is favored or if a parent is unusually sensitive and easily upset by jealous behavior. However, if there are no indications of serious problems in the children or the parents, the clinician should help the parents make a plan. He can encourage the parents by saying that although he can understand there is a problem, the situation does not seem severe. He may remind the parents that both children share responsibility for the problem and that they are often capable of handling these things on their own. (Sometimes, parents are trapped into trying to decide who is right without an unbiased report of the facts.) Finally, the clinician can communicate clearly that both children have a responsibility to handle their quarrels in a way which does not impinge on the rights of other family members. He should never be glib about reassurance and should plan adequate follow-up. If the problem does not improve, additional assessment for more serious difficulties should be undertaken.

2. Toilet Training: Difficulty with toilet training is an example of another "normal" developmental challenge which may present a problem. Mrs. Williams' son is 18 months old, and he is learning to use a potty chair. She is in frequent conflict with him about the toilet training and other issues of control. As a result, she dreads each day's encounters and finds herself becoming increasingly irritable, unhappy, and less patient with her son.

The clinician needs to gather a developmental and social history, assess the relationship of Mrs. Williams with her son, formulate a plan, and arrange follow-up. If the toilet training is not progressing satisfactorily within a few weeks, or if other developmental or social problems become apparent during follow-up visits, the situation will require a more thorough evaluation and a new formulation and plan.

3. New Situation—Kindergarten and Bus: New experiences are frequently quite stressful to entire families. The primary clinician can be a helpful advisor in situations when a child has a difficult adjustment to make.

Joshua is a five-year-old boy who comes for his routine "school check-up" late in September of the year he begins kindergarten. During the history, his father mentions that in the past few weeks Joshua has wet the bed a few times at night and is resisting going to sleep. Also, he has been less willing to play independently, especially outdoors. He had not previously been enuretic, and independent play and a relaxed bedtime had been usual.

It turns out that Joshua's parents have been anxious about how he will adjust to school. They are not comfortable with the marked difference in expectations between Joshua's nursery school and his kindergarten. Joshua tells Dr. Badillo, the clinician, that he is afraid he will miss the school bus and be left alone at school at the end of the day. His parents did not know about their son's fear.

Dr. Badillo should review Joshua's adjustment to other situations such as nursery school and should update the developmental social history. She can talk briefly with his parents about the difficulties children have with new experiences and make a plan to help both Joshua and his parents feel less anxious. A parent–teacher conference seems indicated here, as well as more explicit verbal instructions, a predictable schedule, and clear support from Joshua's teacher. Probably these measures will bring improvement.

It is also important for Dr. Badillo to speak with Joshua directly, perhaps saying, "Children sometimes feel that going to a new school and taking the bus are scary things. It is good that you can tell us what worries you, so that we can help fix things. Your parents will be able to talk to the teacher and they will make sure that you won't miss the bus and will help make it less scary. I will talk to your parents again, and will hear how you are. (pause) Is there anything you would like to ask me?"

A follow-up telephone call or an office visit a few weeks later is certainly called for, with clear instructions for the parents to call earlier if the situation worsens.

4. Budding School Avoidance: Children frequently have difficulties in school, and they depend on their parents to help solve their problems. A pediatric clinician can help parents understand their child's school problem and also support the parents in their discussions with school personnel.

Ann Polansky is a ten-year-old girl who has never had any major physical or psychological problems. When she comes for a routine health evaluation, Ron Wilson, the physician's assistant, learns that she is resisting going to school and that she complains of tiredness and stomachaches. Ann's mother does not know what to do, is quite annoyed at her reluctance to attend school, and is impatient with her daughter's tiredness and stomachaches. Mrs. Polansky asks the clinician whether there is something wrong with her child.

Mr. Wilson knows from the medical history and physical examination that Ann is physically healthy. In addition, he knows that her family life is good, her peer relationships are quite normal, and she has previously been happy and well-adjusted. Her school work generally has been quite good, but arithmetic has always been a difficult subject for her. She is a hard worker and does not want to disappoint her parents with poor grades. Ann tells Mr. Wilson that she works hard to learn her arithmetic but the teacher "is very nasty, and makes fun of my mistakes in front of the other kids." She admits that her tiredness and stomachaches are excuses to avoid her problem with math.

Mrs. Polansky is extremely reluctant to go to school and speak with the teacher. She, herself, had not been a good student and was frequently unhappy as a child because of her own school situation. In addition, she was recently intimidated by the school personnel at a routine conference. Mr. Polansky speaks English poorly, and because of his immigrant background is even more intimidated by the school than his wife. The parents have discussed the situation together, but they feel Mrs. Polansky must handle the conferences at school.

During the clinical summary, Mr. Wilson should encourage Mrs. Polansky to talk to the teacher, and principal if necessary, in order to find out what is actually happening in school. If Mr. Wilson can give Mrs. Polansky some confidence in her ability to handle this situation, he will actually be helping to manage the school problem indirectly by helping her to insist the school personnel work out an effective plan to help Ann. He can give additional support to Mrs. Polansky by saying that Ann should go to school, even if she feels tired or complains of a stomachache. A clear statement by Mr. Wilson that he is confident they can solve the school problem together, will reassure both Ann and her mother of his active support.

In addition, Mr. Wilson should speak directly with Ann. The discussion might include a statement that she should attend school in spite of the stomachaches because she will not really change anything by staying home, and she will miss the other things at school that she enjoys and does well. He should be sympathetic about her worries, but should also be very encouraging that her mother and he can work together to improve the school situation.

It is unlikely that a more serious school avoidance problem will develop if the history is accurate and if the mother can carry out this plan successfully. Nevertheless, the precursors of a more serious problem—school phobia—may be present. Ann's situation, in combination with her parents' handicaps, makes explicit follow-up essential.

CHAPTER 13

The Clinical Summary With Major Problems

Introduction
General Principles
Assessment and Initial Management of Major Physical Problems
    Statement of the Problem to the Parents and Child
    Diagnostic Measures
        1. Four-year-old with Fevers for Four Weeks
        2. Eight-year-old with Headaches and Symptoms of Central Nervous System Mass
        3. Fifteen-year-old with Vomiting for Four Days
    Description of the Illness
    Management
    Response to the Management Plan
    Follow-up
Assessment and Initial Management of Major Psychological Problems
    How the Problems Present
    Preliminary Assessment by the Primary Clinician
    Statement of the Problem to the Parents and Child

Recommendations for Treatment
Parents' Responses to Recommendations for
Consultation and Therapy
Follow-up

INTRODUCTION

Major problems are ones for which complex diagnostic and/or therapeutic procedures are necessary. A major *physical* problem usually involves the possibility of detrimental sequelae and sometimes even shortened life span or life-threatening complications. Examples are a urinary tract infection, rheumatoid arthritis, osteomyelitis, diabetes mellitus, leukemia, slipped femoral epiphysis, appendicitis, and severe trauma.

Initially the examiner may not know the full and exact diagnosis although it is already clear that the signs and symptoms suggest a serious abnormality. Of course, most major problems have the potential for cure or complete control, but one cannot always predict the course at the time of presentation. Thus even the slight possibility of detrimental sequelae, chronic illness, or death makes the problem a major one.

Major *psychological* problems are ones in which the signs and symptoms indicate serious disorganization in psychological functioning, delay in development, abnormal relationships, and/or handicapping emotional discomfort. These problems present the likelihood of detrimental sequelae in the child's psychological development. They require intervention by a pediatric clinician with adequate experience in the management of psychosocial problems and consultation from a mental health professional.

Examples of major psychological problems frequently encountered in children are an infant's inability to be comforted, delayed language development in a three-year-old, poor peer relationships in a seven-year-old, encopresis, school avoidance, and drug abuse. In addition, problems suffered by one or both parents may have a sufficiently great impact on the child that they require assessment and management as well. Examples include defects in parenting, marital crises, alcoholism, depression, and serious physical illness.

GENERAL PRINCIPLES

When a significant problem is discovered in the course of a well-child health evaluation, or when the visit is for evaluation of a complaint, the clinician should use the time set aside for the clinical summary to discuss the problem and to formulate a management plan. The purpose of the discussion is for the practitioner to ensure that the family members reach an understanding about the presence and nature of the problem, to describe the steps necessary for a complete diagnosis, to consider the implications of the problem, and to make a plan for immediate management and follow-up.

The clinician must organize and analyze the data from the evaluation before she or he has the summary discussion with the family. It is important to select the relevant data from the history, physical examination, and developmental assessment, recognize and define the problem, and make a management plan.

Not infrequently, a clinician's own feelings about a particular family may make it difficult to tell them about a serious problem. There are many reasons for this: she or he may strongly identify with the parents if they are all approximately the same age or if they share common cultural, ethnic, educational, or occupational characteristics; and a pregnant clinician may find it very hard to discuss a birth defect. Adults can also identify with a sick child: a young student clinician may identify with the adolescent patient, or a clinician may identify with the child whose parents are in the throes of a divorce. Practitioners should be aware of this problem and recognize that they can be most helpful to a family if they are able to face their feelings and maintain a professional perspective —namely, a well-balanced combination of empathy, encouragement, support, and clarification.

Student clinicians are also reluctant to tell families about a serious problem because they know they are inexperienced and therefore are insecure about their ability to be helpful. The skills of assessment and formulation are complex and develop only with experience and careful review of the student's work. Every student should have access to a senior pediatric clinician before she or he conducts a clinical summary, especially in cases with major problems. This provides an opportunity to discuss both the student's feelings (briefly) and the assessment and plans. A detailed discussion about the student's feelings may be very helpful as well and should take place after the family has completed the visit. Whenever supervising clinicians can share their own experiences in similar situations—including personal reactions—the student can better understand the feelings she or he has experienced, and consequently be more confident in future clinical relationships.

The primary clinician must know several things about a major problem in order to conduct the summary discussion adequately. It is crucial that the practitioner be able to define clearly both what the problem is and what it is not. Similarly, she or he must know if the diagnosis is definite, unconfirmed but likely, or not yet determined. If more diagnostic procedures are required, the clinician needs to know about them in detail. For a physical problem, x-rays, laboratory tests, or a biopsy may be necessary. For a psychological problem, a full developmental evaluation, psychometric testing, and/or a conference with the child's teachers may be indicated.

If the diagnosis is definite, the clinician needs to know as much as possible about the etiology of the problem. Even if a specialist manages the therapy, the primary care clinician should know a great deal about the treatment. It is also important to clarify who will manage diagnostic procedures and therapy: the primary care clinician, a consultant, or both.

The format suggested below will help organize the information that is dealt with in the clinical summary of major problems, to avoid confusion and omissions. The discussion usually includes a statement of the problem, a description of the illness, and plans for management, including diagnostic steps, treatment, consultation, and follow-up arrangements. As mentioned in previous chapters, the practitioner should not adhere to a rigid order in conducting the discussion, but should try to alter it to best suit the needs of the particular clinical situation. When a problem is serious, a complete discussion of the situation may not be possible in the first visit because the parents may be very upset. In this event it will be necessary to continue the discussion at subsequent scheduled visits.

ASSESSMENT AND INITIAL MANAGEMENT OF MAJOR PHYSICAL PROBLEMS

Statement of the problem to the parents and child

One of the most difficult tasks for a clinician is to tell parents that their child has a serious problem. In stating the problem the first task is to present the information clearly and to be sensitive to the family's reaction. At the same time, the practitioner must be aware of his or her own feelings and their effect on the situation.

The clinician should begin by stating clearly that there is a problem; then the problem must be identified (sometimes with a medical term). It is important, in this context, to be sure to use language that the family can understand. Health professionals sometimes forget how much technical language pervades their conversations when they talk with each other about diagnosis and treatment. After this has been done, it is appropriate to pause a bit to let the information sink in and to give the parents and the child ample opportunity to ask questions. It is best if both parents are present for the initial discussion, but if it is not possible, an appointment to see the parents together should be scheduled for the immediate future. It is almost never helpful to "protect" one parent from the difficulty; this is true even when a parent is mentally ill.

Serious problems have an emotional side which experienced clinicians find they must address. At the least, a serious problem will generate some intense anxiety. Most parents experience, in some form, the emotional sequence of denial, grief, mourning, and (it is hoped!) acceptance when they are faced with major problems. It should, consequently, come as no surprise if a sick patient's parents are angry, in despair, or refuse to believe in the diagnosis at first. Hence a clinician may face the task of overcoming defensive denial on the parents' part before treatment can commence. Then there is an obligation to support the family through the sometimes lengthy phase of treatment and adjustment to the illness. This phase may be even more difficult if the parents had no idea that their child had a serious illness before this fact was presented to them by the clinician. For example, when there is a serious, but asymptomatic, condition such as congenital heart anomaly or a metabolic disease, the parents will probably be completely unprepared for the news that a serious physical problem exists. Parents would probably be equally distressed when a child presents a symptom (such as fever) which usually is not an indicator of serious illness, and then a major problem (such as a malignant tumor) is identified.

Occasionally, the parents persist in their disagreement with the clinician about a problem. They may think that no problem is present or that the situation is not serious. Although this occurs more frequently with psychological problems, it can be a major obstacle in the management of a physical problem as well. The disagreement should be noted in the record and the clinician should try to resolve it while continuing to work with the family.

Diagnostic measures

If there is no definite diagnosis that can be made, possible causes of the signs and symptoms should be discussed with the family; then one can explain the rationale for further evaluation. This evaluation will include more data from the interview, developmental assessment, laboratory tests, or other diagnostic procedures. Sometimes consultation is necessary.

It is not always possible to predict, initially, how much time will be necessary to complete an assessment of a serious problem. If it appears that the problem is especially complex, the family should be told that it may take time to figure out what is wrong and that this can be difficult for them. Parents are less upset about a time-consuming evaluation if they know about it from the beginning and if the clinician has explained the rationale for these measures.

It is best to describe all the diagnostic steps that are needed. If one knows the details, it is a good idea to tell the family how long the process will take to perform, whether any of the procedures are painful, when they will be scheduled, what their cost is, when the results will be available, and how to prepare the child for each one. If a consultant will be participating in the diagnostic phase, the primary clinician should explain the rationale for the consulation, and also the role the consultant will take in diagnosis and treatment.

The following three common examples illustrate the diagnostic phase in practice.

1. Four-year-old with Fevers for Four Weeks: Joan Brown comes with her father to see Ms. Somers, their nurse practitioner. Mr. Brown gives the history that his four-year-old daughter has had intermittent fevers ranging from 101°F. to 104°F. (38.3°C. to 40°C.) for the past four weeks. She also has been less energetic than usual and is irritable when febrile. About one week prior to the visit, Joan had a rash on her trunk and upper arms and legs which lasted for five days. It looked "like measles" and was made up of many small red-pink "bumps." The remainder of the history is remarkable in the *lack* of symptoms to suggest involvement of any particular system in the body. Past medical history and family history are unremarkable. Physical examination reveals moderate splenomegaly and generalized lymphadenopathy. There are no other abnormalities and Joan is afebrile.

The nurse practitioner discusses the case with the pediatrician and together they decide to order several laboratory tests to help them make a diagnosis. For the time being, they decide on a working diagnosis of juvenile rheumatoid arthritis. However, it is necessary to test for infections and malignancies, nor should the possibility of a factitious (false) fever be forgotten.

Mr. Brown will benefit from a brief discussion about the rationale for the tests, and a follow-up appointment should be arranged within a few days to discuss the diagnosis further.

2. Eight-year-old with Headaches and Symptoms of Central Nervous System Mass: Steven Hotchkiss, who is eight years old, comes with his mother to see their pediatrician, Dr. Frank Mansurian, because of a four-week history of headaches. It seems that Steven fell from his bicycle around the time the headaches began, but it is not clear which came first, the headaches or the fall. There has been a trend toward increasing frequency and severity of the headaches so that "aspirin doesn't help anymore." Steven has been more irritable and perhaps slightly clumsy in the last two days. The family has a history of migraine headaches.

The physical examination reveals bilateral papilledema and a slight decrease in the child's ability to perform some tests of coordination. Dr. Mansurian is confident there is an intracranial mass and decides that Steven should be seen immediately by a neurologist. He tells Steven that he will need a consultation and then has a more detailed discussion with Mrs. Hotchkiss alone about the rationale for the consultation and its urgency. Of course, this will be a very difficult discussion.

3. Fifteen-year-old with Vomiting for Four Days: Amanda Johnston is 15 years old. She makes an appointment to see her physician's assistant, Ms. Serena Raintree, with the complaint that she has been vomiting for four days. Amanda has also felt unusually tired and has had some increased frequency of urination for the past week. She has had normal bowel movements and has not had any fevers. Further history reveals that her siblings have had the "flu" with vomiting and diarrhea during the past ten days. The review of systems reveals that Amanda's last menstrual period was ten weeks ago and that she has a history of irregular menstrual cycles. She has had sexual intercourse without birth control many times since her last menstrual period. The physical examination is unremarkable, and she refuses to have a pelvic examination.

There are several possible diagnoses, including pregnancy, urinary tract infection, and "flu." Laboratory tests on the urine can reliably support the diagnosis of pregnancy or urinary tract infection. Ms. Raintree discusses the diagnostic possibilities with Amanda, explains the rationale for the tests, and makes a follow-up plan for the next few days. In this situation, particular care is needed in assessing the patient's ability to deal with the possibility of pregnancy. If the primary clinician is not sure she can adequately assess the patient's personal abilities and resources to cope with this eventuality, consultation with another health clinician or a social worker would be appropriate. Further, it would appear that Amanda needs counseling on sex and contraception. Here, too, Ms. Raintree might wish to call in another health care practitioner to provide Amanda with the necessary information and counseling. The issue will become even more pressing if Amanda turns out to be pregnant and the question of terminating the pregnancy is broached.

Description of the illness

When a diagnosis has been established, the clinician should describe the illness to both the parents and the patient (at the child's level of understanding). This description should include etiology, usual course, response to treatment, and ultimate outcome of the disease. However, these statements should not be presented as absolute facts, but rather as the average or usual characteristics of the illness. It is very important, in this context, not to overly simplify the information. The family should have a realistic view of the difficulties in predicting the outcome of a disease; on the other hand, they should not be burdened by all the worst possibilities. The clinician can be hopeful in an honest way, without implying there is no possibility of complications or disappointments.

There are some specific questions that the clinician should answer, which may be asked explicitly by the family or anticipated by the clinician in the discussion of the problem. These questions include whether the condition is serious or life-threatening; if it will leave the child with a disability; what caused the condition; whether it is inherited or contagious; and whether the parent did anything which may have caused or increased the problem or failed to do anything that may have prevented it or made it less severe. Not infrequently, parents have a misconception about the etiology of a problem, and this may contribute to their tendency to blame themselves or someone else in the family unduly.

It is important for practitioners to be aware of their own style when discussing a condition and its etiology, especially when they suspect that the parents have not done all they could have done either to prevent the problem or to seek treatment soon enough. One should, of course, be honest and straightforward, but not harsh or judgmental. Even if the parents have been negligent or abusive, in the long run it is helpful if the clinician will try to understand the parents' situation, while simultaneously identifying their role in the problem. In the clinician's obligatory position as an advocate for the child, it is best to sustain an alliance with the family in order to help them foster the child's best interests.

Management

The first task of management is to propose a plan to the parents and child. The explanation should be simplified to suit the child's language abilities and, consequently, the parents and child often may benefit from separate explanations. All treatment modalities should be described clearly, along with the rationale and specific instructions for medication, diet, exercise, and any other measures to be taken. It also helps to discuss how effective the treatment is expected to be; how long it will be used; how uncomfortable it may make the patient; the probability and severity of side effects; where the treatment is available; and how expensive it will be.

The clinician must assess who will be responsible for implementing the outpatient management plan. If the parent or adolescent patient is unable to take this responsibility, the clinician will have to find a responsible person from the child's extended family or friends; failing in this, it will be necessary to obtain assistance from a health care agency such as the Visiting Nurse Association. A pediatric social worker can be an extremely helpful consultant in this situation.

In each case involving consultation, the primary clinician should clarify who will handle the treatment—the consultant, the primary care clinician, or both of them together. When a specialist does manage the problem, many of the questions about medications and other treatments can be answered by this person rather than by the primary clinician. However, the task of explaining the role of the consultant falls upon the primary care clinician.

Part of presenting the management is taking into account the family's ability to integrate the information. If they are so overwhelmed by the problem that they cannot pay attention and absorb all the information on the first visit, the initial presentation should be limited to the most necessary points. Some people need very simple directions, and some prefer to have information written to supplement verbal instructions. Follow-up visits in the immediate future (within several days) can be scheduled to continue the discussion, to check that the information has been correctly understood, and to answer new questions that may have arisen.

Response to the management plan

When a serious problem occurs, it may take weeks or months for the parents and child to grasp its implications for the entire family as a unit. People's ability to assimilate such information is closely related to their emotional responses to the problem. The clinician should anticipate this, and should be available to the family throughout the process of adjustment. It may be necessary to repeat information conveyed earlier which the family did not fully comprehend. Even when a specialist is managing the case, the primary clinician may have a major role in counseling the family.

Occasionally, parents reject the diagnosis or are dissatisfied with a proposed management plan. They may visit another practitioner or go to another medical center without telling their primary clinician. Alternatively, they may ask their primary practitioner about consultation with another clinician. This may be a reasonable request for another opinion, or it may reflect their effort to avoid the reality of the child's serious illness. Parents may search desperately for a new cure, and they may be attracted to a disreputable clinician whose methods are not accepted in the professional community. When this occurs, the primary clinician should try to maintain contact with the child and family and be assertive in trying to convince them to get other opinions from reputable health care professionals. It is important for the practitioner to be direct with the opinion that the child's health will not be improved by the parent's efforts to "shop around" for a long time and that they are denying the reality of the illness. In this manner, and by continuing to show concern without rejecting the parents, the primary clinician may be able to regain influence with them and convince them to follow a rational plan.

Follow-up

One should always make explicit arrangements for the next visit. If necessary, instructions should be written to help the family know when and where the next visit will be. If diagnostic procedures are required, the next visit may not be scheduled until after the results from those tests are available. In such instances a home visit or planned telephone call will help maintain contact in the interim. The parents should also be reminded that they are welcome to call any time they think of questions after they leave the office or if the course of the problem is different from what they were led to expect. The quality of the relationship established between the family and the primary practitioner during previous health care visits is very important in determining how they continue to communicate; this in turn may play a major role in how well the parents cooperate in the management of the health care plan. Therefore, when major physical problems are managed primarily by a consultant, it is important for the primary clinician to indicate his or her own continuing role in health promotion for the patient and the family.

ASSESSMENT AND INITIAL MANAGEMENT OF MAJOR PSYCHOLOGICAL PROBLEMS

The following discussion concerns situations which the primary care clinician encounters in an office visit for a routine health evaluation or in a visit for evaluation of a concern, rather than true psychiatric emergencies. The actively psychotic child or parent, or one who is dangerous to herself, himself, or others, is not difficult to identify. In these emergencies the pediatric clinician makes the diagnosis and arranges for immediate transfer to a mental health consultant. Careful supervision at home or in a hospital may be crucial to ensure the safety of the patient or others until the mental health consultant takes responsibility for the case. However, these topics are beyond the scope of this book.

How the problems present

There are some situations in which the primary clinician is the first one to realize that a child has a psychological problem. In caring for a child over many months, the clinician may note a series of minor psychological problems. Consequently, thoughtful analysis might indicate that these stresses and crises are symptoms of a problem which is serious and requires intervention. In another situation the clinician may not have known the child and family for a long time, but may nevertheless observe rather quickly during a routine health evaluation that there are signs and symptoms of a serious psychological problem. Sometimes parents will tolerate long periods of abnormal behavior before they comment or ask the clinician for an opinion. Parents who have had minimal experience with children may fail to realize that their child has a problem, and even experienced parents may deny that a problem exists. Then again, a problem may be partly acknowledged and partly denied. Teachers and parents frequently request only a physical examination to determine whether there are any physical or organic factors which could account for a child's behavior or learning problem. Pediatric clinicians should always go beyond that request, gathering a thorough history of the child's psychological and social development and current status in order to make an intelligent recommendation about the problem.

Frequently, however, parents or an older child will approach a clinician for help with clearly acknowledged psychological problems. These concerns usually fall into one of three groups: inadequate school performance or delays in developmental achievements; behavior which alienates parents, teachers, or peers; and behavior which indicates the child's discomfort, such as sleep disturbances, sadness, or unusual fears.

Preliminary assessment by the primary clinician

Whenever the clinician or parents realize there is a problem—even if it is only still understood in vague terms—it is of utmost importance for the clinician to acknowledge the problem explicitly and clearly and to state a plan for action. In most cases, a sufficient plan at the earliest stage is to gather more information about the concern. Precise diagnostic terms are *not* appropriate, and referral to a consultant is probably premature.

On rare occasions the parents present a clearly identified problem and will ask for consultation from a specialist in child development or mental health very early in the evaluation. However, this is quite unusual. (This is different from the situation in which there is a serious physical problem, when consultation and complex diagnostic evaluations are common early in the assessment.) Referral to a consultant for a psychological problem is rarely successful if the primary clinician has not first spent some time evaluating the problem independently. In addition, an apparently hasty primary assessment gives families who are afraid or skeptical about consultation an excuse to reject that recommendation.

In order to make an accurate assessment of psychological problems and to assist in an effective referral, the primary practitioner must devote one or more visits to gathering an expanded psychological, developmental, and social history. Also, the family's motivation to accept consultation from a specialist must be explored. Therefore, the initial clinical summary at the end of a health evaluation in these cases is often, in essence, an introduction to a series of interviews about the problem. This is good to keep in mind when one decides how to present an initial finding of a psychological problem.

The summary, then, should include some outline of the course to be followed in the immediate future. Separate interviews with the child and each parent may be necessary, and in some cases a structured developmental assessment will be called for. The 24-hour day history can also be a useful tool in this context. All this may add up to a lengthy period of pediatric evaluation, involving one to six hours of the clinician's and the family's time. Predictably, some parents will feel impatient when more than one session is required to make a diagnosis. This impatience can usually be diminished by explaining at the beginning the nature of the practitioner's concern for the child and the need for a thorough assessment of the problem.

Not infrequently, parents say they "doubt talking will help." This strong negative sentiment often covers up fears of exploring their child's problem. Very frequently the underlying fear is the dread of uncovering complex family problems, the existence of which has been denied, often at the expense of a child's psychological symptoms. One should not be afraid to push the parents to acknowledge the seriousness of the child's problem and the need for continued work. In most situations, parents think about their child's problem during the time between visits and find that they have more information to tell the clinician and a better understanding of the problem at subsequent interviews. This same process often continues during the waiting period between the primary clinician's assessment and the first visit to a consultant and during the evaluation done by the consultant. However, there can be increasing resistance to the preliminary psychological evaluation as it proceeds. The clinician must not be intimidated. Understanding, persistence, and open acknowledgment of the difficulties may persuade the family to continue in the evaluation of the problem.

Even a preliminary diagnosis of a psychological problem can be quite upsetting to parents and children; therefore, it is important to be careful about the way one carries out the assessment. Above all, confidentiality and a supportive relationship with the family should be maintained.

One particular feature of this type of interview which may interfere with the relationship between clinician and family is note taking. If one needs to take notes during the interview, it is a good idea to explain why one is taking them and what they will be used for; and it is always helpful to reassure the family that strict confidentiality will be maintained. In any event, notes should be as brief as possible, and they should not interfere with attention either to verbal communication or to nonverbal components of the interchange, such as eye contact and body positions. In this context, the 24-hour day format is a very useful tool because it allows a great deal of information to be recorded with a minimum of notes.

Statement of the problem to the parents and child

Practitioners are most constructive when they are honest without being harsh, presenting their opinions clearly and supportively. Whenever possible, both parents should be present when the summary of a preliminary assessment of a psychological problem is presented. Parents deserve the support they can give each other when they learn that their child has a serious developmental or psychological problem. In addition, serious psychological problems are often accompanied by significant family problems, including marital difficulties. By having both parents present at the conference, one can avoid dividing the parents, letting one blame the absent spouse, or further weakening the marriage. Also, if one parent relays the information to the other, there is much more opportunity for distortion and misunderstanding, which may prove very difficult to resolve.

The statement of the problem can begin with information familiar to the parents and child from the history and from behavioral and developmental observations. Much of this will conform to what they have already noted and can be supplemented by information from the clinician's assessment. A balanced presentation of the child's strengths and weaknesses helps parents to experience the statement as less harsh and also as more realistic. Frequently, history about physical problems such as abdominal pain, headaches, enuresis, poor growth, or obesity is relevant to the conclusion that a psychological problem is present; all these facts should be included in the opening statement.

During the presentation of the problem, jargon or diagnostic labels should not be used. Jargon is not precise, even though it may sound so; it frequently intimidates because it is not understood and the listener is ashamed to admit "deficiency." Diagnostic labels are easily misconstrued or misunderstood, usually involve some jargon, may in fact be incorrect, and often serve little more than to categorize patients in an impersonal manner, antagonizing many people. Diagnostic labels should only be used by clinicians who understand them well; and are best reserved for discussions among professional colleagues. They are not appropriate for a discussion with most parents. However, it may be necessary to let parents know that others may refer to this problem with certain diagnostic labels, such as retardation or autism.

A practitioner should resist the temptation to give a complete analysis of the cause of a problem or detailed advice about its treatment. By definition, major problems are complex and require expert evaluation. Simplistic interpretations of incomplete data lead to false conclusions and unfounded certainty on the part of clinicians, and in the end may give the parents an excuse to reject consultation.

Here is an example of how to present a problem after the preliminary assessment:

"I would like to discuss what I know now about John's difficulties. As you mentioned to me, he takes an unusually long time to get used to new situations, and he finds even small changes in his daily routines very upsetting. This has affected his everyday life and interferes with his relationships with adults and children. I have also noticed that John is a very anxious child who is rarely relaxed and comfortable. Although he has good abilities to solve problems, and is competent in his ability to play, his anxiety and tension interfere with these activities."

It is important that the practitioner not end with a negative statement of the reason for further evaluation or treatment. At this point, one should go on to discuss the child's strengths and to recommend a plan to help him. In ending on an optimistic note, however, the clinician should be careful that a balanced report is not misunderstood as an attempt to minimize serious problems:

"John has very good intellectual abilities and he speaks very well for his age. He also can trust adults who he knows, and he does ask for help. These are assets which he can learn to use better and which will be very helpful in the future."

Parents may ask directly why their child is having difficulties, or the practitioner may bring it up. In either case one should not attempt to answer the question completely, and especially should take care not to blame the parents or the child for the problem. The appropriate approach is to try to give the family a general understanding of the origin of psychological problems; the fact that they are often extremely complex may be offered as one reason for referral and treatment. For instance: "I cannot explain all the reasons why John has these problems because the reasons are complicated and require more work to understand. However, I do know that problems such as his are related to a number of factors, including the child's innate qualities, his way of responding to stress, and life experiences he has had. It is usually not one single event or stress that causes a problem, but a combination of many things."

Recommendations for treatment

After the problem has been stated and discussed, parents may ask directly about treatment. If they do not, the clinician must bring up recommendations for intervention. The recommendation should be very clear and the practitioner should be prepared to explain the reasons for the choice. This can be done quite briefly by saying, "I believe that John needs the special help that a person trained in treating psychological problems can offer. I would recommend a child psychiatrist (or other mental health professional) who is skilled in working with young children and their families. If we start treatment now, we can help John feel much better and can also promote healthy adjustments as he grows up."

Parents' responses to recommendations for consultation and therapy

Parents are frequently relieved to hear that the practitioner takes their concerns about their child seriously. They may have been told by relatives, friends, or other health care professionals that the child's problems were "just a stage," that "he'll grow out of it," or "that's really nothing."

They may be eager and ready to accept consultation from a mental health professional.

Frequently parents feel guilty, assuming that they caused their child's problems; consequently, they may assume that the clinician also blames them for the difficulties. If they hint at this or express it directly, it is important that the clinician not deny their involvement in the situation, but neither should their feelings of guilt become the focus of the presentation. One may say, "Parents often feel like they wish they could have prevented the problems their children have. Bringing up children is one of the most difficult jobs we do. I think you should know that your support, combined with an evaluation and treatment, can improve John's situation a great deal."

Some parents may want to know why you, the primary pediatric clinician, cannot treat the problem. This demands an explicit answer—perhaps, "These are complex problems which are best treated by someone with special training and experience. My own work has been in general pediatrics. Although I am interested in psychological matters, treatment of these problems is not my specialty. I will continue to work with you as your clinician as I have done in the past, and I will be available to discuss any concerns or further problems that arise."

Anxious parents understandably want reassurance or even a guarantee that treatment will cure their child's problem. The clinician is in the difficult position of recommending treatment because of the belief that it will help, and yet is not able to guarantee particular results in any specific range of time. If parents do ask directly whether treatment will help, the best answer is, "I really believe that treatment will be helpful for Cynthia and will make her feel much better. I have known other children with similar problems for whom treatment was most helpful. I cannot guarantee exactly how much improvement will occur, nor how fast it will happen. Nevertheless, I can assure you that intervention now would be best for both you and Cynthia."

In many cases, the parents have much more difficulty admitting that their child has a serious psychological problem than a serious physical problem. Experienced clinicians are prepared for this resistance; they try to understand why the parents do not want to accept their recommendation, and also try to convince them of its importance. One can say, "Can you tell me more about why you feel that Cynthia should not see a specialist?" The parents may not be able or willing to answer, but sometimes this line of questioning does prompt them to discuss their concerns.

Parents sometimes acknowledge that their child is going through a difficult period but argue, defensively, that they have seen this problem before and that later it improves spontaneously. One answer to this stratagem is, "There has been temporary improvement in the past, but we have also seen that each stressful period brings more and more difficulties. Without help she will become more anxious and have more problems. Intervention now can save her a lot of unhappiness and prevent the situation from becoming worse."

Some parents vigorously deny that the symptoms represent abnormalities or problems. They may focus narrowly on a symptom such as shy behavior, bed-wetting, or poor school work and say this is a behavior problem that many children have. Here it is useful to point out that there are many possible causes for one symptom, just as there are many causes for a physical symptom such as a fever. Some of these causes are minor, but some require major treatment and this is one of the latter instances. Naturally, some parents will continue their denial, claiming, "It is just a stage. She will grow out of it." This calls for a forceful response from the practitioner: "The reason it is necessary to evaluate the problem now, instead of waiting to see if it will resolve itself spontaneously, is that in my experience these problems tend to become worse and may be even more difficult to treat if they are allowed to continue." In addition, it may be important to remind parents about the child's current suffering and mobilize their concern and desire to be helpful in diminishing it now, regardless of long-range outcome.

If a child is not "bothering" anyone, it is particularly difficult to convince some parents that the child needs evaluation by a mental health professional. The unhappy child, or one whose development is marked by a long series of stresses which has never reached a crisis point but has clearly had a detrimental cumulative effect, may go unnoticed for a long time. Developmental delays which are not very severe and other subtle abnormalities in personality development may not seem very important or alarming to some parents.

Occasionally parents say they know of a friend's child who had a similar problem but who did not see a specialist. One can simply indicate that each person's situation is unique, and it would not be wise to base a recommendation for Cynthia on another child's situation. Also, one can remind the parents that a symptom can have many causes, and sometimes the same symptom in two different children may require different kinds or degrees of intervention.

A common reason why some parents refuse a recommendation for consultation by a mental health professional is that the child's problem is, at least in part, related to problems in their marriage. The parents are afraid to discuss the marriage and even fear that consultation for the child will break up the marriage, although this fear may be entirely unconscious. Similarly, a parent may be afraid that his or her own carefully concealed psychological problems (such as alcoholism, depression, or a phobia) will be uncovered. The health care practitioner should not deny that possibility. Rather, it is helpful to be sympathetic to the parents' concerns; one should state clearly that the person who talks with them and their child will be in a position to help the adults with their problem, too. In most cases, however, this problem will not be mentioned to the primary care clinician, but will have to be inferred. It will only come up after the family has become involved in therapy.

If the parents do not actively refuse the referral, but are visibly quite reluctant, one can focus one's remarks on the evaluative aspect of the consultation rather than on long term therapy. In effect, the primary clinician asks for the parents' support in obtaining the consultant's opinion without asking for a larger commitment. This may be less threatening and allow the parents and older child to be more in control of the long-term plan. It is generally very helpful to say something like, "Parents sometimes feel that if they agree to the consultation, they are accepting a large unknown commitment of time, energy, and money. Would it help if I explain a little more about the referral?" Most parents will accept this. The clinician can proceed to describe how she or he contacts the mental health professional, what the intake procedure is (especially with an agency or clinic), and what is included in the evaluation and family conference with the consultant. It may be useful to emphasize that only after the evaluation and conference will a plan of therapy be made. Parents are often relieved to learn that they will be involved in planning for future management and do not have to feel trapped in a long-term agreement. Nevertheless, if the primary clinician can persuade the family to have the evaluation, this usually does amount to promoting the ultimate decision to accept treatment.

If the parents do not agree to the referral at the time of the clinical summary, the practitioner should make it clear to them that he or she will remain as their clinician and would like to try to help in any way possible. Not infrequently, the parents will return some weeks or months later to request the consultation which they refused earlier. The child's symptoms may have worsened, or the family may have reevaluated the situation in view of the clinician's previous statements. For whatever reason, the clinician should be ready to accept their request without making "I told you so!" remarks or in other ways inducing them to feel guilty about refusing the first recommendation.

On rare occasions, clinicians know that it would be too detrimental to accept the parents' resistance to further evaluation and treatment. If careful explanation of the purpose for the referral and the exploration of the parents' reasons for refusing it are not adequate, the practitioner must make the disagreement explicit and present a persuasive and firm argument about the consequences to the child and family, just as would be done for a physical problem such as meningitis. It may help to suggest that another opinion be sought immediately with regard to the recommendation. However, if all else fails, the clinician has to make it clear that he or she cannot accept the parents' decision. In some cases the involvement of a protective services agency may be necessary; at other times the practitioner may have to make it clear that the recommendation is so important that the parents' will have to choose another clinician if they cannot reach agreement about this matter.

Follow-up

After the family is successfully referred to a consultant, the primary practitioner should continue to provide health supervision and care for acute illnesses, just as before the referral. Parents occasionally complain to the clinician that they are annoyed at the slow and irregular progress of their child's treatment with the specialist. This annoyance can occur with both physical and psychological problems and may become a major factor in the parents' reluctance to continue with treatment. Here the clinician should encourage the family to talk with the specialist about their reservations. It may also be possible to relieve their impatience and unspoken doubts by acknowledging their frustration, repeating the fact that treatment is not "magic," emphasizing the importance of continuing treatment at the current time, and offering encouragement that the treatment will have positive results.

During all routine health evaluations for a patient with a psychological problem, and also in the course of visits for other children in the family, the clinician should be careful to pay attention to the developmental and psychological history in each case. Frequently, the psychological problems of one child affect other members of the family. An older child may feel that the problem child gets all the attention and consequently may be having difficulties with that sibling or with the parents. In addition, tensions with in the marriage frequently become more overt or serious, and the parents themselves may need guidance, counseling, or therapy to solve their own problems. So it is important that the clinician be available to the other children in a family, and to the parents as well, in the role of counselor and resource person for their own difficulties.

CHAPTER 14

Consultation

General Discussion
Some Illustrative Examples
    Consultation Confirms Diagnostic Plans:
    Treatment by Primary Clinician
        Four-year-old with Rash
        Two-year-old with Delayed Language Development
    Initial Management by Consultant: To Primary Clinician for Later Treatment
        Ten-year-old Diabetic
    Consultant Manages Treatment and Primary Clinician Takes Role as Counselor
        Three-month-old with Heart Murmur
        Seriously Ill Child with Trauma: Seven-year-old Child Hit by a Car
    Management and Counseling by Consultant
        Twelve-year-old with Unilateral Knee Pain
        Ten-year-old with Psychological School Problem
        Five-year-old with Cystic Fibrosis
Conclusion

GENERAL DISCUSSION

Primary health care practitioners frequently ask for the opinion of another clinician about diagnosis and treatment of patients' problems. Generally, they do so after having amassed a fairly extensive data base, identifying the problem, and sometimes even making a provisional diagnosis before obtaining the consultation. The nature of the problem and its course will determine the exact point at which a clinician decides to ask for another opinion, as will the primary clinician's training and experience, the resources she or he has available, and the parents' desire or need for another opinion. The consultant may be another pediatric generalist or a subspecialist such as an orthopedist or a child psychiatrist. The nature of a consultation will naturally vary, depending on circumstances; it may be simply a discussion of the situation between professionals, or the consultant may need to see the child and parents more or less extensively in order to gather additional data. In urban medical centers patients are referred more often than is usual in rural areas where the primary clinician is more likely to manage even a quite serious problem, using a specialist only as an occasional resource when necessary.

The primary clinician's choice of consultant is generally based on the area(s) of the specialist's competence, the rapport the specialist is likely to develop with the parents and their child, and the history of previous collaborations. Other factors to be weighed are the cost of the consultant's services, the distance the patient would have to travel, and the length of time before an appointment is available. It is important for the primary care clinician to state the reasons for a particular choice of specialist. However, occasionally a parent has or knows of a particular practitioner whom she or he would like to consult. This may be based on personal experiences or on the recommendations of friends or relatives.

When a primary clinician recommends a consultant, it is often helpful to give a description of the consultant's expertise, one's own relationship and experience with this person through other referred patients, and the lines of communication that one has developed with that person. For example: "Dr. Jones is an orthopedist who sees many children with problems like Robert's. She is experienced with the management of this problem, and she also understands parents' concerns."

The primary practitioner should always communicate frequently with the chosen consultants to ensure the most effective collaboration for the family. Usually, the primary clinician calls or writes a referral letter to the consultant, providing pertinent background data to help give a context for the assessment of the problem. The consultant may call and/or send a report back to the primary clinician after the patient has been seen, a diagnosis established, and a program of treatment instituted. The primary clinician should also expect to receive periodic letters about the child's progress, and should request such updatings if they are not automatically forthcoming.

In contrast with consultation for a physical problem, there is much more concern about confidentiality in the management of psychological problems. Parents and older children are naturally quite concerned about the confidential nature of their communication, both within the family and between the primary clinician and consultant. Generally, the consulting mental health professional will contact the pediatric practitioner after his or her evaluation is completed and will discuss the diagnosis and treatment plan in a general way, excluding any confidential details of the assessment.

If the problem is complex and requires the services of a number of clinicians, a conference may be required to establish adequate procedures for communication among them in order to ensure good team work and comprehensive care. An example is the child with spina bifida whose care may involve a neurosurgeon, hospital and public heath nurses, a pediatrician, an orthopedist, a physical therapist, a nurse practitioner, a social worker, and a teacher.

It is crucial that the primary clinician have a clear idea of his or her own role in relation to the consultants in each case. In some situations the consultant will only give an opinion; in others he or she will also make a diagnosis and institute treatment. Occasionally the consultant will assume ongoing responsibility for the management of the illness and will help the family in their adjustment to the problem. Whatever the arrangement, the primary practitioner should maintain the role of primary pediatric clinician, remain informed about the patient's course, and—perhaps most important—be an advocate for the patient. In regard to the latter point, it is very important to remember that no matter how extensive the involvement of subspecialists, the primary health needs of the child should be met and protected by the primary clinician.

Too frequently, the family of a child with a serious chronic illness attempts to circumvent the referring primary practitioner and move all of the child's health care to the specialists. This may be because the parent, under the stress of the chronic problem, simply does not take the time to arrange for visits to the primary clinician for health care maintenance, or, on the other side of the coin, because the primary clinician has indicated some reluctance to care for the child with a chronic illness. This is not a good development, since other important aspects of the child's health and development may be neglected. The primary care clinician should be explicit at the time of a referral in reminding the patient and parent that during subsequent primary care general health maintenance of the child remains extremely important—especially for a child with a chronic problem; subspecialty care therefore cannot be seen as a substitute. In addition, it should be explained that the primary practitioner can reinforce the therapeutic plans of the consultant; play an essential role in providing counseling for the family about the chronic problem; and provide a broad range of other services while the specialist manages the more immediate problems directly related to the illness. Sometimes it is necessary to encourage the consultant to support the family's continuing relationship to the primary care clinician.

SOME ILLUSTRATIVE EXAMPLES

The following cases illustrate the varied relationships that can evolve between consultants and primary care practitioners in the care of both physical and psychological problems.

Consultation confirms diagnostic plans

In some cases the consultant provides initial confirmation of the primary clinician's diagnosis and proposed plan of management and the case is then managed by the primary practitioner.

1. A four-year-old girl is seen by her pediatric nurse practitioner because her father noted a rash on her face and trunk. The practitioner makes the diagnosis of eczema; since its distribution is somewhat unusual, she consults the pediatrician with whom she works about the diagnosis and management of the problem. The condition is not particularly severe, and the pediatrician decides that the distribution does not alter the diagnosis or treatment plan. The nurse practitioner manages the problem and discusses the case with the pediatrician only if she needs further advice about treatment. When a case of eczema is very severe, unusual in its manifestations, or resistant to the usual forms of treatment, the nurse practitioner and pediatrician probably will consult a dermatologist. After the consultation, the nurse practitioner again will manage both the treatment and follow-up of the problem.

2. A two-year-old boy receives his primary care from a physician's assistant (P.A.) who works in a group practice. The P.A. notes during a routine health visit that the child has a mild but significant delay in his language development. Further information is obtained by interviewing the parent, observing the child in conversation, and talking to the staff at the child's day-care center. The P.A. then discusses the information with one of the pediatricians in the group to decide what other data are necessary in order to determine the etiology of the child's language delay and to formulate a treatment plan. Their conclusion, in this case, is that the child has normal hearing, functions well and without delay in all other developmental and psychological areas, and that his language delay is probably related to inadequate stimulation in his home. Consequently the primary and consulting clinicians devise a program for language stim-

ulation at home (with one or both parents participating) and also in the day-care center. During the next three months the child will be reevaluated by the physician's assistant; if he has not progressed adequately in his language development, a subspecialist will be consulted.

Initial management by consultant

In other cases initial management is provided by the consultant, but the primary clinician is responsible for care after the initial phase of treatment. The consultant remains available to the primary clinician for further consultation and may resume responsibility for management of complications. This pattern is more common when the patient lives far from an urban medical center and consequently only sees the consultant for reevaluation or management of complications at infrequent intervals.

A ten-year-old boy receives his health care from a rural group practice which includes a nurse practitioner and a pediatrician. The pediatrician is asked to see the patient because his parents note that he is lethargic, has been drinking and urinating more than usual, and has lost weight over the past three weeks. The pediatrician makes the diagnosis of acute diabetic ketoacidosis and immediately arranges for hospitalization at an urban medical center. Although the primary clinician maintains contact with the patient and his family, an endocrinologist takes responsibility for the child's care. At the time of discharge from the hospital, the ongoing management plan is for both the child's routine health care and management of the diabetes to be the responsibility of the primary pediatric nurse practitioner and pediatrician who are near his home. In this case, the pediatric nurse practitioner is an especially important figure in the follow-up. The child will return to the endocrinologist only for an opinion about complications or difficulties in management.

A similar distribution of responsibility may also occur for a child with a seizure disorder, sickle cell disease, or severe asthma.

Consultant manages treatment and primary clinician takes role as counselor

There are also many situations in which it is appropriate for the consultant to manage the problem, but where the primary practitioner can provide a valuable concurrent service as a counselor to the family.

1. A three-month-old girl comes to the medical center for a routine health evaluation. The medical student who is providing primary care for the child notes a previously unrecognized heart murmur during the physical examination. She and the supervising physician decide that the child should be seen by a cardiologist even though the child is asymptomatic. The medical student takes on the task of describing to the parents the initial evaluation in the cardiology clinic, including the examination by the

cardiologist and any laboratory tests such as the chest x-ray and electrocardiogram.

After the initial consultation, the medical student continues to provide primary health care. Since she is often more easily accessible to the family than the consultant, she may be able to provide the valuable service of reinforcing what the cardiologist already has discussed with them. She may answer questions, advise the parents what to expect from the child in view of the cardiac problem, and, if necessary, recommend an earlier than scheduled visit to the cardiologist.

2. In the event that a child suddenly develops a life-threatening illness or experiences a severe trauma, the primary practitioner may take the role of a counselor and advocate for the family even though she or he is not directly involved in the child's medical management. Primary clinicians who have counseling skills are the best counselors when a child becomes ill, because they have known the family before the illness, often have an understanding of the family's strengths and vulnerabilities, and already have built a trusting relationship with them.

The following is an example of this situation.

A seven-year-old boy is hit by a car. He sustains several fractures and has a severe concussion which necessitates hospitalization, several operations, and a long convalescence. In this situation, the hospital staff and several subspecialists manage the medical problems. However, during the period of acute intervention, the primary practitioner can have a major role in supporting the family through the crisis. Interpreting the medical findings to the family and counseling the parents, the sick child, siblings, and other relatives are important functions. Collaborating with a social worker may be valuable if one is associated with the pediatric inpatient service, or the social worker alone may provide counseling.

In many cases of acute crisis, sources of support for the patient and the family are mobilized. But then, after the crisis itself is over, the support dissipates or diminishes and the family may often be neglected. This can occur while the child is convalescing in the hospital or may not happen until after discharge. When support does diminish, the role of the primary clinician becomes even more important. Aside from providing emotional support, the clinician will also need to counsel the family about rehabilitation facilities, special school arrangements, and the long-term psychological effects of the illness.

Management and counseling by consultant

In some situations both management and specific counseling about a disease are the responsibility of the consultant. The primary clinician may be called on to support the family's cooperation with the treatment, however, even though there is no direct management responsibility.

1. A twelve-year-old boy with a history of unilateral knee pain of two

months duration is seen by his nurse practitioner. The practitioner evaluates the problem and confers with the pediatrician with whom he works. The pediatrician examines the child and recommends specific x-rays, which lead to the conclusion that the knee pain is due to Osgood-Schlatter disease of the knee. The boy is then referred to an orthopedist for management of the problem. However, the nurse practitioner will continue to provide primary health care for the child. If the family has numerous other problems, the nurse practitioner's involvement may be essential to ensure that the parents follow the orthopedist's recommendations for treatment.

2. A ten-year-old girl who has not attended school for six weeks because of fatigue is seen by her primary clinician, a physician's assistant. The history reveals severe family problems, but an extensive history and thorough physical examination reveal no physical problems for the girl. The physician's assistant consults with the pediatrician in the practice and together they decide that only a few simple laboratory tests should be done in order to rule out possible organic disease. These prove to be normal. The physician's assistant and pediatrician present this case to the consulting child psychiatrist, who recommends psychiatric treatment. The physician's assistant then presents this recommendation to the family and helps them obtain psychiatric care. Subsequently, primary care continues to be provided by the physician's assistant; but the management of the psychological problem is the responsibility of the psychiatrist.

3. A five-year-old girl with cystic fibrosis is followed for primary care by a pediatrician in her home town. The diagnosis of cystic fibrosis was made when she was six months old; she has received care for this problem, at a medical center, from a pediatrician and nurse practitioner whose expertise is in respiratory diseases of children. Together they are responsible for and care for both the medical and psychosocial problems related to the child's disease. They regularly communicate with the primary pediatrician by letter so that he or she knows about the child's physical and emotional status and can use this information in the primary care of the patient and her siblings.

CONCLUSION

The clinical summary is a critical aspect of the clinical assessment; it is often undervalued or even overlooked by pediatric clinicians. It has a number of very important uses, and it deserves the same thoughtful consideration as the data gathering part of the interview, the developmental assessment, or the physical examination. Full use of the clinical summary can achieve most or all of the following desirable consequences.

1. Enhancement of the rapport between clinician and family members (including the patient).

2. Conveyance of important, specific information to the patient and parents in a manner increasing the likelihood of its being understood and acted upon.

3. Formulation of health maintenance, evaluation, or treatment plans that are likely to be adhered to because the family was involved in their design.

4. Discovery of additional information about family strengths and liabilities, needs for additional services, and related problems. Once these are found, further plans can be formulated for dealing with them.

5. Encouragement of family members to be active participants in the health management program of the patient, and perhaps in their own health management as well.

Rushing a clinical summary or treating it haphazardly in order to "save time" is a false economy. It is wrong both in philosophy and in practice. Patients and their parents deserve respect and a conscientious effort on the part of the practitioner to communicate with and understand them as fully as possible. The careful work from the earlier assessment is utilized in the summary. Clinical experience has demonstrated over and over again that people are able to act positively to promote their health and the health of their children when they are well informed and feel concern and respect from the professionals on whom they depend. This is the cornerstone of successful health care.

Suggested Readings
Unit IV:
Clinical Summary

Chapter 11: General Principles and the Typical Clinical Summary with No Problems

Feinstein, A.R. *Clinical Judgment*. Baltimore, Williams & Wilkins, 1967, pp. 24–25.

Chapter 12: The Clinical Summary with Minor Problems

Carey, W.B., and Silunga, M.S. Avoiding pediatric pathogenesis in the management of acute minor illness. *Pediatrics* 49:553–562, 1972.

Chapter 13: The Clinical Summary with Major Problems

Kennell, J.H., Soroker, E., Thomas, P. and Waisman, M. What parents of rheumatic fever patients don't understand about the disease and its prophylactic management. *Pediatrics* 43:160–167, 1969.

UNIT FIVE

The Annotated Interview and Write-up

CHAPTER 15

The Annotated Interview and Write-up

The Annotated Interview
The Write-up of the Interview

THE ANNOTATED INTERVIEW

The following interview transcript illustrates a clinician conducting an initial history and clinical summary. The interview is verbatim, from a tape recording involving a two-and-one-half-year-old girl's first visit to her nurse practitioner's office. It is not simulated to illustrate the ideal interview. The names are fictitious to maintain confidentiality.

The annotative notes set off in the text indicate the rationale for including particular questions, the significance of selected comments from the father, and guidance on the order of the interview which the examiner is trying tactfully to maintain.

This interview illustrates how to combine open-ended techniques with specific questions in order to gather a detailed history of the child in his or her family. The reader should note some of Ms. J.'s technical shortcomings, such as grouping several questions together and saying "okay" after the parent's responses. By no means does this represent the full history, which is assembled over many visits to the practitioner as the child grows and develops and the clinician gets to know the family better. Naturally, there are many areas that could have been explored in greater depth, including the parents' relationship with each other, the father's concerns about his daughter's sensitivities and lack of large muscle skills, the past psychosocial history of the family, the mother's attitudes toward the child, and the family's religious affiliations and their meaning to the family. Since the information which was discussed presents a picture of a competent, intact family who seem to get along well, and since it is very likely that the relationship with the practitioner will continue, it was reasonable for the clinician in this case to decide *not* to pursue those areas further during this visit.

Actually, this interview was followed by a brief developmental assessment using selected toys and also by a physical examination. Both were normal. They are not recorded but are alluded to in the ensuing clinical summary which is in the annotated transcript.

Ms. J.: Good morning Mr. Franklin. How are you?

Introductions should always include mention of the family name to make sure you have the right family.

Mr. F.: Fine, thank you.
Ms. J.: My name is Emily Jones and I'll be your pediatric nurse practitioner here at the health plan. Is this Diane?

The clinician should identify himself/herself by name and role.

Mr. F.: Yes.
Ms. J.: Hi, Diane. How are you? (then to Mr. F.) I expect that Diane might be kind of shy and not want to talk to me too much.
Mr. F.: She is kind of shy of strange people and new places.
Ms. J.: I see. Since this is the first time that we've had a chance to meet and it's your first visit to the health plan, I'll begin by asking whether you are familiar with pediatric nurse practitioners and what they do?

Making an opportunity to explain one's role. This is important, although it will not always be necessary to explain it.

Mr. F.: Yes, I am. We had a nurse practitioner in Chicago. But who will be our pediatrician, and how do you arrange our visits?
Ms. J.: Dr. Gordon Steinberg, Dr. Alice White and I work together. You will have a chance to meet Dr. Steinberg later this morning. We will alternate routine checkups between myself and Dr. Steinberg for your children. For any acute problem either I or Dr. Steinberg will see you. We decide which one of us, depending on the problem and our schedules. Dr. White sees our patients when we are not available; also, she is available as my consultant when Dr. Steinberg is not here.

Today I'll be asking you a lot of questions, both about Diane's current health and development as well as things in the past. After that, we'll do the check-up and then we can take care of any screening tests or immunizations that she might need. Before I begin, are there any things that you want to ask me?

Providing an opportunity for the parent to ask questions at the beginning of the interview. This supports the open-ended technique and allows the parent to talk about areas which may be of particular concern.

Mr. F.: Well, Diane's two and a half years old now, and we've begun to become a little concerned about the fact that she's so attached to her bottles. You know, we haven't really been able to decide to take it away from her, though sometimes we think that it's probably the right time or maybe even a little too late. I'd be interested in your opinion about that.

Ms. J.: Maybe you can tell me a little bit first about how long she's had her bottle and how important it's been to her.

Going from the general to the specific, but not being totally directive; this format allows the clinician to learn how the parent thinks and feels about the issue at hand.

Mr. F.: She has had her bottle since she was little, but it's been very important to her for at least a year.

Ms. J.: Did she have a bottle as an infant or was she breast-fed?

More specific questions to help elicit the history.

Mr. F.: Well, my wife nursed her for the first four or five months, but I guess in the first month or two she developed a mastitis which was very painful and it required surgery, actually, and so Diane started on the bottle very early. But then she, see even after she was drinking from her cup, the bottle became something that she kind of held on to when she was unhappy.

Ms. J.: Can you explain to me, or give me some example, of how she uses the bottle now? What kind of unhappiness, how often she uses it?

Still more specific questions to learn about the situation in which Diane uses the bottle for comfort.

Mr. F.: Well when she's tired she always likes her bottle. She kind of takes her bottle into bed with her before she goes to sleep, and she takes her bottle when she feels a little scared of something or when she has cried when she's had a fight with us about something we tell her not to do. And when she's on a trip she'll want her bottle with her to make her feel more secure it seems.

Ms. J.: Are there any other things she uses for comfort? Does she suck her thumb, have a pacifier, a favorite stuffed animal?

Information about other transitional objects.

Mr. F.: She doesn't suck her thumb but she has a special what she calls a "blanky" and a "beary" that are very close to her. You can see that she has those with her now. (Points to small blanket and teddy bear.) We take those places when we go out of the house.

Ms. J.: But she still prefers her bottle or uses it with those other things?

Mr. F.: She um . . . I wouldn't say she prefers her bottle but she uses it together with those other things but she's very upset if we tell her she can't have it. Well, maybe she does prefer it.

Ms. J.: Can you also tell me what is usually in the bottle, what does she usually drink?

Information related to nutrition and dental caries.

Mr. F.: Well, she drinks apple cider. We get this apple cider from the orchard near where we're living now, and she used to drink apple juice when we were in Chicago and strained orange juice. She used to drink milk but she doesn't drink much milk anymore. Sometimes we water it down a little, 'cause she drinks so much of it.

Ms. J.: Yes. Can you tell me how your wife feels about it?

Both parents' views are necessary parts of the data base—not only for complete information, but also to assess whether there is conflict over the problem and to plan future management.

Mr. F.: I'm not really sure. I think she feels both ways like I do, that we don't want to take it away from her because it will make her unhappy, but yet we're worried about it, you know. Um, my father was a dentist and I worry about her teeth sometimes too.

Ms. J.: And has anyone else told you that it's probably not a good idea for her to still have the bottle, any other doctors or nurses, or family or friends?

Particularly in child rearing situations, it is helpful for the clinician to know about advice and opinions which the parents have heard. It also tells about significant other people for the family.

Mr. F.: Well, the dentist is very much against it and our . . . my mother of course is very much against it, and I think that my wife's mother . . . I think everybody is against it as a matter of fact, except for maybe the babysitter who kind of has the same attitudes toward children that we have.

Ms. J.: What do you think about these opinions—except for the sitter's?

Mr. F.: I think they may be right, but I'm not sure what to do.

Ms. J.: It's a complicated issue, but I'm sure we can make a sensible plan. Let me ask you a few more questions, first. Do you have any other children?

It is important to acknowledge the parents' difficulty, and also to indicate a positive approach to a solution. By explaining that there will be a few more questions, the interviewer tells the parent that the problem will not be ignored.

Mr. F.: Yes, I have an older daughter who is six years old.

Ms. J.: And how did you work it with her and her bottle?

Mr. F.: Well, we took her bottles away when she was about Diane's age or maybe just a month or two older and um . . . but she had a pacifier and wasn't that attached to the bottle as Diane is. But she also seemed like, I don't know, in some ways she was a less sensitive little girl than Diane.

Ms. J.: What do you mean by "sensitive"?

Mr. F.: Oh, she's more easily upset by change than her older sister was at this age.

This "sensitive" label could be a very loaded comment. The interviewer can ask for more details, as she did here. In this situation she chose *not* to pursue it further. However, the question of Diane's "sensitivity" is a point that should be remembered; and it probably should influence the clinician's impression of this child and her father.

Ms. J.: Okay. I think I share the general feeling that when children are about two and a half or so it's time to give up the bottle. It's hard to know what to do for the particular child and the family, and I'd like to work out a plan with you and your wife that's comfortable for everyone. The teeth are a major concern, and nowadays there is a lot more in the pediatric journals about how the bottle, and particularly juice and even milk can cause very early cavities in teeth. So I think that we probably should try to work out a plan to stop the bottle.

Return to the concern about the bottle. The clinician shares her thoughts about bottles in general.

> I would like to come back to this at the end of our talk when I know Diane a little better and know some more about your family. Would that be okay?

It is premature to give advice, but it is appropriate to indicate that a plan will be formulated at the end of the complete assessment.

Mr. F.: Sure, that would be fine.

Ms. J.: Okay. Are there any other areas that you would like to discuss?

Mr. F.: No, I think she's really a healthy little girl and doing very well in other ways. We feel good about her.
Ms. J.: Good. You say she's healthy. Has she been healthy in general as she's grown up?

Open-ended question about general health.

Mr. F.: Yes. She's been a very healthy little girl.
Ms. J.: And where did she get her health care when you lived in Chicago?

Past medical history begins.

Mr. F.: We had a pediatrician—Dr. Klein.
Ms. J.: Uh-huh. And had Diane lived in any other places or was all of her care in Chicago?
Mr. F.: No, all of her care was in Chicago with Dr. Klein and also a nurse practitioner—Ms. Harrison.
Ms. J.: Okay. Maybe you can tell me something about her birth. What that was like, how much she weighed and so forth.

Mixture of open-ended and specific suggestions.

Mr. F.: Actually, I don't remember exactly what she weighed, but she weighed six pounds something and there were no real problems that I can remember. She was alright.
Ms. J.: Did she come on time, or was she early or later than expected?
Mr. F.: She was about on time.
Ms. J.: And was she born head first?
Mr. F.: What do you mean?

It is not uncommon for a parent to be unable to answer a technical question, even in lay terms.

Ms. J.: Regular vaginal delivery—came out head first—not feet first or butt first?
Mr. F.: There were no problems, I guess. I was there. She came out head first.
Ms. J.: Okay, fine. And did your wife have any prenatal care?
Mr. F.: Sure.
Ms. J.: Do you remember from approximately what time in the pregnancy?
Mr. F.: I guess from pretty much as soon as we thought she was pregnant.
Ms. J.: And how pregnant was she at that time? For instance, was it one month or three months or six months?

A more specific question is needed to ascertain at what month of gestation prenatal care began.

Mr. F.: Oh, it was a lot less than six months. It was more like one or two months.
Ms. J.: Did you plan to have a child at that time?
Mr. F.: Yes, we wanted a second child and thought that three and one-half years would be a good spacing.
Ms. J.: Okay. How long did your wife and the baby stay in the hospital after the baby was born?
Mr. F.: Actually just about a day or two.
Ms. J.: Uh-huh.
Mr. F.: She wasn't very happy there. She persuaded her doctor to let her go home.
Ms. J.: In what way was she unhappy?

"Not very happy" could mean nothing onerous or it could mean serious physical or psychological problems.

Mr. F.: Oh, too hot and too noisy. She figured she'd rest better at home.
Ms. J.: I see. And I assume both your wife and Diane were healthy at the time they left.
Mr. F.: Yeh, she felt pretty good. And the baby was fine.

Ms. J.: How were things after that, after the baby came home and your wife came home?

Mr. F.: Well, it was kind of a hard time. We had just moved into our new home a few weeks before, and it was a hard time, but I think things were pretty good. The baby was doing well and, until my wife developed that mastitis, things were pretty good.

The historian appears reluctant to say how bad things were. The answer is a mixture of "hard times" and "pretty good." Here again, the *quality* or *tone* of the answer should alert the interviewer to the tendency of the father to minimize the stress of both the child's birth and the move to a new home.

Ms. J.: And can you tell me a little more about that? You mentioned there was surgery. Did that involve a hospitalization? Did she have to stop nursing? How was that for the two of you—and Diane?

Mr. F.: Well, she nursed less but I don't think she actually stopped nursing. I think she stopped on the infected side and there was a lot of soaking and there was a lot of . . . she was very uncomfortable. She had antibiotics and it was finally incised and a lot of pus came out of it.

Ms. J.: Did she go to the surgeon's office to have it drained or did she have to go into the hospital?

Mr. F.: Well, she didn't stay over night in the hospital. I don't remember if it was in the hospital.

This answer is a bit garbled and vague. It may reflect a style of inattention to detail, but may also reflect how stressful that period was.

Ms. J.: And after that how did things go? Was she able to resume nursing completely—how did it work out?

Mr. F.: She still nursed a lot, but the baby was on bottles, too. Actually, our first baby was on some bottles too, 'cause my wife works.

Ms. J.: What kind of work does your wife do?

Follow the lead of the historian.

Mr. F.: She's a secretary.

Ms. J.: Does she work full time or part time?

Mr. F.: Part time.

Ms. J.: And around the birth of Diane, did she take any time off?

Mr. F.: About . . . I guess, it was four weeks. It might have been a little longer than that because it was summertime.

Ms. J.: Who took care of the baby and your other child after she went back to work?

Mr. F.: The same woman who had been our sitter since our older child was a baby. Also, I take off one afternoon a week and also set aside Saturday mornings to care for the kids. It's good for all of us.

Ms. J.: So, that worked out alright?

Mr. F.: Very well.

Ms. J.: Good. Is there anything else you want to tell me about that early period?

Return to the history of early infancy with an open-ended question.

Mr. F.: No. I guess this baby was a lot more fussy than our other baby. We held her a lot and we had the baby swing to crank up. She was kind of a sensitive, fussy baby, we thought. She didn't like loud noises—still doesn't. But a happy baby and an alert baby. She was more and more content and happy after the first month or two.

The father's initial response is "No." However, he continues to talk, perhaps encouraged by the interviewer's unhurried and interested manner. The father's concern about Diane's sensitivity recurs.

His reference to "happy and alert" suggests he does not want to make Diane sound too unpleasant. Perhaps he is asking the clinician for help with this worry. The interviewer decides *not* to pursue this now. But she should note it in her impression about the father.

Ms. J.: A few more questions about her growing up. How has her health been since the infant period?

A structured return to the past history.

Mr. F.: Very good.
Ms. J.: Has she ever been hospitalized for anything?
Mr. F.: No. Oh, yes—actually there was one hospitalization when she was four or five months old that frightened us quite a bit. She had a cold and she, I guess, developed pneumonia. Once she got treated she was alright.

Again, the initial "No" followed by affirmative information.

Ms. J.: Where was she hospitalized?
Mr. F.: At the university hospital in um . . . Chicago.
Ms. J.: And how many days was she in the hospital?
Mr. F.: She was in the hospital five days, I guess, four or five days. We stayed with her most of the time.
Ms. J.: Was your wife still nursing her at that time?

Of some significance in learning about the parent's attitudes and commitments to breast feeding. It may be generalized to other child rearing practices.

Mr. F.: Yes, some of the time, yes.
Ms. J.: What did you think about the breast feeding?

It is very important to learn how the father feels (felt) about the breast feeding. Not infrequently, a father is jealous or annoyed or wishes his wife would not nurse. If this was the case, it would be useful to learn how and if they resolved this conflict.

Mr. F.: I think it was a good thing. It got to be a burden on my wife when Diane was in the hospital with pneumonia, though. My wife usually was there to nurse Diane, and I was at home with Rachel or at work. If Diane had been on bottles, I could have helped more with Diane in the hospital.
Ms. J.: How long did your wife continue to breast feed Diane?
Mr. F.: Until she was 11 months old. She just weaned herself—lost interest.
Ms. J.: How was that for your wife?
Mr. F.: Fine. It seemed like the right time to stop. It had been pretty much the same with Rachel, when she changed to bottles at nine or ten months.
Ms. J.: And after Diane came home from the hospital, how was her health?
Mr. F.: She seemed fine.
Ms. J.: Did she have any other serious chest infections or pneumonias or any other difficulties since?
Mr. F.: No.
Ms. J.: So, that seemed to be a one-time thing?
Mr. F.: I hope so, yes. But I do worry about her getting pneumonia again. It was scary for all of us.
Ms. J.: Usually, if children have one episode like that, and they are completely healthy otherwise, they don't have further difficulties. So, it's not like a child who has had two or three episodes of pneumonia at a very young age. This is something we can talk about more at the end, but the fact that she's been well since infancy is really quite a good sign, and the one episode of pneumonia is not anything to be particularly alarmed about. I realize it was scary for you at the time, and parents normally are upset by things like that.

It is appropriate to take the time to address the parent's worry. This takes a few minutes, but it is the humane way to respond and communicates a real effort to support the parent.

Mr. F.: Is it true that children who have early chest infections sometimes have asthma later on? Because my wife has some problems with asthma.

The father spontaneously tells why he is particularly worried: the family history of asthma.

Ms. J.: I see. Has Diane ever had episodes of wheezing or asthmatic attacks herself?
Mr. F.: No. In fact, my wife and I have remarked how few colds she's had and how quickly she gets over them. Never any wheezing.
Ms. J.: Well, in answer to your question, Diane's history, even though it includes one episode of pneumonia in infancy, does not suggest that she is a child with respiratory problems. If you had told me that Diane has had wheezing, or other chest problems, then I would say the chances were higher that she might develop asthma. The fact that there is a family history of asthma on your wife's side means that Diane is more likely to develop allergies and even asthma than someone without that family history. However, it's not something we can predict and it's not something we can prevent in any way. Are there other questions you have about that? (pause)
Mr. F.: No. That answers my question fine.
Ms. J.: Has Diane had any accidents? For instance, needing stitches or broken bones?

Return to the past medical history.

Mr. F.: No.
Ms. J.: Any serious illnesses where she had to stay at home for a long stretch?
Mr. F.: No.
Ms. J.: Any childhood illnesses, like chickenpox, measles, German measles, or mumps?
Mr. F.: Yes. Chickenpox last winter—with her sister.
Ms. J.: Was it a bad case?
Mr. F.: No. She only had a few spots and a little fever.
Ms. J.: And has she had all her baby shots?
Mr. F.: Whatever the pediatrician told us she needed, she had.
Ms. J.: And when you moved from Chicago did you either bring an immunization record or a letter with that information written down?
Mr. F.: No. That was silly, but I . . . we could get that I think.
Ms. J.: Okay. Before you leave today, I'll ask you to sign a permission slip and we can send for those records.
        Now, if you can tell me a little bit about your household—who lives there, what its like and so forth.

Continue with social history.

Mr. F.: Well, we just moved a month ago, so that things are kind of settling in, but I think we have a real nice place. It's just my wife and I and our six-year-old daughter, Rachel, and Diane.
Ms. J.: Any other family members or anyone in your household?

It is important not to assume that the nuclear family always comprises the household. Very often, extended family or friends temporarily or permanently live with the patient.

Mr. F.: No.
Ms. J.: Okay. And can you describe your house a little bit?

A useful open-ended question which provides information not only about the house but also about the family's social and economic situation.

Mr. F.: It's a nice house. It's a ranch house with three bedrooms, living room and dining room and kitchen, backyard, and it's in a nice area with other one-family houses, a lot of trees around—we like that.
Ms. J.: It sounds lovely. How was the move for the children?
Mr. F.: I think both children were upset in their own way. Rachel was concerned about leaving school. Diane really was quite whiney and cranky, and we were a little short with her a good part of the time. It was hard for us and hard for them. But we feel good about having moved, now that it is done.

Mr. F.'s pattern is to be sure to note the resolution of difficult situations into more positive outcomes.

Ms. J.: Moves can be particularly hard. Everybody does react in their own way as you said. Do you think the children are now adjusted and back to their regular routine?
Mr. F.: I think they are doing pretty well.
Ms. J.: And what was the reason for your move here to New Haven?

The interviewer should ask the reason for major changes in the patient's environment. These reasons tell a great deal about the social and economic conditions under which a family operates. A family who moves frequently from one apartment to another because of failure to pay the rent, for instance, is in a very different situation from Mr. F.'s family whose move was prompted by the parents' wish to be nearer to extended family, combined with an attractive work opportunity.

Mr. F.: Well, my job really.
Ms. J.: I see. What do you do?
Mr. F.: I'm a junior high school teacher.
Ms. J.: And what do you teach?
Mr. F.: I teach math.
Ms. J.: And how did you happen to come from Chicago to New Haven?
Mr. F.: Well, we were thinking about moving East and I'd grown up in Rhode Island. So had my wife. We have lots of family around here—and I landed a job here.
Ms. J.: How has the move been for you and your wife?
Mr. F.: Hard—like most moves. We still are getting to know our way around and making acquaintances with our neighbors and people at work.
Ms. J.: Um-hum. And is your wife working?
Mr. F.: She's not working yet, but soon she will look for a part-time office job. She enjoys the work and we can use the extra income.
Ms. J.: Has your older daughter gotten settled in school?
Mr. F.: Yes.

The question is so specific that the affirmative answer "yes" gives us little information about the school. Therefore, the interviewer chooses to continue with more open-ended and planned questions.

Ms. J.: Which school is she attending?

Since the older child will have a health assessment with Ms. Jones later, the practitioner does not have to ask about Rachel's school work at this time. However, the school which Rachel attends does tell a little about the family's standards of acceptable schooling and gives Mr. F. an opportunity to discuss the school if he perceives any problems there.

Mr. F.: The elementary school near our house.
Ms. J.: How is that school?
Mr. F.: Pretty good—we're pleased with what we've seen and heard about the schools in the area.
Ms. J.: Can you tell me something about your health insurance?
Mr. F.: Yes, we have membership in my health plan and major medical through the city, at work.

It is even more important to ask about health insurance when the family is *not* a member of a prepaid health plan. The type of insurance a family has may influence their ability to use health services: lack of adequate insurance for office visits may lead to overuse of the emergency room for acute illnesses (but nonemergency ones) because hospital visits are covered by insurance. Sometimes inadequate insurance will lead to poor compliance in buying medication, obtaining consultation, or keeping follow-up appointments.

Ms. J.: I'm going to switch gears now and ask you some questions about Diane and her growing up and what she's like. You've already told me that she's generally been quite a happy child. How would you describe her, in more detail, to someone who didn't know her?

Return to the developmental history, beginning with an open-ended question.

Mr. F.: I would say that she's a really smart kid. She's a very good-natured kid although she's sensitive and during this move she became irritable, and she's frightened of noises and frightened of some other things that other kids take in their stride. But when she's comfortable, she's a delight—she's funny and good-natured. She has cheered us up a lot when we're feeling bad. She's a really nice kid.

The idea that a child gives something to the parents is important. It is always present, whether in a positive or negative way. Mr. F. expresses this feeling positively, and in a way that shows Diane is not considered a chronic burden. This is especially important in this child's history, since the description of her early infancy greatly emphasizes her irritability and sensitivity.

Ms. J.: These times when she is irritable, sensitive, or uncomfortable, what do you do? How do you handle that?

It is important always to ask how parents handle a difficult situation. The answer tells a great deal about their attitudes toward child rearing.

Mr. F.: She likes books especially. They help calm her. We read to her, we hold her, and we can talk to her. She's got a fantastic vocabulary—we're really surprised. I mean, I guess we're a little proud of her and everything but she can . . . her grammar and her articulation and her syntax is, I think, very advanced, very advanced.

Mr. F.'s answer goes off on a tangent. However, the content includes useful data for the developmental assessment.

Ms. J.: Maybe I'll get to hear her talk after a while. I see she's playing comfortably with those toys over there—and in a little bit, I'll go over and play with

	her, too. How does she get along in the family? With your wife? You? With her sister?
Mr. F.:	She gets along well.
Ms. J.:	Has she had opportunities to play with other children?
Mr. F.:	Not too much, but when she does she seems to get on alright with them. You know, she doesn't share too much but she'll share some. Sometimes her sitter in Chicago would take her visiting to friends with children. And she plays with the younger brothers and sisters of Rachel's friends. She likes to be with other children.
Ms. J.:	Have you thought at all about a babysitter or nursery school or day care for when your wife goes back to work?
Mr. F.:	We're worried about babysitters already. We're looking. That's always a big problem.
Ms. J.:	What kind of a problem?
Mr. F.:	Well, it's hard to find a good sitter. We were lucky, back in Chicago, to find such a good sitter. I'm sure we can find a capable person who will take care of Diane like we want, but it takes time and energy to arrange it all.
Ms. J.:	Yes, I understand the problem. Tell me about the things Diane likes to do. You mentioned that she really likes books. What other things?

Return to current developmental history.

Mr. F.:	Well, she likes to play with some puzzles we have. She likes to string beads. She has this Chinese checkers game where she arranges the different colored pegs into designs. She likes to listen to music. Actually, she's been kind of attached to one record, lately. Driving us crazy since the move this is—a Sesame Street record.
Ms. J.:	Do you let her listen to it as much as she wants?
Mr. F.:	As much as she wants, usually. But occasionally we insist on having a little break from it . . . and then she gets upset, but she tolerates it.
Ms. J.:	Does she fall apart or just protest?

"Gets upset" may mean a transient protest or it may represent a more severe and prolonged situation. It is helpful, here, to give Mr. F. an opportunity to elaborate.

Mr. F.:	It varies. Usually she just protests and sometimes she'll cry real hard. But it is always over quickly and she goes back to playing happily.
Ms. J.:	Have you noticed any stubborn behavior, or naughty things that Diane does?
Mr. F.:	We sure do! I'd say that on and off over the last year, she's had a lot more stubborn spells than when she was younger. I remember it from Rachel's growing up—one part I could do without!
Ms. J.:	What does she do?
Mr. F.:	Oh—say "No" or "Why?" when she knows the answer perfectly well. Or she'll take what seems like hours to get into her car seat, just when we're in a rush.
Ms. J.:	What do you do about it?
Mr. F.:	Well, it depends on our mood and how rushed we are. Sometimes we cajole her, or just wait. Occasionally we'll pick her up and *put* her in the car seat. She protests, sometimes cries, but calms down in a couple of minutes.
Ms. J.:	Do you think this is more than it should be, or that we should talk more about it?
Mr. F.:	No. I don't like it, but I don't feel it's a big deal. Most of the time Diane is quite decent to be with. This oppositional stuff isn't a big deal for us.
Ms. J.:	Fine. Now a few specific questions about things Diane does. How does she do with climbing? Running? Things of that nature?
Mr. F.:	Not so hot. I think she's more of a girl.

Mr. F.'s sexist views are apparent. Ms. J. does not argue with him but neither does she agree. In addition, she does not assume she knows what he means by these comments; she asks him to elaborate.

Ms. J.: What do you mean by that?
Mr. F.: Well, she walked late, and she uses her head (I mean her brain) mostly, and she's a little awkward with things like the tricycle and running, and she falls a lot.
Ms. J.: Is that something you've noticed all along or is that something you've thought of only recently?

This question helps Ms. J. know if this is an acute problem which may reflect recent central nervous system disease or whether this "clumsiness" is a developmental characteristic.

Mr. F.: I think all along. She's not half as competent, physically, as my other daughter, who's a real gymnast. A real difference.

Excessive comparison between children can be a sign of serious disappointment with one child. In this situation Ms. J. will note this comment. But she need not discuss it, unless a pattern of negative comments emerges.

Ms. J.: How old was Diane when she first sat by herself?
Mr. F.: Seven months, I believe.
Ms. J.: And how old was she when she took her first step without holding on?
Mr. F.: I think it wasn't 'till 14, 15 months.

Developmental landmarks have limited usefulness. In this case landmarks do add objective information to the father's report of clumsiness and relatively slow gross motor development. However, his memory may not be accurate and may even be prejudiced by his view of this child as "more of a girl" and unathletic.

Ms. J.: When do you think it was that she was walking pretty well and not using the crawling any more? It's a little hard to remember that far back but maybe you have some idea.

It is helpful to encourage the parent to give more details.

Mr. F.: I think she was still crawling some when she was a year and a half, for instance, while Rachel really wasn't crawling any more at that age.
Ms. J.: Yes. Does she seem interested in doing things like climbing on a jungle gym, or going on a slide, or riding a tricycle?
Mr. F.: She tries, and she does enjoy those things. She's wary though. She's careful, more careful and more afraid than the other kids I see at the playground.
Ms. J.: If you give her extra attention and support, will she tackle things and learn new things like that even though she's afraid?
Mr. F.: Yes, she tackles them and she'll learn and she's just not a very fast learner or very well coordinated. I think she's something of a "klutz."
Ms. J.: How are you and your wife at things like athletics?
Mr. F.: I was very athletic when I was a kid. I don't do much anymore. I do a little jogging now, but my wife, I don't know, she doesn't do much sports.
Ms. J.: I think we'll come back to this at the end. I'd like to do a good check-up and, you know, take a look at Diane's body before I say anything, and then we can talk some more and answer any other questions you might have about it.

Ms. J. is appropriately careful to delay giving an opinion until she has been able to evaluate the entire situation, including the physical examination. However, she also indicates interest in the questions about Diane's development and explicitly says she will return to this subject later.

Ms. J.: Can you tell me something about Diane's routines? For instance, sleeping—how does that go?

Continues with the routine history. The introductory comment "about her routines" helps to orient Mr. F. to the content of the next group of questions.

Mr. F.: She sleeps fine.
Ms. J.: Any problems going to sleep?
Mr. F.: Not really.
Ms. J.: Does she generally sleep through the night?
Mr. F.: Yes. Well, we get her up to urinate when we go to bed around midnight. That's because of the bottle.
Ms. J.: Uh-huh. Is that because you don't want her to wet the bed?
Mr. F.: Yes. She wets the bed right through her diaper. We put a diaper on her at night because of her bottles, and she'll wet right through the diaper.
Ms. J.: And when you wake her up to urinate, she goes?
Mr. F.: Yes.
Ms. J.: And goes back to sleep?
Mr. F.: Yes.
Ms. J.: Any trouble with that?
Mr. F.: No problem.
Ms. J.: How often did she wet the bed before you began waking her?
Mr. F.: Oh—two or three times a week.
Ms. J.: Does your system of waking her eliminate the bed-wetting?
Mr. F.: Yes, almost completely. Sometimes she'll wet (once in two or three weeks) early in the morning—around 5 or 6 A.M.—and will wake us up to change her.
Ms. J.: Okay. And how does she normally wake up? What kind of state is she in when she gets up?
Mr. F.: She's usually pretty good—a pleasant mood, happy.
Ms. J.: Tell me something about her, also where she sleeps. Does she have her own room?
Mr. F.: Yes.
Ms. J.: And does she sleep in a bed or a crib?
Mr. F.: She sleeps in her own bed. She switched from a crib before we moved, and it went very well.
Ms. J.: Good. Tell me something about Diane's diet and eating. For instance, what's her average diet like?

Open-ended questions are particularly useful around eating behavior, since there are so many opinions about the "right way" to feed children. The open-ended approach leads to more honest answers and, hopefully, to a relaxed discussion about sensible eating habits. The average diet gives room for normal variations from day to day.

Mr. F.: She eats pretty well. She'll eat Cheerios for breakfast, and she'll eat maybe some oranges, or orange juice, and she'll eat maybe some cheese. She'll eat a little bit of everything. She won't sit on her chair. Her eating habits are not so hot, but I think she probably gets enough food into her.
Ms. J.: Uh-huh.

Mr. F.: At lunchtime, it varies, sometimes a hard-boiled egg, sometimes some tuna fish and stuff. And at dinner she'll eat what we eat, but it never seems like she eats very much; but somehow she's growing and we don't make a fuss over food if we can help it. Sometimes I make a fuss over food, when she leaves it on her plate, but it doesn't help anyway.

The comment "it never seems like she eats very much" occurs frequently in parents' histories for toddlers and preschool-age children. Mr. F. provides his own reassurance, but he would probably feel better if Ms. J. were to make a clear statement about Diane's growth at the end of the visit.

Ms. J.: Do you remember any of this with Rachel when she was two and a half?
Mr. F.: Yes. Diane and Rachel are alike in this.
Ms. J.: Is it something that aggravates you a lot?
Mr. F.: No. In fact, I'd rather she be skinny. I had trouble being fat when I was a kid.
Ms. J.: What was that like?
Mr. F.: I had to be careful, especially as a teenager, not to eat too much.
Ms. J.: How do you think of Diane: skinny, fat, medium?
Mr. F.: She's fine—medium.
Mr. J.: Good. Okay. Do you and your wife ever argue about her eating habits?

Child rearing issues are often a focus of disagreement between parents.

Mr. F.: No, we don't. However, she is more relaxed about it, and doesn't worry like I do. She knows I worry because I was chubby as a child.
Ms. J.: I think it helps a lot if parents do not differ too much about eating habits. If they do differ and can't work out a solution, it really makes a hassle for everybody and it can make it worse for the child.
    About how much milk to you think Diane gets in a day?

The history continues with the content of Diane's diet.

Mr. F.: She's not drinking much milk.
Ms. J.: Does she have any cheese?
Mr. F.: She has it . . . she'll have some cheese. . . . yeh. . . . on her bread. She'll have some of our cottage cheese and maybe some hard cheese in the morning.
Ms. J.: And she has milk in her cereal?
Mr. F.: A little.
Ms. J.: Ice cream?
Mr. F.: Yes, she has more ice cream than she should. My wife and I do argue about that. I kind of sympathize with the kids and want them to have as much ice cream as they want. My wife really doesn't think they should have that kind of junk in the house.
Ms. J.: How do you resolve it?
Mr. F.: We compromise, and it seems reasonable. We have ice cream some of the time.
Ms. J.: About how many times a week does Diane eat meat or fish?
Mr. F.: Every night we have some meat, fish, or chicken—most every night.
Ms. J.: And one other question: do you have a well at your house or do you have city water?
Mr. F.: We have a well at our new house.
Ms. J.: I don't know what it was like in Chicago, but the natural water around here doesn't have adequate flouride in it, and so we usually recommend to folks who have their own wells that the children do take fluoride tablets.
Mr. F.: Where do you get those?
Ms. J.: I'll give you a prescription for them. Does she take any vitamins?

Mr. F.: No.
Ms. J.: Fine. Generally if a child has a good diet at this age—and Diane's sounds fine—vitamins aren't necessary.
   Can you tell me a little bit about Diane's toileting? You mentioned she wears diapers at night.
Mr. F.: But she's really toilet trained. She probably could go at night too sometimes; it's just that it's inconvenient for us. Sometimes she does wet her diaper.
Ms. J.: How old was she when she was toilet trained?
Mr. F.: She's only been toilet trained for about four months.
Ms. J.: And how did that go?
Mr. F.: I think it was alright. Not much problem.
Ms. J.: And she's trained for urine and bowel movements?
Mr. F.: Yes.
Ms. J.: Does she ever have any of what they call "accidents"?
Mr. F.: No.
Ms. J.: She doesn't wet her pants or things like that?
Mr. F.: No.
Ms. J.: It sounds like Diane's toileting is quite accomplished. I'll come back to the nighttime wetting later.
   We had talked earlier about Diane's relationship with the family, and I was wondering how she does when she's with other people, the sitter, either the regular daytime sitter or an evening sitter. How does she do with other people?
Mr. F.: She's pretty good.
Ms. J.: Does she ever protest when you or your wife leave?
Mr. F.: Rarely, if her sister is with her and the sitter, or if it is a babysitter she knows. We're pretty careful about it. She may fuss, now, since the move. We have to introduce her to a new daytime babysitter, and an evening sitter for when we go out. But I think we'll try and do so gradually, before my wife goes back to work.
Ms. J.: Right. That's a good idea. It will help a lot if you can make the changes gradually. And how does she react to strange people? I know how she reacted to me. She was clearly shy, which is appropriate. Is that typical?

It is good to acknowledge that shyness is appropriate. Some parents feel that shyness is unfriendly and they are uncomfortable when their children are shy.

Mr. F.: Yes.
Ms. J.: And does she stay shy for a long time? Does she get warmed up? How does she approach new people?
Mr. F.: She stays shy for a while. It may take her ten minutes or two hours for her to talk to strangers. She's careful. Some people she never warms up to.
Ms. J.: Did Rachel react the same way to other people?
Mr. F.: Oh, much more. Rachel was *really* shy.
Ms. J.: Is she still shy?
Mr. F.: I don't think so, no.
Ms. J.: While we're mentioning Rachel, have you made plans for her health care as well?
Mr. F.: Well, I'd like you to see her, too.
Ms. J.: Okay. Good. I like getting to know the whole family. It will be my pleasure to meet her. Is she well?
Mr. F.: Yes.
Ms. J.: Right now I'd like to ask you a few questions about your family medical history. How old are you?
Mr. F.: Thirty-three.
Ms. J.: How is your health?

Mr. F.: Fine. Oh, I do have occasional back pain—which goes away with aspirin and a heating pad.
Ms. J.: Anything else—things for which you take medicines or consult a clinician?

Since Mr. F. tends to minimize things and perhaps to ignore significant history, Ms. J. gives him an additional opportunity to recall his own health history.

Mr. F.: No.
Ms. J.: How old is your wife?
Mr. F.: Thirty-three.
Ms. J.: How is her health?
Mr. F.: Fine. The only thing is the allergies I mentioned and asthma years ago.
Ms. J.: Can you tell me a little more about that?
Mr. F.: Well, my wife is allergic to some medicines, I guess, and she has a mild case of . . . what-do-you-call-it in the late summer with her nose.
Ms. J.: Hay fever?
Mr. F.: Hay fever, yes. I guess that's worse here even than it was in Chicago. We'll see what happens. She also had some wheezing attacks when she was a child and teenager.
Ms. J.: Yes.
Mr. F.: She's had some shots for the hay fever, and that helped, and then she stopped taking them about ten years ago. Sometimes she gets a cough and a tight feeling in her chest from what happens with her nose during hay fever season.
Ms. J.: Okay. Anybody else in the family have any allergies?
Mr. F.: Not that I know of.
Ms. J.: Any other medical conditions that you can think of either on your side or her side?
Mr. F.: Not that I can think of.
Ms. J.: Any history of high blood pressure?

Although Mr. F. says there is no other family history, Ms. J. pursues selected medical conditions which may influence Diane's health maintenance plans. For example, serious hypertension would indicate more careful and frequent blood pressure measurements for Diane as she grows up, and possibly caution about excessive salt intake. This practice of asking selected specific information in the family history is useful in most health assessments.

Mr. F.: No, no.
Ms. J.: Any heart trouble?
Mr. F.: Yeh, my dad actually had a heart attack when he was quite young—10 years ago when he was about 50. It wasn't too serious and then he had another one not too long ago, actually just before this move. I hope he's alright.

Mr. F. is clearly (appropriately) concerned about his father's health. Therefore it is sensible to continue the discussion to learn if this is a significant family problem.

Ms. J.: Was he hospitalized for this last heart attack?
Mr. F.: Yes, he was. I didn't get to see him 'cause we were busy with the move. I'm going to have to go visit him next week—he lives in Atlanta—and see how he's doing. I hear from my sister and mother that he's doing quite well, but I'm concerned about him.
Ms. J.: I can understand that. Is there any history in the family of diabetes?

Mr. F.: No.
Ms. J.: And do you know anybody, family or friends, who has TB?
Mr. F.: No.
Ms. J.: Okay. Now I have some more questions to ask you about Diane. It's kind of going from top to bottom, and it helps me make sure we haven't forgotten any pieces of the history that might be helpful. Does Diane have any problems with her skin that you know of?

Ms. J. continues with the review of systems. The questions proceed from the general to the specific within each area of the review of systems. As will be apparent here, it is adjusted for the pediatric patient.

Mr. F.: No.
Ms. J.: Okay. And any problems with her ears?
Mr. F.: Oh, yes, she had . . . twice she had infections in her ears and one time she was up crying through the night, and we had to give her medicine for ten days.
Ms. J.: Antibiotics?
Mr. F.: I guess so.
Ms. J.: How old was she, approximately, when she had those ear infections?
Mr. F.: One when she was about one and a half and one just not too long before the move.
Ms. J.: Right. And after the antibiotics were begun, how soon did the pain and whatever other symptoms there might have been stop?
Mr. F.: I believe that in a day she was better.
Ms. J.: Do you think that she hears well?
Mr. F.: Yes, I think she hears very well.
Ms. J.: I always ask that in general, but I also always ask it after an ear infection in case there's any residual fluid in the ears. We can check that out when I do the physical examination. Does she have any problems with her eyes?
Mr. F.: No.
Ms. J.: Have you ever noticed that she had crossed eyes?
Mr. F.: No.
Ms. J.: Okay. Any problems with her nose?
Mr. F.: No.
Ms. J.: Nosebleeds?
Mr. F.: No.
Ms. J.: Okay. Any difficulties with her mouth?
Mr. F.: No.
Ms. J.: You had mentioned your concern about her teeth and mentioned the dentist. Has she actually seen a dentist?
Mr. F.: No, she hasn't.
Ms. J.: Did Rachel go to a dentist when you were back in Chicago?
Mr. F.: Yes.
Ms. J.: Do you remember about what age she started going?
Mr. F.: I think the pediatrician sent us for a visit, just to get to know the dentist and have her teeth cleaned and checked for cavities, sometime when she was in nursery school.
Ms. J.: That was at three years of age?
Mr. F.: I'm not sure if she was three or four.
Ms. J.: Okay. That's something we can talk about also, when Diane's a little bit older; it's a good idea to start around that time.
Mr. F.: We will need a recommendation if you know somebody good in town here.
Ms. J.: Yes, we know some very good people who really like to work with children, and we'll be able to help you out with those names and addresses. Has Diane had any problems with her chest, other than what you told me about the pneumonia?

Mr. F.: No.
Ms. J.: Cough, difficulty catching her breath?
Mr. F.: No.
Ms. J.: Any problems with her heart?
Mr. F.: No.
Ms. J.: Ever have any heart murmurs?
Mr. F.: No.
Ms. J.: I usually like to ask about the child's digestion. Any troubles with nausea, vomiting?
Mr. F.: No.
Ms. J.: And her bowels—any difficulty with diarrhea?
Mr. F.: No.
Ms. J.: What about constipation?
Mr. F.: She's had some, yeh, she's had periods actually where she cried, her stools were so hard and they seemed very big. We were worried about them, especially when she was drinking a lot of that bottle and she wasn't eating any food.
Ms. J.: How old was she then?
Mr. F.: Actually, it wasn't that long ago, but she's had it on and off since she was a year old, I guess.
Ms. J.: And what do you do about it?
Mr. F.: Pretty much leave it up to my wife, but I think she tries to get her to eat more vegetables and more fruit. For a while she was drinking a lot of milk, and we cut down on some of the milk or watered it down, I think. One time the doctor gave us something to give her but I don't think we used it very much. Lately her stools have been fine.

If Mr. F. had not given such a complete answer about the constipation, Ms. J. would have had to ask specifically about medication, course of the symptom, current situation. The information provided by Mr. F. indicates that Diane's parents know how and when to seek help with a problem and that they know how to use and follow a management plan. This is as important as the constipation itself, and is useful in learning about how the F. family uses the health care system.

Ms. J.: I think we'll leave it that if you notice she has more difficulties with constipation, you or your wife should call me, and we'll see what we can do. I think it is probably related to diet and the milk in the bottles, and we're going to get back to that at the end of this afternoon's talk. Does she ever have any blood in her stools?

This question provides information which tells Ms. J. whether there is likely to be a fissure, with a cycle of painful stools and voluntary stool retention.

Mr. F.: No.
Ms. J.: Okay. And what's the longest she goes without having a bowel movement?

Again, a question to determine whether Diane is voluntarily withholding stools. If she were, a more vigorous program to soften the stools would be indicated.

Mr. F.: She pretty much has one every day or every two days.
Ms. J.: You mentioned that Diane has been toilet trained for urine for a while. Has she ever had any problems with burning on urination?
Mr. F.: No.
Ms. J.: Do you think she has a good stream?
Mr. F.: Yes.

Ms. J.: Have you ever seen her urinate?
Mr. F.: Sure. She stands up sometimes on the lawn to pee.
Ms. J.: Okay. Any problems with her arms or legs or joints?
Mr. F.: No.
Ms. J.: Okay. And has she ever had any problems like seizures or convulsions?
Mr. F.: No.
Ms. J.: Good. Do you think she's been growing?
Mr. F.: Yeh, she's growing fine.
Ms. J.: She grows out of her clothes?
Mr. F.: Sure.
Ms. J.: And the pediatrician was never worried about her growth?
Mr. F.: No. He had this chart. She was alright.
Ms. J.: Right. I have a chart also, and I'll show that to you at the end of the check-up. Has Diane ever had any problems with her blood, like anemia?
Mr. F.: No.
Ms. J.: And do you notice if she eats things or puts things in her mouth that are not food?
Mr. F.: No. She used to but not anymore.
Ms. J.: Has she ever been in a place that had a lot of peeling paint?
Mr. F.: Not that I know of.
Ms. J.: How old was your house and the babysitter's house back in Chicago?
Mr. F.: Both were very old.
Ms. J.: Very old—before World War II?
Mr. F.: I guess, yeh, they were both old apartments.
Ms. J.: The reason why I ask is lead paint was used in those days, and we're concerned if children do eat paint chips with lead.
Mr. F.: I don't think she did.
Ms. J.: Were the houses in pretty good repair?
Mr. F.: Yes—very good shape.
Ms. J.: Okay. And is your house a new house now or is it also an old house?
Mr. F.: It's a new house.
Ms. J.: A new house. Fine. As far as you know, does Diane have any allergies?
Mr. F.: No.
Ms. J.: And I take it she probably had some form of penicillin for those ear infections?

If a child has had penicillin or any other drug without adverse reaction, it is safe to assume there is no allergy to those drugs. However, allergy can always develop in the future.

Mr. F.: I don't know.
Ms. J.: You don't know. Okay. Is she on any medicines now?
Mr. F.: No.
Ms. J.: Do you have any pets?

Pets can be sources of infectious diseases, such as salmonella from turtles and parasites from dogs and cats.

Mr. F.: We have a fish and a guinea pig.
Ms. J.: And has Diane ever traveled to places outside of Chicago, aside from New Haven and this part of the country?
Mr. F.: Yes, she's traveled south.
Ms. J.: Can you tell me where?
Mr. F.: We visit my mother-in-law in Florida.
Ms. J.: She lives in the city?
Mr. F.: Pardon me?
Ms. J.: She lives in the city rather than the country? I ask because there is more chance of contracting gastrointestinal parasites in rural areas with poor sewage and lots of contact with the soil.

Certain conditions are much more frequent in certain geographic areas, such as gastrointestinal parasites in the tropics, coccidioidomycosis in the San Joaquin Valley of California, and histoplasmosis in the midwestern part of the United States.

Mr. F.: Yes. I see. They live in the city.
Ms. J.: Okay. Fine. I think I've pretty much finished my list of questions. Are there any things that have come to mind that you would like to ask me about?

Sometimes the parent thinks of other questions during the interview. In addition, parents and older children may need the interview to assess whether they feel comfortable enough with the clinician to ask more personal or emotional questions. This extra opportunity to ask questions only takes a few seconds of the clinician's time, but provides a valuable opportunity for the parent and older child to continue the interview if they need to do so.

Mr. F.: No, I don't have anything to ask.
Ms. J.: Okay. What I'd like to do now would be to have Diane play with a few of these puzzles and things that I have, and I think since she's comfortably playing on the floor, I'll go over to her. If she seems a little uncomfortable, you can come join us or put her on your lap. After that I'll do the check-up and then we can talk again.

Since Ms. J. will do a very informal developmental assessment of Diane's problem-solving skills and language abilities, she does not make any statements about developmental screening. She will discuss Diane's development in the clinical summary, referring both to her own observations of Diane's skills during the entire visit and to information taken from the history.

Mr. F.: Okay.

Clinical summary
(after the physical examination)

Ms. J.: I think maybe Diane will be comfortable playing with some of these toys while we talk about the things that we already discussed earlier and my observations from the check-up. First thing I'd like to tell you is that Diane is really a very healthy girl. She's in good shape. I'll show you the growth chart. This is where she is for her height and her weight (pointing to the growth chart).

It is helpful to give an adequate explanation about growth charts at the first visit for health assessment. This short discussion is a simple but significant way to communicate to the parent and older child that you value their understanding of the health assessment; you (the clinician) are not only *telling* them what you think, but are *sharing* information.

Ms. J.: You mentioned you'd seen these before. Her weight at this age is 32 lbs. which is very, very good. She's about the 75th percentile, which means that if you took ten children, two would be heavier than her at her age and seven would be thinner than her at her age. Her height is also in proportion to her weight, and here she is at 36 inches and around the 50th percentile for height. Also, the physical examination itself was completely normal. Everything was fine.

The subsequent lengthy discussion is worthwhile because, once again, it helps Mr. F. to understand the rationale behind Ms. J.'s advice. Advice is appropriate here, but it should not be handed down as the law. This approach, combined with later opportunities for Mr. F. to ask questions, will lead to better rapport with Ms. J. and hopefully to better compliance with management plans.

Ms. J.: I'd like to go back and talk a little bit about some of the things you had mentioned earlier. The first was the issue about the bottles. I think that my general position still holds, which is that children by about one and one-half to two years of age should really not be having their bottles. I'm concerned in relation to their teeth and in relation to social pressures. It usually starts to get uncomfortable for the parents or the child when she begins nursery school, and other people comment in a negative way about the bottle. The difficulty, as you said, is that Diane's really attached to her bottle, and it's not just a source of something to drink—it's a very important comfort to her. I think you ought to talk to your wife about what I've said, and we can talk about it again. In view of the fact that you've just moved and that your wife probably will be going back to work and Diane will be adjusting to a new sitter, you should not make the big change of giving up the bottles now. There will be a lot of other things going on in her life, and the fact that she still has her bottle another month or two or three isn't really going to make any big difference. I think that psychologically, the bottles will be of help during these changes. After she gets settled and those major changes are completed, then we can consider how to help her give up the bottles.

I also want to say one other related thing which has to do with the diapers at night. Some people would say that she is actually able to wake and urinate even though she has the bottles and all this urine in her bladder. It is under her conscious control. I believe that. The question is whether you and your wife will be comfortable with that, put her in pants, and tell her that she will wake to urinate in the potty. You could still wake her before you go to sleep just to save any worry. I don't think it's terribly important which way you do it.

Again, the points Ms. J. makes are not law—they are opinions. Child rearing issues are best handled with honest attention to how both parents feel in a particular situation. If Ms. J. gives advice that is contrary to what the parents can accept, the advice will either be ignored or cause unproductive conflict.

Ms. J.: I think the most important thing is that you're both comfortable. If you'll be anxious about the wet linens, and if Diane will feel guilty or bad, leave her in diapers. But if you think that you can be comfortable and, what should I say, confident that she will urinate on the potty, go ahead and put her in pants all the time. I think it will be very important to make sure she stays in pants in the day because if you go back to diapers in the day, it gives her a very mixed message about whether she's able to control her urination. How does that all set with you?
Mr. F.: That's fine. It's very similar to our own discussions at home.
Ms. J.: Okay. It's the kind of situation where I can't tell you what to do in your family. So, I'd like you to go home, talk about it, and feel free to give me a ring. Let me know how it's going or call if you have any questions at all. Also, I expect I'll be seeing your older daughter, and we can chat more about Diane's toileting at that time.

If the constipation recurs, let me know. I think it probably is related to the diet from what you tell me, and one way to manage it is to make sure that her milk intake does not exceed a quart a day. Also, make sure she does have some roughage, some salads, some bran cereals in her diet. She'll probably do alright.

Now, you had mentioned that you were concerned about Diane's clumsiness. From the history, it does sound like she's a child who has been more into talking, quiet playing, and personal relationships than into gross motor activities. But as I did the check-up, I saw that she is okay. Her bones and her muscles are fine. Her coordination is not bad at all for a two-and-a-half-year-old. There was one period where she got very excited, and I noticed that she stumbled on her feet. But that was only once toward the end of the check-up when she was really into playing with the ball with me. She climbed nicely on the slide in the waiting room, and she's been able to climb around on the grown-up chairs very well. She threw the ball nicely. Her feet are straight. So I think that this really is just Diane's way of developing and doesn't represent any significant medical or physical problems.

Mr. F.: Do you think she'll be an athlete?

Ms. J.: Well, you can't tell. She might fool you yet. At this point she certainly is within the average range.

At this point it is not appropriate to delve into the meaning of Mr. F.'s question about Diane's future as an athlete. Ms. J. will include it in her impression of Mr. F.'s overall level of concern about his child, and may discuss it further if it remains a problem for him.

Ms. J.: You had mentioned the allergies, and I think in that regard I need to tell you that her chest is completely clear. There are no wheezes. Also related to that, there is no sign of allergy elsewhere. Her ears look fine, and there's no sign in her nose, mouth, or lungs of any respiratory allergy that's currently active. With her past history, I'm not concerned about it. If something pops up, if she gets a cold and wheezes, we can take care of that. But there's nothing that you could do at present that could prevent allergies or asthma from developing. It's one of those things. You just have to sit tight.

Okay. We had mentioned dental care. I recommend fluoride supplements to your well water. At this age, Diane would take a half a milligram of fluoride a day. Fluoride pills are not a terribly dangerous pill to have around, so that even if she took four or five at once, it wouldn't really harm her. But if she got into the whole bottle, or for some reason was eating them regularly in excessive amount, it could be harmful to her teeth and to her body. So, I would treat this just like you'd treat any other medicine, which is to keep it out of reach, keep it in the original container and nowadays, of course, they're prescribing the child-proof containers.

Vitamins, fluoride, and other preparations taken for health maintenance (rather than for treatment of an illness) are frequently left accessible to children. They should be in child-proof containers and should be stored with awareness of their potential harm.

Ms. J.: A related subject at this age is that although you tell me that Diane doesn't put a lot of things in her mouth, every once in a while a child who has previously been very reliable will become very curious, and pills, medicines, and other things that you wouldn't think a child would put in her mouth, pop in. So I really encourage folks to be very careful about where they store things—like detergent, dishwasher soap, pills, and so forth. And it's a good idea to keep things in their original containers and keep them out of the reach of the children.

Mr. F.:   This brings to mind the use of Ipecac for poisonings. Are you familiar with it?

Mr. F.:   Yes. We have some with our first aid stuff. We used it once for Rachel—she ate some of my mother's arthritis pills when she was 18 months old.

Ms. J.:   It's good to have around. However, always call us here before you use it. There are some situations where you should *not* use it, and we can give you advice about it if the need arises.

If Mr. F. was not familiar with Ipecac, Ms. J. would either give him a one-ounce bottle of Ipecac or a prescription, along with instructions for its use.

Ms. J.:   Now then, I'd like to get back to your children's dental care. Your big girl will also need fluoride, and I can write up a prescription today for her for fluoride also. She'll take a whole milligram every day.

    Which brings me to the subject of dentists. We have a list which the secretary can give you on your way out. These are dentists who do well with children, and we've had very good success referring our families to them. For your older daughter, you can just make an appointment at your convenience. For Diane, again I think I would wait until she's really well settled into her new routine, and sometime after her third birthday. At that time the dentist will clean and check her teeth for cavities.

    Also, before you go out, I'll ask you to sign a form so we can get the records from your pediatrician back in Chicago.

    When I first meet folks, it seems like I have a lot to talk about with them. I have a few more things on my list I'd like to mention. One question I didn't ask yet was what your family does about car seats or car restraints for the children.

Mr. F.:   We have a good car seat.

Ms. J.:   Do you know what kind you have?

Mr. F.:   Those white ones that you get from the Chevrolet place.

Ms. J.:   The GM love seat?

Mr. F.:   Yes.

Ms. J.:   Okay. And does Diane use that?

Mr. F.:   We're strict about it. She *always* uses her car seat.

Ms. J.:   How many cars do you own?

Mr. F.:   Two.

Ms. J.:   And do you have two seats, one for each car, or do you . . .

Mr. F.:   We switch them back and forth. Each car has the special hook in it.

Ms. J.:   Okay. I think it's very, very important. It's probably one of the best things you can do for your child's health—to regularly use the car seat. Does your big girl use seat belts?

Mr. F.:   Yes.

Ms. J.:   The last thing I want to talk to you about is some of the changes that you might find with Diane. You're already experienced because you've had another child, but each child is a little different. You probably will find that in the next stage, Diane will be interested in becoming more independent, exploring things around her house, maybe being a little reckless, running out in the street. And you'll just have to keep a watch on those things. The other big question in her development will also be nursery school or day care or a babysitter, whatever. And I have some thoughts about that and I know a little bit about the schools in the area. So when you are ready to consider that, you could give me a ring, and we could set aside some time to talk about that. Are there any other things you want to ask me about?

Mr. F.:   No. This has been very helpful. I've never been to a practitioner or a doctor who spent this much time.

Ms. J.:   Well, I'm glad you feel like that. And it's been very nice for me to get to know you in this way. I'm also interested in meeting your wife, and I was also interested that you came alone with Diane for our visit today.

Mr. F.: I came alone so that my wife could have some relaxed time alone with Rachel. With this move, we haven't had much leisure time with the kids. I think she will bring Rachel for her check-up, and you'll meet her then.

Ms. J.: Fine. Generally I see children at Diane's age every four to six months for a routine check-up. But since you may want to talk sooner about weaning her from the bottle—and also about nursery schools and day care—you might want to make an appointment earlier, mostly to talk about those things. Now I'll introduce you to Dr. Steinberg and then you can be on your way.

THE WRITE-UP OF THE INTERVIEW

Health records are an extremely important part of the health care delivery system. Clinicians on a team use the information supplied by their colleagues, and the health care they provide is affected by the completeness, readability, and organization of the patient's health record.

The following write-up is for the interview transcribed earlier in this chapter. This write-up is quite complete and is not necessarily what a clinician in practice would always record. Frequently, forms are used to expedite note-writing, and a more abbreviated record is often used. Handwritten records tend to have far more abbreviations and shortcuts than dictated and typed records. I have used the abbreviations and short phrases typical of my own records. Naturally, this varies among clinicians.

This write-up follows a modification of the Problem Oriented Medical Record (POMR), representing a major change in health records over the past decade.* The POMR facilitates a well-organized series of notes, with each problem handled separately and clearly. Our own patient, Diane, had only two major problems: *General Care* (used in pediatrics to include all the routine information of the interest to the clinician) and *Status Post-pneumonia*. Several significant but minor concerns—including bed-wetting, constipation, her father's concern about excess weight gain, and slow gross motor development—were grouped under general care so that they would not be lost at future visits and would be discussed again. They were not made into separate major problems with their own numbers because they are considered temporary and within the range of normal variation. If any of these problems were not resolved, or if their significance increased, the clinician would make a new problem: for instance, #3. Constipation.

The stylistic variations among records should not prevent their usefulness to other clinicians. Even this write-up, with its individual format, phrases, and abbreviations, would be comprehensible and useful to another clinician who was not familiar with the patient.

---

* L.L.Weed. Medical records that guide and teach. *New Eng. J. Med.* 278:593 and 652, 1968.

ID: 2½-year-old girl—first health assessment here; with father, reliable.
1. *Current Health*
   A. *Generally* well child; past care Dr. Klein, Chicago.
   B. *Diet:* adequate in four major food groups, with adequate iron and vitamins. Milk, about 4 to 8 oz. per day, and cheese and ice cream. Well water. Uses cup, fork, and spoon well.
   Father concerned child should not get too fat; he "had a tendency to be fat as a child" and had to diet as a teenager. He is also more permissive (i.e., re: ice cream) than mother. Parents seem to make satisfactory compromises.
   C. *Sleep:* own bed, own room; no difficulties.
   D. *Elimination:* toilet trained four months ago without difficulty; trained for both BM and urine; still wets several times a week at night, so in diapers at night. Parents in routine of waking her at 11 or 12 at night to urinate—works well and virutally eliminates bed-wetting. No significant serious conflict over toileting.
2. *Past Medical History*
   A. *Birth:* 6 lbs. plus; normal, full term, vaginal, vertex; neonatal period okay; home at 2 days.
   Mo. with prenatal care from about 2nd month gestation.
   B. *Infancy:*
   1. Breast fed combined with bottle until about 11 months, then to bottle only. *Mo. with mastitis* when *child 2 mos.* old; treated with meds and incision by surgeon for breast abscess; mo. continued to nurse on other side and resumed both sides when infection cleared; clearly emotionally stressful, but father reports only positive outcome.
   2. *Pneumonia, age 5 months;* hospitalized at University Hosp. in Chicago for 5 days, one parent always there, mo. breast-fed throughout. No subsequent resp. problems, but father concerned about future resp. problems because maternal history of asthma and allergies.
   C. *Childhood:* chickenpox, age 1½ years—no complications.
   D. *Immunizations:* "Okay"—record in Chicago, to be sent here.
   E. *Allergies:* none.
3. *Patient Profile*
   A. *Current life situation:*
   Household: mother, father, 6 yr. sister Rachel.
   Mo.—looking for part-time work as secretary; sitter with children.
   Fa.—Junior high school math teacher.
   Primary care from mo., fa., sitter. Fa. very much involved with child care.
   Home: 3-bedroom ranch in suburbs.
   Economic: steady job, health insurance adequate.
   Support: extended family in New England. None in this vicinity. With move from Chicago last month, have few friends and little support.
   B. *Development:* description of sensitive, sometimes irritable, usually

happy and delightful. "Sensitive" means afraid of loud noises, fussy as an infant. Nothing major as a concern now. Good relationship with mo., fa., and sib. Described affectionately. Reasonable amount of oppositional behavior for age. Fa. proud of Diane's good vocabulary and intellectual abilities, but concerned about clumsiness and relatively slow gross motor development.

    1) Large muscle skills: climbs well, uses slide and tricycle; occasionally clumsy when hurries.

    2) Small muscle skills: good manipulative skills with beads, puzzles, crayons, and blocks.

    3) Problem-solving: very good with puzzles and block building.

    4) Language: quite advanced in both comprehension and production; large vocabulary; speaks in complex sentences, explains pictures and events; speech unusually clear for $2\frac{1}{2}$-year-old.

    5) Play—by report has good play skills for age.

4. *Family Medical History* (incomplete data)

Father: 33 years old, "well"; occasional mild back pain.

Mother: 33 years old, "well"; history of allergies, hay fever, asthma; no current resp. problems.

Sister: 6 years old, "well."

Paternal grandfather: heart attacks at age 50 (10 yrs. ago) and this year.

Negative for TB, diabetes.

5. *Review of Systems*

    A. *Ears:* 2 episodes of otitis media, age $1\frac{1}{2}$ and $2\frac{1}{2}$ years; Rx. with antibiotics, cleared well, no sequelae.

    B. *Constipation:* probably dietary, Rx'd with diet and a medicine for short time; currently BMs normal.

    Otherwise noncontributory.

6. *Physical Examination*

General appearance: Slightly shy, bright, healthy-looking preschooler; cooperative with support from father.

    V.S.: Pulse 96/min. Resp. 20/min.
        Wt. 32 lbs., 75%
        Ht. 36 in., 50%
        H.C. 49.5 cm., 50%

Skin: clear

Nodes: normal

HEENT: Ears: normal TMs with normal movement
        Eyes: no strabismus, fundus normal
        Nose and throat clear

Chest: clear, normal breath sounds

Heart: clear heart sounds, no murmurs, good femoral pulses bilaterally, without lag

Abdomen: no tenderness or organomegaly

Genitalia: normal female child; no hernias

Extremities: normal anatomy and function; gait normal

Neurological: cranial nerves, motor, and sensory grossly intact. DTRs —2+ bilat, patellar

Impression:

I. General Care: Healthy child, normal growth and development
              Family competent
              Incomplete data: immunization record
                            family medical history
                            profile of family relationships
            Father's concerns: child should not be overweight
                            child's sensitivity
                            child's "slow" motor development
            Family recently moved, making adjustments

II. Status Post-pneumonia at 5 months of age: completely resolved

Plan:

I. General Care:

  A. Write for immunization record.

  B. Discussed weaning from bottle: fa. to discuss with mo. and call me; I suggested to wait until new sitter and other adjustments made around move.

  C. Discussed growth (normal)—not excessive weight.

  D. Discussed gross motor (normal).

  E. Today needs: Hemoglobin/hematrocrit
                   Urine analysis and culture

  F. Prescribed Fluoritabs 0.5 mg/d, #100

  G. Return in 3 months for:
    1) follow-up (will see mo. with sib earlier) on adjustment to move.
    2) concerns re: sensitivity, excess weight gain, motor development, constipation, bedwetting.
    3) give any immunizations needed.

                                              Diana Jones, PNP

Suggested Readings
Unit V: The Annotated Interview and Write-up

Chapter 15: The Annotated Interview and Write-Up

Weed, L.L. *Medical Records, Medical Education, and Patient Care: The Problem-Oriented Record as a Basic Tool*. Cleveland, Case-Western Reserve University Press, 1969.

Weed, L.L. Medical records that guide and teach. *New Eng. J. Med.* 278:593 and 652, 1968.

Index

Abdomen, examination of, 57, 219
Abdominal pain, 117, 119, 122, 124, 127
   of appendicitis, 117
    lactose intolerance and, 123
    mittelschmerz and, 120
    peristaltic waves and, 120–21
    rectal examination and, 220
Abducens nerves, physical examination and, 60
Abortion, adolescent, 33–34
    counseling about, 67–68
    Tay-Sachs disease and, 66
Accessory nerves, physical examination and, 60–61
Accident prevention, advice about, 248–49
Acne
   adrenal system and, 48
   advice about, 248
   patient's history and, 46, 48
   patient's worry about, 252
Adaptive skills. *See* Problem-solving (adaptive) skills, development of
Adolescent(s)
   advice about, 247
   advice to, 248
   clinical relationship and, 105–6, 110–11, 244
   examination of, 56, 193, 201–3
   female, eye irritation and, 123
   female, flank pain and, 120
   as historian, 28, 110–11
   language and communication skills of, 162
   muscle skills of, 161–62
   as parents, 114–15, 143, 243
   personal-social skills of, 162
   personality of, 161
   problem-solving skills of, 162
   questions of, during interview, 91–92
   relationship to parents, 161, 229, 244
   stress and, 122
   work relationships and, 146
   See also Abortion, adolescent; Puberty; Sexual activity, adolescent; Sexual maturation
Adrenal system, review of, 48
Advice, about health. *See* Clinical summary, typical elements in; Diet, advice about
Advocacy, of clinician for child, 4, 9, 114, 269
Agencies
   child's health problems and, 244, 269
   family relationship to, 146–47
   patient's records and, 38
Agenda, for interview, 84
Age, patient's
   on records, 22
   as screening criterion, 64–65, 69
Aggravation, of symptoms, 122
Allergic problems, 254–55
Alleviation, of symptoms, 122–23
Anemia
   iron deficiency, 69
   screening and, 69, 74
Antibiotics, 5
Anus, physical examination and, 59, 203, 220
Appendicitis, 117
Asthma, 254–55
Athletics, participation in, 150
Attitude, of staff, 11
Audiometry, pure tone, 74, 159
Auricular (otic) nerves, physical examination and, 60
Auscultation
   of abdomen, 57, 121
   of thorax and lungs, 56–57
Authority figures, 146

Band-Aids, use of, 230
Barlow's sign, 221

Bed wetting. *See* Enuresis
Birth control, 34
   counseling about, 67–68, 248, 268
   religion and, 23
Birth history, on patient's records, 28–31
   labor and delivery, 29–30
   maternal obstetric history, 29
   neonatal period, for infant, 31
   patient's condition, at birth, 30
   postpartum period, for mother, 30–31
   pregnancy, 29
   prenatal care, 29
Blood pressure
   physical examination and, 52, 222–23
      parents' questions about, 189–90
      young child and, 193, 211, 222–23
   tests, value of, 75
Blood type, screening test for, 74
Body language. *See* Communication, nonverbal
Body-mind interdependence, 7–8, 124
Bowel movements, as symptoms, 126
Breasts
   physical examination of, 55–56
   review of, 47
Brudzinski's sign, physical examination and, 61

Canals, ear, physical examination of, 54
Cardiovascular system
   examination of, 57, 216–18
   review of, 47
Caregivers, 4, 7
   ascertainment of primary, 114
   child's relationship to, 142–45
   at clinical summary, 243–44
   description of, on patient's records, 37
   observation of, at home, 163
Cerumen, removal of, 213, 233–34
Chest, examination of, 216–18
Child abuse, 4, 9
   detection of, 25
   reporting of, 86
Childhood and adolescent health, on patient's records, 32–35
   accidents and injuries, 34
   allergies, 34–35
   common illnesses, 32
   immunizations, 35
   obstetric history, 33–34, 47
   psychological problems, 33
   serious illnesses, 32–33
   surgical procedures, 33
Child rearing
   advice about, 95, 174, 248–49
   consistency in, 96
   disagreements about, 96–97, 144
   questions about, during interview, 93–96, 174
Children
   examination of, 185–87, 199–203, 206–11
   health needs of, 3–4
   relationship to adults, 4–5, 7

   role of, during interview, 102–6, 112–13
   See also Personal relationships
Chronology, of symptoms, 119–22
Clinical summary, 241–61, 263–79
   conduct of, 244–45
   about development, 172
   follow-up of, 256, 270–71, 279
   major physical problems and, 263–71
   major psychological problems and, 263, 271–79
   minor physical problems and, 251–56
   minor psychological problems and, 256–61
   participants in, 242–44
   purpose of, 241–42
   setting of, 242
   statement of problem, 265–66, 273–75
   time constraints during, 245–46, 287
   typical elements in, 246–50
   use of, 286–87
Clinicians, 6, 14
   developmental assessment and, 132–36
   feelings about parents and child, 9, 97–98, 264
   responsibility for genetic counseling and, 67
   role of, in consultation, 282, 285
   role, discussion of, 83
   screening, in judgments of, 63
   style of, in discussing problem, 269
   See also Communication; Health care professionals; Interview, clinical; Personal relationships; Team, health care
Clinicians, student, 9–11
   clinical summary and, 264
   developmental assessment and, 136, 151
   emotional distance and, 115
   in interview, 87
   during painful procedures, 229
   record-keeping and, 12, 19
Clitoris, 59
Cognitive development, 4, 7–8
Colds, as symptoms, 121–22
Colic, renal, 117
Colors, understanding of, 171
Communication
   with children, during examination, 191–95
   during clinical summary, 244, 265–66, 273–75
   of clinician to family, 94–95, 133, 249–50, 265–66, 268–69
   clinician's need for skills of, 4, 8
   of data, in screening programs, 72
   denigration of, 13
   among health care professionals, 71
   nonverbal, in interview, 17, 80, 83, 100–1, 104, 142, 245
   during painful procedure, 227–28
   during physical examination, 185, 191–95
   See also Confidentiality; Language of patient; Privacy

Communication and language, development of
  adolescent, 162
  assessment of, 74, 134
  child under five years, 147–48, 171–72, 283–84
  description of, for history, 42–43
  infant, 42, 155
  preschool child, 158–59
  school-age child, 160–61
Community, in health care, 7
Comprehensive primary care, 6
  defined, 6–8
  personal relationships in, 8–9
Confidentiality
  of information, 9, 164
  of interview, 86
  psychological problems and, 282
  in screening programs, 73
Computers, screening and, 72–73
Consultation, 270, 281–87
  with mental health professionals, 276–78
Continuity of care, 10–11
  economic factors and, 13
  See also Health care, society and
Coombs' test, 74
Coordination, physical examination and, 61
Cost, of screening programs, 72–73
Cough, as symptom, 122–24, 127, 129
Counseling, pediatric, 256
Country of origin, patient's, 23–24
Cranial nerves, physical examination and, 60–61
Cretinism, screening and, 69
Cystic fibrosis
  consultation about, 286
  on patient's records, 23

Daily life. See History, patient's, 24-hour
Data base
  definition of, 17
  obtaining of, 18–19, 174
  organization of, 12
  See also Development assessment; History, patient's; Screening
Day care centers, 179
Deafness
  in children, examination and, 196
  in infants, 155
Decision-making
  about birth control, 68
  of educationally disadvantaged persons, 110
  in pediatric practice, 9–10
Dental care, 7, 75
  advice about, 247–48
  poor, 253
  screening and, 75
Dermatitis, contact, diagnosis of, 126
Developmental assessment, 17–18, 132–72
  achievements, 147–50
  adolescent, 161–62
  child under five years, 147–49

child over five years, 149–50
clinician's statements about, 247–49
on history, 39–43, 136–50
home visit and, 134, 162–63
infant, 152–56
preschool child, 156–59
school-age child, 159–61
school visit and, 134, 163–64
of structured tasks, 164–72
See also Personal relationships; Personality characteristics
Developmental problems of children, 4–5, 174
  adaptive ability, 43
  clinician's statements about, 245–47, 250
  communication and language, 42–43
  discussion of, 245–47, 250
  family and, 7
  feeding habits, 41
  general description of, 39–40
  management of, 8
  moods and anxieties, 40
  motor skills, 43, 147
  on patient's records, 36, 39–43
  play habits, 42
  serious illness and, 23
  sleeping habits, 41
  toilet habits, 41–42
  See also Communication and language, development of; Personal relationships
Diabetes insipidus, symptoms of, 128
Diabetes mellitus
  review of, 48
  screening and, 69
  symptoms of, 124, 128
Diagnosis, 266–68
  consultation and, 283
  errors in, 127, 256
  family history and, 65
  technology and, 5
  See also Psychological problems, detection of
Diagnostic labels, use of, 274
Diarrhea
  handling of, 252
  as a symptom, 126–27
  treatment for, 126
Diet, 177, 182
  advice about, 247, 249, 253
  diarrhea and, 126–27
  review of, 41, 46
Diphtheria, immunization for, 35
Disagreements, between clinician and patient or parent, 96–97, 144
Discipline, methods of, 144
DPT immunizations, on patient's records, 35
Drawing, in developmental assessment, 171
Dressing procedures, 176
Drugs, pregnancy and, 29
Duchenne's muscular dystrophy, screening and, 65

Ears
  cerumen removal from, 213, 233–34
  physical examination of, 54, 196, 211, 213–15
  review of, 46
  See also Hearing
Eating patterns, 176–78, 181–82
Economic situation, of patient's family, 38. See also Socioeconomic class
Eczema, 254, 283
Emergency rooms, 25
Emotional problems of children, 4, 7
  identification of, 8
  See also Psychological problems
Emotions
  adolescent's, in interview, 161
  of children, during interview, 102–3, 112–13, 156, 160
  of clinician, 97–98
  of historian, 98–99
  See also Clinicians, feelings about parents and child
Endocrine system, review of, 48
Enuresis
  etiology of, 124, 127–29
  renal disease and, 130
Environment
  of child, 4, 7
  description of, on history, 36–38
  developmental history and, 136–37
  family and social, 146–47, 173–83
  feeding, 41
  observation of, 162
  of pediatric health care, 11
  See also Setting, clinical
Epididymis, physical examination and, 58
Equipment
  physical examination and, 193, 195–96, 199
  in health care system, 13
E test, illiterate, 74, 213
Ethical beliefs, medical treatment and, 67–68
Ethical implications, of screening tests, 73
Ethnic groups
  nonverbal communication and, 101
  screening and, 66
Evaluation of complaint, 117–30, 263–65
  ascertaining location, 117–18
  associated phenomena, 123
  chronology of symptom, 119–22
  context of symptom, 122
  course of symptoms, 121–22
  duration of symptom, 120
  factors affecting symptoms, 122–23
  intensity and quantity, 118–19
  onset of symptom, 119–20
  periodicity and frequency, 120–21
  psychological complaints, 124
  quality, 118
  scope of inquiry, 123–24
  use of interview in, 124–30
Evaluation of health. See Clinical summary; Diagnosis

Examination, physical, 17, 19, 51–61, 185–225
  abdomen, 57, 219
  anxiety of child during, 191–201
  art of, 51, 185–225
  blood pressure, 189–90, 193, 211, 222–23
  bones, joints, and muscles, 52–53
  breasts, 55–56
  cardiovascular system, 57
  chest, 190, 192, 216–18
  clinician's talk during, 191–95
  cooperation during, 113, 185–87, 197, 200–1
  diagnosis and, 124
  ears, 54, 196, 211, 213–16
  equipment for, 193, 195–96, 199
  extremities, 59
  eyes, 53–54, 209, 212–13
  fontanelle, 212
  general appearance, 51–52
  genitalia, female, 59
  genitalia, male, 58–59
  head, 53, 74, 208, 224–25
  heart murmurs, 74
  height, 224
  hips, 74, 221
  of infant, procedure for, 204–6
  integument, 52
  lymph nodes, 53
  mouth, 55, 207, 209–10
  neck, 55
  nervous system, 60–61, 221–22
  nose, 55
  order of, 198–99, 206
  parent's behavior during, 187–90
  pelvic, 201
  procedure for, 201–3, 206–11
  rectum and anus, 59, 203, 220
  screening and, 62–63
  separation from interview, 80–81
  siblings, presence of, 190–91
  skull, 53
  thorax and lungs, 56–57
  throat, 55, 213–16
  vision, 54, 74
  vital signs, 52
  weight, 224
Eye(s)
  drainage from, as symptom, 123
  physical examination of, 53–54, 209, 212–213
  removal of foreign body from, 234
  review of, 46
Eye contact, during interview, 100–1

Facial nerves, physical examination and, 60
Family
  assessing problems of, 12, 107, 111
  description of, on patient's records, 36–38
  in health care, 7–9
  medical history of, 43–45

screening and, 65
See also Personal relationships
Family planning, genetic counseling and, 65
Fantasy play, development of, 148–49
Fatigue, consultation about, 286
Fears, developmental assessment and, 141
Feeding environment, of child, 41
Fetal diagnosis, 68
Fever, as symptom, 124, 127, 129, 252, 267
Finger-stick test, 232
Flexibility
  in child rearing, 96
  of clinician, 14
  of interviewer, 86–87
  during physical examination, 51, 186, 197–98
Fontanelle, 212
Foster parents
  clinical summary and, 244
  health evaluation and, 84
Frequency of condition, screening and, 68

Gait, physical examination and, 61
Galactosemia, screening and, 64, 69, 73
Gastrointestinal disease, 124, 127
Gastrointestinal tract
  parasites of, 127
  review of, 47
Genetic counseling, 63–67
  religious beliefs and, 67
  sickle hemoglobin and, 64–65, 74
  Tay-Sachs disease and, 65–66
Genitalia, physical examination and, 58–59
Genital tract
  female, review of, 47
  male, review of, 47
Geographical regions, screening and, 67
Glasses, review of, 46
Glossopharyngeal and vagus nerves, physical examination and, 60
Glucose-6-phosphate-dehydrogenase (G-6-P-D) deficiency, 22
Gonads, review of, 48
Grandparent(s)
  of adolescent parents, 114–15
  child's relationship to, 146, 163
  at clinical summary, 243
Grasping behavior, of infant, 154–55, 168
Greeting, in interview, 82–83
Growth
  clinician's statements about, 247
  deviation from normal, 253
  discussion of, 46
  poor, as symptom, 124, 129
  rate of, 48
  review of, 46
Guidance, anticipatory, 247–49

Hair
  adrenal system and, 48
  physical examination and, 52–53
  review of, 46

Hand(s)
  use of, by adolescent, 161
  use of, by infant, 154–55, 168
  See also Muscle skills, development of
Headaches, as symptoms, 120–21, 124, 267
Head and face
  circumference, measurement of, 52, 74, 208, 224–25
  physical examination and, 52
  restraint of, during painful procedures, 229, 233–34
  review of, 46
Health care
  funds for, 13
  primary, inadequate, 252–53
  quality of, 13
  resources, allocation of, 4, 13
  society and, 13
  sources of, 27
  See also Pediatric health care; Preventive health care
Health care professionals, 6
  communication with parents, 94–95
  confidentiality and, 86
  public information and, 62, 71–73
  questions about, 90
  responsibility of, 86
  screening and, 62–63, 73
  See also Clinicians; Nurse(s)
Health, general, review of, 46
Health maintenance, 6–7, 132
  birth history and, 28
  data base and, 17
  definition of, 24
  plans for, 250
  questions about, 90
Health records, 250, 314. *See also* Data base; History
Hearing
  examination of, 54, 74, 159, 215–16
  tests of, information about, 250
Heart, physical examination of, 57, 190
Heart disease, screening and, 65
Heart murmurs
  physical examination and, 74
Height, physical examination and, 52, 74, 224
Hematocrit, screening tests and, 69, 74, 250
Hematopoietic system, review of, 48
Hemoglobin, screening tests and, 74. *See also* Sickle cell hemoglobin
Hemoglobin electrophoresis, 64, 74
Hereditary disease, 67. *See also* Genetic counseling
Hernia(s)
  patient's history and, 47
  physical examination and, 58
Hips
  pathology, and knee pain, 117
  physical examination and, 74, 221
Hirsutism, 48
Histoplasmosis, 48
  screening and, 67

Historians (sources) of medical information, 25–27, 45
  adolescent, 110–11
  emotions of, in interview, 98–99
  evasiveness of, 108–9
  foreign-language-speaking, 111–12
  inaccurate, 134
  nonparental, 84
  psychiatric problems of, 109
  questions of, to clinician, 85–86, 89–92
  reliability of, 25–26
  retardation of, 110
  tension of, 106–7
  types of, 86, 97
  unfocused, 107–8, 174
History, patient's, 17, 22–49
  birth, 28–30
  chief complaint on, 24–25
  of childhood and adolescent health, 32–35
  developmental status for, 39–43
  in diagnosing psychological problems, 274
  evaluating problems for, 27–28
  family medical history for, 43–45
  identifying data for, 22–24
  of infancy, 31–32
  in medical records, 19
  patient profile for, 36
  review of systems for, 45–49
  screening and, 62–63
  social, 36–38
  style in recording, 28, 314
  24-hour, 173–83, 272
  See also Developmental assessment
Hobbies, of child, 150
Home visits, 134, 162–63
Homosexuality, patient's concern with, 114
Hypertension, discussion of, 190
Hypoglossal nerves, physical examination and, 61
Hypothyroidism
  congenital (cretinism), screening for, 69
  screening for, 64, 73

Immunization, 5, 7
  advice about, 249–50
  children's cooperation with, 113
  on patient's records, 35, 250
  questions about, 90
  See also names of specific diseases
Infants
  advice about, 248
  body-mind interdependence of, 7
  examination of, 190, 192, 199, 203–6, 224. *See also* names of specific bodily parts
  fine motor-adaptive skills of, 168
  injections for, 230–31
  during interview, 104
  language and communication skills of, 155
  looking behavior of, 155
  muscle skills of, 154–55, 167–68
  personality characteristics of, 152–53
  personal and social skills of, 155–56
  relationship to parents, 153–54
  screening of, 64–65, 74
  thrush, discussion of in, 253–54
Infectious diseases, 5
  screening and, 66–67
Injections
  child's fear of, 103, 197
  restraint of child during, 230–31
  side effects, caution about, 249
Inspection
  of abdomen, 57
  of thorax and lungs, 56
Institutions, record forms of, 36
Intelligence tests, 73, 75
Interpreters
  clinical summary with, 243, 245
  use of, in interviews, 111–12
Interview, clinical, 17, 46, 80–115
  adolescent parent and, 114–15
  agenda for, 84
  annotated, 291–314
  child rearing, questions about, 93–96
  child, role of during, 102–6, 112–13
  communication, nonverbal, 100–1
  components of, 81–86
  confidentiality of, 86
  developmental, 138–39
  disagreements during, 96–97
  emotions, handling of, 97–99
  in evaluating complaint, 124–30
  flexibility during, 86
  historian, problems with, 106–12
  interpersonal functions of, 80–81
  opinion, presentation of, 94–96
  physical problem, concern about, 113–14
  questions, from historian, 89–91
  questions, clinician's, 92
  sex of clinician and, 114
  technique of, 87–89
  for 24-hour history, 175–83
  write-up of, 314–17
  See also Clinical summary
Intestinal obstruction, diagnosis of, 121

Jewish population, Tay-Sachs disease and, 66
Joints, physical examination and, 53

Kernig's sign, physical examination and, 61
Ketoacidosis, acute diabetic, 284
Kindergarten, adjustment to, 259–60
Klinefelter's syndrome, 48
Knee(s), pain in, 117, 122–23, 285–86

Labia, female, 59
Laboratory procedures, 17, 19
  children's cooperation with, 113
  diagnosis and, 124
  interview and, 80

Laceration, suturing of, 234
Lactose intolerance, 123
Language development. *See* Communication and language, development of
Language of patient
  foreign, and interview, 111–12
  health care and, 23
Lead ingestion
  screening for, 64, 72, 74–75
  socioeconomic class and, 66
Lead time, screening and, 69
Lessler, K., 63
Leukemia
  concern about, 45, 120, 252
  symptoms of, 120
Limbs, physical examination and, 53
Lipid metabolism, disorders of, 65
Looking behavior, in infant, 155
Lungs. *See* Respiratory infections; Thorax and lungs
Lymph nodes, 48

Maltreatment. *See* Child abuse; Neglect
Management, of health problem, 269–71
Marital problems
  discussion of, 243
  effect on child, 257, 274, 277, 279
Marital status, patient's, on records, 23
Measles, 123
  immunization for, 35, 75
Medical terminology, use of, 244, 265
Menstrual cycles
  flank pain and, 120
  review of, 47
Mental health care, 7. *See also* Psychological problems
Mental status, physical examination and, 60
Metabolic diseases, screening tests for, 73–74
Mittelschmerz, diagnosis of, 120
MMR immunizations, on patient's records, 35
Moniliasis, oral ("thrush"), 253–54
  symptoms of, 125
Monovac test, for tuberculosis, 75
Motor nerves, physical examination and, 61, 221
Motor skills. *See* Muscle skills, development of
Mouth and throat
  examination of, 55, 207, 209–10
  review of, 46
Mucous membranes, physical examination and, 52
Mumps, immunization for, 35
Muscle(s), physical examination and, 53
Muscle skills, development of
  adolescent, 161–62
  child under five years, 147, 168–69
  description of, on history, 43
  infant, 154–55, 167–68
  preschool child, 157–58
  school-age child, 160

Muscular dystrophy, 65
Musculoskeletal system, review of, 47–48

Nails
  physical examination and, 52
  review of, 46
Neck
  examination of, 55
  review of, 47
Neglect, 9
  reporting of, 86
  See also Child abuse
Neoplastic disease, 123
Nervous system
  physical examination and, 60–61, 221–22
  review of, 48
Nose, review of, 46
Nurse(s), pediatric, 5–6
  developmental assessment and, 134
  as practitioner, 83
  role of, 6
Nursery, special care, 31
Nursery school. *See* School, nursery
Nutrition
  education about, 7
  infant, 5
  See also Diet
Nystagmus, physical examination and, 53–54, 61

Observations, 133, 150–52
  structured, 164–72
  unstructured, 151–64
Obstetric history. *See* Birth history, on patient's records; Childhood and adolescent health, on patient's records
Oculomotor nerves, physical examination and, 60
Olfactory nerves, physical examination and, 60
Ophthalmoscopic examination, 54
Opisthotonus, physical examination and, 61
Optic nerves, physical examination and, 60
OPV (oral polio vaccine), on patient's records, 35
Ortolani's test, 221
Otoscope. *See* Ear(s)
Ovary, 120

Pain
  depth of, 118
  intensity of, 118–19
  location of problem and, 117–18
  periodicity and frequency of, 120–21
  stress and, 122
Painful procedures, 226–35
  conclusion of, 229–30
  cooperation of child during, 197, 227
  interview and, 113
  parents, role of during, 228–29

restraint during, 228–29, 231–34
siblings and, 191
Palpation
  of abdomen, 57
  of thorax and lungs, 56
Panhypopituitarism, 48
Parasites, intestinal, 48
  screening and, 67
  symptoms of, 127
Parents
  behavior during child's examination, 187–90
  birth experience and, 29–31
  reliability of, as historians, 26–27
  response to child's psychological problems, 265–79
  serious illness, attitudes toward, 33, 266
  See also Caregivers; Family; Marital problems; Personal relationships
Patient profile, on records, 36–43
  agencies, 38
  caregivers, at home, 37
  economic situation, 38
  family, description of, 36–38
  family relationships, 36
  home, physical characteristics of, 37
  school, 37–38
Pediatric health care
  characteristics of, 3–5
  history of, 3, 5
  setting in, 10–12
  See also Comprehensive primary care; Health care
Peer group
  child's relation to, 145, 150
  influence on child, 7
Pelvic examination, 59, 201, 203n
Penicillin, 123
Penis
  patient's history and, 47
  physical examination and, 58
Percussion
  of abdomen, 57
  of thorax and lungs, 56
Peritoneal disease, 117
Personality characteristics
  of adolescent, 161
  ascertaining, in interview, 139–42
  infant, 152–53
  of preschool child, 156
  of school-age child, 160
Personal relationships
  child-authority figures, 146
  child-family environment, 146–47
  child-parents, 136–37, 142–45, 151, 156–57, 160
  child-school, 42
  child-siblings, 145, 190–91, 258–59, 279
  clinician-family, 8–9, 11, 18, 80, 82–83, 132–35, 165
  clinician-patient, 134–35
  infant-parents, 153–54
  patient-family, 36, 40

See also Environment, family and social; Parents; Peer group
Personal and social skills, development of
  adolescent, 162
  child under five years, 148–49
  infant, 155–56
  preschool child, 159
  school-age child, 161
Pertussis, immunization for, 35
Pets, patient's health and, 48
Phenylketonuria (PKU)
  questions about, 90
  screening for, 64, 68–69, 72–73
Physical contact, during interview, 100
Physical problems
  major, 242, 244–45, 256, 263–71
  minor, 242, 251–56
Pica, 64, 75
  socioeconomic class and, 66
Pituitary system, review of, 48
PKU. See Phenylketonuria (PKU)
Play
  developmental assessment and, 148–49, 178
  questions about, 42
Pneumonia, diagnosis of, 124
Poisoning, accidental, 248. See also Lead ingestion
Polio, immunization for, 35
Polyuria, as symptom, 128
Poor children, health care of, 6
Posture
  of clinician during interview, 100
  of infant, and developmental assessment, 154, 167–68
  physical examination and, 61
PPD test, for tuberculosis, 75
Pregnancy
  adolescent, 33–34
  on birth history of patient, 29
  diagnosis of, 268
Prenatal care. See Birth history, on patient's records
Prenatal visit, 248
Prevalence, of condition, screening and, 68
Preventive health care, 4–5
  education about, 7
  funds for, 13
  See also Health maintenance; Screening
Primary care. See Comprehensive primary care
Privacy, 8, 160
  adolescents' concern with, 9
  for clinical summary, 242
  physical examination and, 200–1
  See also Confidentiality
Problem Oriented Medical Record (POMR), 11–12, 314
Problem-solving (adaptive) skills, development of
  adolescent, 162
  child under five years, 147, 169, 171

infant, 155
  preschool child, 158
  school-age child, 160
Psychological health, of children, 4-5
  on patient's records, 33, 36, 48-49
Psychological problems, 256-61, 271-79
  consultation and, 282
  definition of major, 263
  detection of, 132-33, 244-46
    major, 271-73
    minor, 257-58
    observation and, 151
    in parents, 189
    24-hour history and, 174
  discussion of, 102, 245-46, 250, 273-75
  enuresis and, 128-29
  evaluation of, 246
  follow-up of, 258, 279
  of historians, 109
  major, assessment and management of, 271-79
  management of, 257-58, 264
  minor, 256-61
  parents' reaction to, 271-79
  symptoms of, 48-49, 124, 271, 273, 277
Psychological tests, 135, 151
Puberty, 47-48. *See also* Sexual maturation
Pubic hair
  patient's history and, 48
  physical examination and, 58-59
Public education, about screening programs, 71-72
Pulses, physical examination and, 52, 57

Questions, during interview, 87, 247
  "by the way," 91-92, 246
  challenges to clinician's, 92
  about child rearing, 93-96
  to children, 103-6
  about clinician, 92
  clinician's language and, 88
  general, from historian, 89-90
  initial, 85-86
  open-ended, from clinician, 81, 107
  about pain, 117-18
  specific, from clinician, 108
  specific, from historian, 90-91
  third party, 91
  See also Evaluation, of complaint

Race
  diseases and, 22
  nonverbal communication and, 101
  patient's, on records, 22
  sickle cell disease and, 22, 64-66
  screening and, 66
Rash(es)
  papular vesicular, as symptom, 122
  as symptom, 124-26
Record system, 11-12
  immunization, 35, 250
  importance of, 19

See also History, patient's
Rectum, physical examination and, 59, 203, 220
Reflexes, physical examination and, 61, 205, 221-22
Reliability, of historians, 25-27
Religion
  medical treatment and, 67
  patient's, on records, 22-23
Renal disease, symptoms of, 129-30
Resources, provision of, for persons screened, 72
Respiration(s)
  physical examination and, 52
  as symptoms, 122
Respiratory infections, 121-24
  diarrhea and, 127
  physical examination and, 198
  symptoms of, 129
Respiratory system, review of, 45, 47
Restraint. *See* Painful procedures, restraint during
Retardation, of historian, 110
Review of systems, on patient's record, 45-49
Rhinnorhea, as symptom, 122, 124, 129, 254
Romberg test, 61
Rubella, immunization for, 35

Scalp, physical examination and, 53
School
  adjustment to, 42, 149-50, 259-61
  child's performance in, 149-50, 181
  influence on child, 7
  interview about, 180-81
  nursery, 179, 260
  psychogenic problems and, 122
  visit to, by clinician, 134, 163-64
School bus, adjustment to, 259-60
Screening, 62-75
  advice about, 249-50
  conditions to be included in, 68-69
  definition of, 63
  developmental, 134-35
  factors in success of, 71-73
  methods of, 70-71
  patients, criteria for, 64-68
  tests, 17, 63, 70-75, 250
    acceptability of, 70
    accuracy of, 70-71
    ethical implications of, 73
    example of schedule for, 73-75
    reliability of, 71
    use of, 135-36, 185
  time and frequency of, 69-70
  use of, 62-63
Scrotum
  patient's history and, 48
  physical examination and, 58
Self-awareness, development of
  child under five years, 148
  infant, 148

Self-help skills, development of, 148
Sensory nerves, physical examination and, 61
Setting
    for assessing structured tasks, 165–67
    clinical, 10–12, 186
    for clinical summary, 242
Sex
    patient's, on records, 22
    of practitioner, patient's concern with, 114
Sexual activity, adolescent, 34, 47, 110, 268
    physical examination and, 201
    responsibility for, 249
Sexual maturation, 47–48, 110
    advice about, 248
    breasts and, 55–56
    examination and, 201
    male, 58–59
Sibling rivalry, 258–59. See also Personal relationships, child-sibling
Sickle cell hemoglobin, 22
    adolescents as carriers, of, 65
    screening for, 64–66, 73–74
Sitters, 180
Skin
    physical examination and, 52–53
    review of, 46
    thyroid system and, 48
    See also Acne; Dermatitis; Rash(es)
Sleeping arrangements
    enuresis and, 130
    questions about, 93–94, 96
Sleep patterns, 176, 182–83
    questions about, 41
Snellen test, for vision, 74, 213
Social environment. See Environment, family and social
Social skills. See Personal and social skills, development of
Society, health care delivery and, 13
Socioeconomic class, screening and, 66
Speech problems, diagnosis of, 160–61
Spinal cord irritation, physical examination and, 61
Spine, physical examination and, 52
Stenosis, distal meatal, 128
Stomachaches, as symptoms, 119, 121
Stools, as symptom, 125–27
Stranger anxiety, 187, 199–200, 203
Stress
    adolescents and, 122
    on child, during examination, 187, 199
    on child, in illness, 141, 187
    on child, in maturation, 141
    direct questions about, 36
    on family, 133
    psychological problems and, 257
Structured tasks. See Developmental assessment, of structured tasks
Student clinicians. See Clinicians, student
Suturing, 234

Symptoms
    duration of, on records, 24–25
    evaluation of. See Evaluation of complaint
    See also specific symptom

Table, examining, 196
Tay-Sachs disease, 65–66
    screening and, 66
Team, health care, 6, 10, 115
Technique, of interview, 87–89
Teeth. See Dental care
Television viewing, of child, 175, 178–79, 182
    advice about, 248
Temperature
    elevation, as symptom, 122
    physical examination and, 52
Terminology. See Medical terminology, use of
Testes
    patient's history and, 48
    physical examination and, 58
Tests. See Intelligence tests; Psychological tests; Screening tests
Tetanus, immunization for, 35
Thalassemia, 22
Thorax and lungs, physical examination of, 56–57
Throat
    physical examination of, 55, 213–15
    sore, as symptom, 123
Throat culture, 235
Thrush
    clinical summary and, 253–54
    symptoms of, 125
Thyroid system, review of, 48
Time
    clinical summary and, 245–46, 287
    of patients' visits, 12
    See also Chronology, of symptoms
Tine test, for tuberculosis, 75
Toilet training, 41–42
    difficulty with, 259
    enuresis and, 129
    questions about, 41–42, 91
Touching. See Physical contact
Toys
    in clinical setting, 11
    in developmental assessment, 166, 178
    See also Problem-solving (adaptive) skills, development of
Travel, patient's health and, 48
Trigeminal nerves, physical examination and, 60
Trochlear nerves, physical examination and, 60
Tuberculosis
    questions about, 88–89
    screening and, 45, 66–67, 70, 72, 75
Tympanic membranes, physical examination of, 54

Undressing, physical examination and, 190, 193, 200, 206–7, 209–10
Urinary tract
  discussion of, with interpreter, 112
  infection of, 124, 128–30, 252
  review of, 47
Urine, control of. *See* Enuresis
Urine culture, screening test and, 75, 250
Urine protein, screening test and, 75

Vagina, 59
Vagus nerves, physical examination and, 60
VDRL, screening for, 74
Venipuncture, 232
Vessels, physical examination and, 57
Vision
  examination of, 54, 74, 213
  tests of, information about, 250
Visits, to health care site
  length of, 12
  prenatal, 248
  reason for, 24–25
  See also Clinical summary; Home visits; School, visit to by clinician
Visual fields, examination of, 54, 213
Vomiting, as symptom, 123–25, 127, 268

Weight, physical examination and, 52, 74
Weight measurement, 224
Well-child care, 28
  clinical summary and, 242, 263
  definition of, 24
  developmental assessment and, 133, 141
  physical examination and, 185, 189